Services for Sale

Services for Sale

Purchasing Health and Human Services

HAROLD W. DEMONE, JR.
and MARGARET GIBELMAN

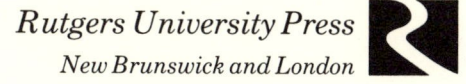

Rutgers University Press
New Brunswick and London

THE PUBLISHERS of the following journals have granted permission to reprint materials that originally appeared in their publications:

Kettner, Peter M., and Lawrence L. Martin. "Making Decisions about Purchase Service Contracting." *Public Welfare* 44 (1982):30–37, 46. Used by permission of American Public Welfare Association.

Richardson, David A., Jr., "Purchase of Service, Third-Party Payments, Market Conditions and Rate-Setting." Based on an article in Project Share's *Rate-Setting in the Human Services: A Guide for Administrators* 24 (September 1981): 97–102.

Sharkansky, Ira. "Policy Making and Service Delivery on the Margins of Government: The Case of Contractors." *Public Administration Review* 40 (March/April 1980): 116–123.

Terrell, Paul. "Private Alternatives to Public Services Administration." *Social Service Review* 53 (March 1979): 56–74.

Library of Congress Cataloging-in-Publication Data

Demone, Harold W., Jr.
Services for sale.

Bibliography: p.
Includes index.
1. Social service—United States—Contracting out. 2. Medical care—United States—Contracting out. 3. Public welfare—United States—Contracting out. I. Gibelman, Margaret. II. Title.

HV91.D463 1988   350.84′0973   88-18443
ISBN 0-8135-1361-8   ISBN 0-8135-1362-6 (pbk.)

British Cataloging-in-Publication information available

To Our Parents, In Appreciation

Contents

Contributors

EARLENE BAUMUNK Supervising Contract Administrator, Office of Recycling, Department of Environmental Protection, State of New Jersey, Trenton, New Jersey.

NANCY CHESS Director of Social Services, McCarty Center, Norman, Oklahoma.

HAROLD W. DEMONE, JR. Professor, School of Social Work, Graduate Department of Sociology and Center for Alcohol Studies, Rutgers University, New Brunswick, New Jersey.

ROBERT A. DORWART Executive Officer, Mental Health Policy Working Group, Division of Health Policy Research and Education, Harvard University, and Assistant Professor of Psychiatry, Harvard Medical School.

ADELL P. FINE School Social Worker, Upper Saddle River School District, and Psychotherapist, Social Work Associates, Glen Rock, New Jersey.

SEYMOUR H. FINE Associate Professor of Marketing, Rutgers University, and President, Fine Marketing Associates.

BARRY FRIEDMAN Lecturer, Florence Heller School for Advanced Studies in Social Welfare, Brandeis University, Waltham, Massachusetts.

MARGARET GIBELMAN Executive Vice President, Asthma and Allergy Foundation of America, Inc., Washington, D.C.

JEANNE M. GIOVANNONI Professor, School of Social Work, University of California, Los Angeles.

ARNOLD GURIN Dean and Profesor Emeritus, Florence Heller School for Advanced Studies in Social Welfare, Waltham, Massachusetts.

BRUCE S. JANSSON Associate Professor, School of Social Work, University of Southern California, Los Angeles.

PETER M. KETTNER Associate Professor, School of Social Work, Arizona State University, Tempe.

RALPH M. KRAMER Professor, School of Social Welfare, University of California, Berkeley.

PATRICIA McGOVERN State Senator, and Chair, Senate Committee on Ways and Means, Commonwealth of Massachusetts, Boston.

LAWRENCE L. MARTIN Director, Office of Management Analysis, Maricopa County, Arizona.

EVELYN KAYS PETTIFORD Associate Executive Director, National Association of Social Workers, Silver Spring, Maryland.

MARIA ROBERTS-DEGENNARO Associate Professor, School of Social Work, San Diego University.

DAVID A. RICHARDSON, JR. Project Share, Rockville, Maryland

IRA SHARKANSKY Professor of Political Science, Hebrew University of Jerusalem and the University of Wisconsin-Madison.

MARK SCHLESINGER Research Coordinator, Center for Health Policy and Management, Kennedy School of Government, Harvard University.

STEVEN RATHGEB SMITH Assistant Professor, Institute of Policy Sciences and Public Affairs, Duke University, Durham, North Carolina.

TOSHIO TATARA Director, Research and Demonstration Department, American Public Welfare Association, Washington, D.C.

ELSA TEN BROECK Administrator, Children's Services, Department of Social Services, San Mateo, California.

PAUL TERRELL Coordinator, Academic Programs, and Adjunct Lecturer, School of Social Work, University of California, Berkeley.

KENNETH R. WEDEL Professor, School of Social Work, University of Oklahoma, Norman.

ISABEL WOLOCK Professor, School of Social Work, Rutgers University, New Brunswick, New Jersey.

DAVID W. YOUNG Professor of Accounting and Control, Boston University School of Management.

Foreword

Throughout American history, the relationship between the public and voluntary health and social welfare sectors has had an enormous impact on what kinds of services have been available, to whom, and of what quality. Political, economic, and social forces shaped preferences for one sector over the other. In the health and social welfare systems of the 1930s and 1960s, for example, public responsibility was met primarily through public agencies; in the 1950s and 1980s, emphasis was on voluntary sector service provision.

Perhaps more important than the preference for one sector over the other has been the historic comingling of functions and responsibilities. In many ways, the two parallel systems created a workable accountability system; the failures of one system might be corrected by the other. Primary responsibilities could be shifted, and, indeed, they have been. The use of public funds has proven to be a most durable and viable means to control which sector delivers what services to whom and to encourage a unique form of accountability to meet public purposes.

The purchasing of services (POS), practiced almost since the inception of this nation, grew in scope and influence to become the primary modern means to utilize the expertise of the voluntary sector. We are fortunate that the voluntary service system was sufficiently developed at the community level to provide essential backup support for the public sector. The use of POS, now and in the past, also guaranteed the ongoing interdependence of these systems. As we can testify from our experience within the United Way system, the influence of POS in molding our health and social welfare system cannot be understated. This influence continues to be wielded.

Given the magnitude and significance of purchase of service, what is perhaps most surprising is how little we know about it. In this volume Demone and Gibelman examine purchase of services from its past and current sociopolitical theoretical base and explore its applications to a wide range of health and human services. To human service policymakers and administrators, the authors' exploration of the "why" and "with what results" of purchase of service provides critical information with which to assess and reevaluate our assumptions about the desirable mix of public and private services and the implications of current delivery patterns on service quality and accountability. It also provides an essential context in which to view the evolving policy of privatizing public functions. In this context purchase of service is viewed as but a rudimentary and early form of a major conceptual and practical change in the responsibility for and financing and administering of health and human services.

The search for answers contributes much to our understanding of the relationship between public and voluntary health and social welfare systems and the consequences arising from public policy decisions. The authors show that the nature of our service delivery system is in part based on happenstance but is also reflective of how values, politics, and economics come together to define and dictate not only how services are to be delivered, but their quality and responsiveness to human needs.

December 1987

William Aramony, President
United Way of America, Inc.
Alexandria, Virginia

PART ONE

Introduction

This book is divided into seven parts. Part one provides an overview of the philosophical and pragmatic issues and factors that underlie the growth of purchase of service, the major arguments advanced in favor of and against this service delivery mechanism, and variations in the types of purchase arrangements and their fiscal, regulatory, and legal base. The goal of this chapter is to provide a contextual framework to connect the perspectives and specialized content presented in each of the subsequent chapters.

Part Two is concerned with theoretical orientations to purchase of service, including public-private roles and relationships, the emerging dominance of the privatization theme, and organizational and service delivery implications of purchase of service arrangements.

Part Three focuses on the technology of contracting, including the applicability of marketing principles, unit pricing, cost comparisons between alternative delivery mechanisms, cost sharing, the components of a contract, and the mechanisms of the contracting process itself, including negotiation.

Part Four is devoted to exploring actual experiences with contracting. Two articles focus on the use of purchase of service from the perspective of the public agency. Other articles within this section examine the implementation of purchase arrangements, including their impact on organization systems, service delivery patterns, and clientele.

Part Five examines the impact of purchase of services from an empirical stance. Data from several studies are presented to demonstrate the effect of contracting on public-private interactions, client services, perceptions of quality of services, and other relevant variables.

Part Six examines issues of monitoring and evaluation from several perspectives. In Part Seven, the editors conclude the volume by examining current trends and likely future developments with regard to the use of purchase of service arrangements.

Case examples and implementation experiences are taken from the health and social services. This emphasis reflects the state-of-the-art of research, theory building, and emerging practical experience with purchase of service. That contracting arrangments are relatively new within the human services, at least in scope and breadth, provides fertile ground for those wishing to study the impact of alternative methods of organizing and delivering services. The Reagan administration gave significant attention to privatizing many social welfare functions previously considered solely within the jurisdiction of government, bringing added attention to the potential and realized uses of purchase of service. A second focus of this volume is on contracting with the not-for-profit, voluntary sector. Though this sector is considered under the umbrella term of "private," it is distinct from for-profit, proprietary organizations. Emphasis on the voluntary sector reflects the major traditions and precedents of public-private contracting relationships.

The philosophical and practical bases for the expanding use of contracting within the social services are numerous and reflect prevailing attitudes within this society about the appropriate delegation of roles between the public and private sectors. Commonly held perceptions about the weaknesses associated with public service provision, the believed superiority of private delivery, and growing interest in forging linkages between public and private concerns all contribute to a sound rationale for contracting out social services. This interest is shared by public and private sector administrators, managers, fiscal officers, lawyers, researchers, and others concerned with performance and outcome measures. Concerns about the costs of social services and questions about their effectiveness also bear relevance to the growing number of empirical studies and theoretical examinations of the use of purchase of service within this field.

Purchasing social services is a logical extension in related health and human services fields, such as vocational rehabilitation, job training, and residential treatment for the emotionally disturbed and mentally retarded. Although the degree of experience with purchase of service is greater in some other fields, the rationale, emerging patterns, and issues have been remarkably similar. Thus, the focus upon social and health services, although necessarily limited, does not preclude generalization of questions and issues and future forecasting.

Potential users of the volume include public policymakers, public and private human service managers, social service practitioners, and educators who seek to prepare students for the realities of current practice. Procurement agents, grant managers, and financial officers will also find this book to be of relevance. Finally, interested citizens concerned with current trends in the use of public funds may find this volume instructive.

1

In Search of a Theoretical Base
for the Purchase of Services

Harold W. Demone, Jr., and Margaret Gibelman

Purchase of services (POS) has been a widely used mechanism to procure goods and services throughout the history of the United States, even prior to its status as an independent nation. The general level of satisfaction with these arrangements is evident in their continued use, despite occasional attention to contracting abuse initiated by the media, government, or organized labor. Even with the increase in the number of alleged and verified contracting abuses by such sources as military contractors and the "Beltway Bandits" (for-profit enterprises based in the Washington, D.C., area that rely on government contracts for their financial sustenance), government's preference to purchase a large portion of its goods and services remains intact.

For a tradition as well established as purchase of service, the scholarly base is remarkably thin. The literature on the subject tends to be ad hoc and sporadic in nature, and few scholars have written more than once on the subject. Kramer (1966, 1979), Savas (1977, 1982), Hatry (1982), Young (1977), Hoogland DeHoog (1984), LeGrand and Robinson (1984), and Kettner and Martin (1987) are among those who have contributed to the scholarly base, and several chapters of this volume represent the work of some of these authors. There have also been some relatively recent dissertations, including those by Gibelman (1981) and Roberts (1981), both of whom have excerpted from their studies for inclusion here. The federal government has sponsored a few studies on the process and outcome of contracting, including those conducted by Urban Institute (Fisk, Kiesling, and Muller, 1978), Pacific Consultants (Weinstein 1979), and the Florence Heller Graduate School of Social Welfare at Brandeis University (Gurin and Friedman 1980), the latter included herein in chapter form. Further, one volume of conference proceedings focused on the policy implications of Title XX purchasing (Wedel, Katz, and Weick 1979).

Privatizing the Public Sector (Savas 1982) is one of the three book-length publications dealing with matters of purchase of service. As its title suggests, it also focuses on many other issues pertaining to the shift of functions and responsibilities from government to the private sector. The subtitle of Savas's book makes clear his objective: "How to Shrink the Government." Human services contracting is only one of many government responsibilities that may be delegated to voluntary or private providers.

More recently, Ruth Hoogland DeHoog has produced a volume on *Contracting Out for Human Services* (1984). Using a conceptual framework drawn from economics, political science, and the multidisciplinary study of organizational theory, DeHoog offers a case study of one state's experiences with purchasing services under two pieces of federal legislation—Title XX and the Comprehensive Employment and Training Act. Similarities and differences in organizational structure, contracting procedures, and service outcomes were explored among and between state departments and programs. The author focuses primarily on establishing a framework for understanding the contracting phenomena, a creative first step. This effort is limited by the intrastate approach and the inherent limitations of generalizing to other state situations and contracting experiences under different program auspices.

Without exception, the researchers and commentators have been consistent in expressing concern about the dearth of empirical information. Given the state-of-the-art, it is not surprising that there are many opinion pieces: pro, con, and in-between. Remarkably, the themes are similar and as data trickle in, speculation has not always been found to be wrong.

The two editors of this volume joined the exchange with their own perspectives on purchase of service. Earlier in his career, Harold W. Demone, Jr., served as a public administrator overseeing the direct operation of a statewide direct service alcoholism program. Several years later, he assumed responsibility for a program in another state that contracted for all direct services. These experiences in two state health departments stimulated a long-standing interest in the merits and pitfalls of direct versus indirect service delivery approaches and the related variables.

6

Margaret Gibelman directed several government-funded contracts, including a state-sponsored training program under university auspices and a national demonstration project on staff development and training. With some clear opinions about contracting, she decided to test the premises empirically, conducting a study on the relative impact of purchase of service versus direct public service delivery on client services within the field of child protection. Demone and Gibelman found that they agreed on the importance of purchase of service as a major trend affecting the process and outcome of public and private organizational roles and responsibilities and the interaction between the two. They contend that the growth of purchasing represents one of the most significant trends in human services delivery and suggest a fundamental and pervasive alteration in the government's role and the nature of public-private sector relations.

More often than not, a theoretical base for purchase of service is preceded by a pragmatic approach. Wedel (1976), Wedel and Hardcastle (1978), Kramer (this volume), and Demone and Gibelman (1983) offer some preliminary thoughts about a theoretical framework. Wedel talks about normative guidelines and Kramer and Hardcastle about pluralism, but strong advocacy on behalf of these perspectives is not characteristic. Since Demone and Gibelman originally shared their pragmatic perspectives, it is with some deference that they now suggest that such atheoretical judgments may have been premature. The problem is that there is no single explanation for the multidimensional phenomena of contracting, but rather several possible theoretical bases. Which, if any, framework is correct is not yet apparent. More likely some new combination of existing theoretical principles is necessary. What is clear is that for a service delivery mechanism so widely used, some greater understanding of its principles, assumptions, practices, rationale, and basis in history and tradition is required.

To best understand this increasingly complex mosaic, sets of constraints have been identified as if to represent pure either-or polarities: public versus private, not-for-profit versus profit. Marxists, Keynesians, liberals, traditionalists, pragmatists, neoconservatives, and conservatives are seemingly locked into rhetorical battles about the various merits of direct public service delivery versus partial or full purchase of service, each convinced of their own perspective. For example, Stoesz (1981) describes the prevalence of contracting for service as the "end of the welfare state." Dichotomies abound. The issue of what form of service delivery works best for what problem and population-at-risk seems at times less relevant than ideological formulations. Demone and Gibelman, along with many public administrators and some program evaluators, have opted for an empirical stance, relatively void of ideological commitment in the search for a theoretical base. The matter is much too complex for simplistic explanations.

There is another, totally divergent, perspective. Purchase of services is seen as merely one of several means to "privatize" the public sector. Given this view, the search for a theoretical base might better be targeted at privatization. Although these authors do not reject the overarching nature of privatization, they suggest that POS is both an important building block of privatization and a free-standing technology often widely used even when not driven by ideological zealots. It was well established long before the concept of reprivatization was first articulated by Drucker in 1968.

Moving from the theme of the relative merits of purchase of service as a mechanism for delivering goods and services, some scholars have been concerned with, and focus upon, the implementation of contractual arrangements, including performance, role delegation and delineation, and interorganizational relationships. Within this framework, concerns have centered on traditional government functions and discernible differences, if any, in the performance of public agencies versus not-for-profit and for-profit organizations.

A number of service delivery problems plague both public and private agencies as they attempt to respond to the range of responsibilities they are expected to fulfill, including comprehensive planning, service provision, and service monitoring and evaluation. The difficulties inherent in the breadth of functions delegated to providers of human services are evident across sectors and are compounded, in some cases, by contractual arrangements. For example, state public health agencies may serve as allocators, contractors, service providers, comprehensive health planners, regulators, and overseers of services delivered by external sources. Similarly, the United Way has attempted to play comparable roles, exclusive of direct service delivery. In both examples comprehensive planning has suffered. Negative results are not surprising as role conflict becomes more evident. Studies by several management consulting firms underscore the point. McKinsey and Company concluded that conglomerates, companies that merge and operate a number of mandated businesses, do poorly compared with those more limited in scope. McKinsey concludes: "Conglomerate managements have shown they cannot manage their businesses well" (Madrick 1983, F7).

Two other examples, one from mental health and one from higher education, reiterate the theme. The president emeritus of Illinois College, I. V. Caine (in a letter to the editor of *The Chronicle of Higher Education*), urged that colleges and universities remember their follies of twenty years earlier. He recommended that college administrators contract for such services as food, endowment, management, student loans, and janitorial services. "It is hard enough to manage effectively the educational mission of the college, which is the only part of the world's work where administration is necessarily competent" (Caine 1983, 34). He urges fewer, not more, internal business operations.

The complimentary example in mental health comes from two reports on the status of mental health services (Massachusetts, 1981, and New York, 1983). The conclusions of both reports urged structural shifts that indirectly suggest the viability of purchase of service. Typically, the closure of some or all of the state mental hospitals was recommended, with responsibility for patient care placed at the community level. The conflict of interest in which the state mental health authorities find themselves is decried. The New York report stated it thus: "The Office of Mental Health carries a divided responsibility in New York State (leading to) . . . a conflict of interest in that it both administers its own direct services and at the same time monitors, evaluates and licenses its own and the community-based services, and distributes funds to both" (*New York Times,* 6 March 1983). The Massachusetts report, funded by the National Institute of Mental Health (Report of the Blue Ribbon Commission 1981) recommends that states should finance, monitor, and regulate mental health care and relinquish their operational responsibilities.

As we become increasingly sophisticated about organizational behavior, blatant structural/functional constraints, such as those identified above, have come to be of increasing concern to many public administrators. In the search for options, purchase of service has been seen as one solution to ease conflict of interest. Others, looking for increased efficiency, cost reduction, improved quality, and diminished bureaucratic constraints, have similarly looked to purchase of service. Thus, over the last decade or so, interest in purchase of service by the public sector has

9

accelerated to an unprecedented level. This volume focuses on the public purchase of human services and addresses the issues that underlie this development, actual experience with these arrangements, and their impact on interorganizational relations, role delineation, voluntarism, and client services.

Although extensive literature on the purchase of human services is lacking, the range of participants and interests is substantial. Public administrators seek to improve public sector performance. Public employees' unions are concerned with the potential loss of members that may accompany the purchase of services. Accountants and economists, legislators and administrators are concerned with economy and cost benefits, e.g., efficiency and expenditure control. Political scientists inquire about structure and function. There are concerns about the potential effect of purchase of services on clients, e.g., has the use of contractual arrangements made possible the more effective provision of quality services and more positive client outcomes? Others are concerned with the elusive public interest.

For many adherents of increased use of purchase of services, the issue is not whether "the least government is the best government," but how government can best achieve its objectives in the public interest. It is this point that will likely separate the neoconservative from the truly conservative. The former are still committed to meeting essential human needs, but are increasingly disenchanted with the means. The conservatives reject both ends and means; they want the government out of the human services "business." A nominal "safety net" is permissible. Then there are the pragmatists, those persuaded of the legitimate need for human services and structures to deliver these services. They merely want to know how best to achieve ends within realistic economic and social limitations. There are multiple rationales that provide for the use of purchase of service arrangements.

THE BOUNDARIES OF PURCHASE OF SERVICE

Definitions of purchase of service have clearly lagged behind discussions of the subject. When definitions are found, they reflect the narrow range and special interests so dominant in this field. The government purchases services from for-profit organizations, from individuals who aspire to be profitmaking, from groups of practitoners, from other governmental units, and from not-for-profit organizations. Exclusive of the U.S. Department of Defense, the largest proportion of those services purchased are arrangements between one public agency and another public agency.

Purchased services may be provided to targeted groups of people—a corporation, a neighborhood group, or special populations such as child abusers or runaway youth. Public responsibility for universal services and concerns about equity will influence some of these choices. In some cases the type or number of people to whom services may be rendered within a group may be limited by statute, regulations, or agreement, or be open-ended.

Purchase of service is, in fact, one part of two larger categories. One is concerned with the transmission of public funds to private bodies, individually or collectively. The other concerns the delivery of services. Throughout this volume, focus is on organized procedures by which an entity of the government enters into a formal agreement with another entity—public, private for-profit, private not-for-profit, or individual purveyor of services. The purchase may be for goods or services, but the focus here is on services and, almost exclusively, those services provided to individuals, groups, and communities to prevent, ameliorate, or resolve environmental, physical, or psychosocial problems.

Thus purchase of service represents one arrangement by which the government may relate to the nongovernmental sector. There are several other commonly used mechanisms, however, for linking public and private interests. Government may induce change by using tax concessions. The use of tax inducements has a long tradition in the United States and has been of significant importance to organized religion, voluntary associations, foundations, and others. During the last two decades, various tax reforms have been proposed and some enacted by Congress. In each instance there has been some tightening of the freedom of individual not-for-profit organizations to receive tax benefits. The 1986 Tax Reform Act significantly decreased the direct and indirect tax benefits to which not-for-profit organizations are now entitled. Most hard hit are the United Way and its affiliates, other human service organizations, and colleges and universities that depend in large part on funds derived from individual contributions or fund-raising campaigns. It is estimated that the repeal of the "contributions to charity" deduction for those who do not itemize their income tax returns would cost nonprofit groups $11 billion

(*Washington Post,* 9 July 1985). Analysis of later versions of the bill found that museums, hospitals, and the like, generally the recipients of larger gifts, would suffer even more.

Tax benefits for the profit sector have a more pendulumlike history than is the case for nonprofits. Clear trends are generally lacking. Use of tax inducements to produce desired goods and services may be considered an indirect intervention into the private marketplace. Purchase of service, in contrast, involves a direct buyer–seller relationship.

It should be emphasized that purchase of service constitutes only one of several ways to plan and deliver services. Savas (1982) identifies nine alternative mechanisms: (1) service rendered by a single governmental agency, (2) agreements between governments, (3) purchase of service by contracts, (4) franchises, (5) grants, (6) vouchers, (7) free market, (8) voluntary services, and (9) self-service. These mechanisms, in implementation, may and do overlap. One government unit may even elect to purchase a service (seldom a good) from another government unit and, in fact, the public purchase of other public services has been quite pervasive within the human services. Agencies (public and private) may be recipients of grants and contracts. Their clients may also be eligible for vouchers. Some of these same agencies may also compete in the open market to attract clientele and "sell" their services while providing voluntary services to others.

Despite the permeability of boundaries, the nine alternative mechanisms described by Savas represent a useful analytic tool that allows comparative assessments of the process and outcome of service delivery under each. From the perspective of public administrators, the following twelve planning issues can be delineated:

Identification of the problem or concern needing remediation
Determination of whether or not to purchase
Specification of what service(s) are to be purchased
Provision of information to service providers about the service need
Evaluation of proposals/options for service delivery
Negotiation of the contract
Price determination
Payment procedure determination
Contract implementation and monitoring
Product evaluation

12

Determination of whether to recontract with the same or different
agencies or to select an alternative service delivery option
To continue to provide the services

Purchase of service can take several forms, with variations in type of
contractual arrangements often depending on the desired buyer-seller relationship and the nature of the service(s) to be purchased. One method is
to purchase the service(s) for particular individuals or classes/categories
of individuals. The premise here is that there are certain individuals,
with identified problems or needs, who are deemed eligible by virtue of
their problem or need to receive services. The service provider, be it an
organization or individual, determines whether or not to sell the service.
The Vocational Rehabilitation Administration, through its state agencies, is a classic user of this kind of arrangement. They often pay market
prices to educational institutions and medical rehabilitative facilities to
provide services to particular clients who have specific, identified needs.
Such contractual arrangements may be long- or short-term. The seller
may offer services based on selective screening or serve all who are referred by the public agency who fall within a particular category or type
of problem. The amount of discretion that may be given to the voluntary
or proprietary service provider has, historically, raised concerns that they
may "cream" the "better" clients, those who are likely to achieve positive
results from the service and are thus easier to "treat."

Time-limited, task-oriented contracts constitute another form of purchase of service. Such arrangements are generally initiated to prepare a
product or deliver a service of a one-time nature; i.e., once the service is
delivered or the product completed, the contract will be terminated.
Health research and defense contracts best illustrate this model. In the
case of defense contracts, the U.S. Department of Defense may contract
with a corporation, such as General Electric or Lockheed, to produce a
new engine for an airplane. Once the engine is completed in the specified
quantities, the contract is concluded. Most often, time frames for the completion of the work are built into the contract itself. In research contracts
a medical school, research firm, or health association might be contracted
to conduct an assessment of patient characteristics in public and private
hospital emergency rooms.

The time-limited contracts, characterized by a high degree of specificity in terms of the product and production deadlines, may have a number

13

of substantial effects on the seller. One disadvantage from the perspective of the service provider is that a substantial start-up period is often necessary to initiate the contracted tasks, with the possibility that the contracted organization will have to disband if the contract is not renewed, when the task has been completed, or if public interests and priorities have shifted. The costs to the seller of implementing and disbanding may be substantial and not necessarily covered by the contract budget. For example, the costs of hiring a staff of experts or expanding the physical plant may not be fully compensated or may be of dubious value in terms of time and effort. However, from the point of view of the public agency, these task-oriented contracts are extremely cost effective and imply a responsible use of public funds in that no long-term commitments are implied. These contracts also allow for assessment and evaluation of the value of the service and contractor on the basis of specific and isolated pieces of work and places the major burden of start-up, personnel dislocation, and project termination on the service provider.

Another common purchase arrangement is for government to write a contract on a more extended time basis. These longer-term commitments assume that the service or product will be needed indefinitely.They also assume that the vendor will sustain high service delivery capability over time. Components of these longer-term contracts may be quite specific, e.g., the populations to be served, the types of services to be offered, and eligibility criteria. Similarly, the focus of the service may be narrow or broad in scope, such as diagnosing health problems or providing treatment and cure.

Deficit financing, as an alternative to purchasing units of service, is also a feasible model. In this case a contracted individual or agency has an agreement to provide a service to a specific population or to all of those applying for service with a particular kind of problem. The service provider is seen as the primary financier of such services, the dollars of which may come from a variety of sources. Assuming that the service is consistent with public priorities and that the provider has met the conditions of imposed or applicable quality assurances, the government makes up the deficit between what the provider is able to secure from other sources and the actual cost of operating the program/service. For example, a half-way house may be able to secure 80 percent of its annual operating budget from United Way contributions, payment of fees by the residents of the house, and fund-raising activities. The government

14

agency, such as alcoholism, drug abuse, or mental health department, awards a generic contract to make up the difference between operating costs and agency income related to the service in question. Most frequently, the amount of the deficit is limited to a figure falling within a designated range. This form of contracting contrasts sharply with the blanket purchase of specific numbers of service units, as in that most often used for purchasing day-care services.

The boundaries of purchase of service arrangements are continually expanding. Service areas that were exclusively within the province of government are now being reexamined to identify alternative delivery forms. The maintenance and ownership of jails is one example. Community fire and police services are two other areas in which heretofore public functions are now being delegated to the private sector by use of the contract method. Almost the only exception to the utilization of contracting is in the area of national security or individual protection. In the former instance, it is only government that can protect the national security and provide for defense systems. With individual protection, some states may legislate that adult and child protective services are exclusively a public function. However, in the latter instance, there are already several precedents for the use of a private sector delivery model.

Although national defense is exclusively a governmental function, the armed services are among the most frequent users of purchase arrangements to obtain a broad array of support services, as well as hardware. The prominence such purchasing practices have received by the media, particularly during the 1980s, will be discussed later in greater detail. Despite some serious problems in the procurement practices of the Department of Defense, the fact remains that almost all of its goods are purchased and more. For example, a private firm under contract operates and staffs the Distant Early Warning Line to detect missiles and airplanes flying over the Arctic Ocean toward North America. The surveillance and monitoring of the Sinai cease-fire agreement between Israeli and Egyptian forces in the 1970s was supplied by a private firm under contract to the U.S. government (Savas 1982).

The extension of the purchase of service boundaries is particularly notable in the area of community security and policing functions. By 1975 there were more private security personnel in the U.S. (435,000) than public police (411,000). In Canada the proportion of public police to private security personnel was nearly equal in number (51,000 versus

48,000, respectively [Shearing and Stenning 1983]). Private policing is far from new and, in fact, has a long and honorable history. Pinkerton, the first such private security organization, was founded in 1830 (Ghezzi 1983). The development of a public police oligopoly occurred later in the nineteenth century. The more equalized number of public and private personnel performing security functions is a relatively modern development and, although substantial growth has occurred in the number of security personnel in both the public and private sectors, since 1965 the growth is most pronounced in the private realm. Thus, even the maintenance of order shows considerable privatization.

Another recent example of privatization can be found in the development of insurance investigation units (Ghezzi 1983). A study of three Massachusetts automobile insurance companies found a burgeoning, privately-funded, fraud detection industry. Special investigation units under private auspices are now appearing nationwide.

In these introductory statements, a variety of terms have been introduced that are in need of definition: *purchase of service, contracts, voluntarism, private sector, not-for-profit, for-profit, privatization, fees for services,* and *deficit financing.* They will be discussed throughout the volume.

2

The Evolving Contract State

Margaret Gibelman and Harold W. Demone, Jr.

The use of purchase of service is not a new phenomenon. A review of historical trends in the delivery of health, welfare, and rehabilitation services in the United States shows this type of arrangement to be pervasive. Traditionally, state and local governments have elected to meet a part of their responsibilities through financing the provision of care and services by local, nongovernmental organizations. In fact, as one views the three-hundred-year development of social welfare in the United States, the interaction between the private and public service delivery systems provides an important vantage point (Cruthirds 1972; Kramer 1964; Randolph 1976).

It has been estimated that over half of all public social service dollars are spent for the purchase of services (Pacific Consultants 1979). Within the field of vocational rehabilitation, the proportion is even greater. Although the health industry is a primary user of third-party mechanisms, it, too, engages in significant contracting. Even the criminal justice system is exploring the application of the concept. The extent to which purchase of service dominates a particular health and human services field is subject to a wide range of influences, including political and philosophical forces and social values and preferences. Purchase of service is reflective of, and integrally related to, changing conceptions of the roles and functions of the public and private sectors of this society. Increases or decreases in the use of purchase of service must thus be understood within the context of prevailing priorities, values, and preferences affecting social welfare policies and programs. Far from a static phenomenon, "contracting out" for the delivery of services may, at different times, be viewed within a continuum of a preferred solution or new type of accountability and administrative problem.

PURCHASING SERVICES: HISTORICAL ROOTS

Purchase of service has its origins in the very first systems established in the United States to provide for the public welfare. During the Colonial era, a rudimentary form of public relief, based on the English Poor Laws, provided a type of last resort assistance when family and individual resources were exhausted. Expectations concerning the extent of governmental intervention on behalf of the needy were limited, as were the resources to meet social and individual needs. The public sector was slow to accept responsibility for maintaining adequate social welfare supports and services, particularly in comparison with other Western industrialized nations (Wilensky and Lebeaux 1965). That government would assume a monopoly on service provision to those with problems associated with economic, physical, or social dependency was simply antithetical to prevailing views. Accordingly, voluntary forms of assistance developed through the church, mutual benefit societies, and private philanthropy, concurrent with a very modest assumption of government responsibility in this early period (Kramer 1964).

The complexities and variations in the interrelations between these two systems has been a dominant theme throughout this country's history. Despite emphasis on the relative merits of one system over the other at various times, there is repeated evidence of governmental bodies electing to discharge their responsibilities through nongovernment service provision. Purchase of service has been a major mechanism for linking public and private systems. Historical examples of the interrelationships between these sectors can be identified in the early arrangements for the provision of public relief. The rudimentary system of outdoor relief administered by some local public authorities as far back as the colonial era was augmented by a system of "contracting out" and a related practice of "auctioning off" the aged, orphaned, and poor to private individuals for care (Cruthirds 1972; Wedel 1976).

In reaction to the many abuses that became evident in the early system of private contracting, reformers in the first part of the nineteenth century urged changes. Successful in their pleas, this reform effort resulted in a movement toward a policy of public indoor, or institutional, relief and the initiation of a subsidy system for private institutions. These earlier contractual agreements took the form of direct subsidies to voluntary welfare organizations. Although governmental subsidies have been

18

traced back as far as 1751 in Pennsylvania, it was only in the last quarter of the nineteenth century that this practice became a common method of discharging government's responsibility for social welfare (Coughlin 1965). Its use also coincided with the evolving growth of public responsibility for social welfare, thus creating parallel or dual service systems. The health industry presented comparable public-private features.

The financial support of the private sector, through subsidies, was seen as less costly than building new public facilities; subsidized institutions could be free of political interference and capable of maintaining high standards without government control (Burian 1970). Kramer (1964) further notes that the readiness to use tax funds to subsidize existing private institutions may also relate to pressures exerted by voluntary agency leadership, which had a vested interest in utilizing its own facilities to the fullest.

Subsidy arrangements, however, were not without their critics. Kramer (1964), for example, points to the long controversy over the practice of public subsidies as exemplifying prevailing sentiments about the respective character and roles of government and voluntary agencies. According to Kramer, those arguing against the public-voluntary agency partnership, through the mechanism of the subsidy system, identified the following flaws:

Voluntary agencies encouraged pauperism by disguising it;
It was not real economy because so many duplicate institutions were
    necessary, one for each sectarian group, and since intake poli-
    cies were not controlled, tax funds were used to support the
    care of the "inmates" at private institutions;
Special pressures were put on legislatures to influence appropriations;
It tended to dry up other sources of private funds; and
It destroyed the freedom of the voluntary agency.

One of the first comprehensive studies of public subsidies to private charities was carried out by Amos Warner in the 1890s. Based on survey data, Warner and his associates summarized the arguments for and against the use of public subsidies. Among the arguments in favor of their use were financial savings when care for dependents is provided by a private voluntary organization, better quality care, more professional business operations, and less stigma attached for the poor and aged. The arguments cited against subsidies included loss of public control, waste-

19

ful duplication of institutions, encouragement of vested interest pressure on legislatures, tendency to dry up the sources of private benevolence, and loss of freedom for the subsidized organization (Warner, Queen, and Harper 1930). Many of the arguments concerning the subsidy system for social welfare services, as advanced at the turn of the century, linger to this day and continue to influence the range and scope of purchase of service arrangements between the public and private sectors.

Nor were the debates limited exclusively to matters of public-private relations. They also concerned the quality of care, sometimes quite vigorously, eventually leading to more experimentation. One purported advancement was the establishment of local public almshouses for paupers. The almshouses, operated by public officials, were, for a while, considered to be a cheaper and better deterrent of malingering and more efficient than other forms of care (Mencher 1967). Despite such "innovative" practices, varying degrees of contracting continued to be practiced. Most popular was the public purchase of special care, particularly in regard to the care of dependent children. Ironically, it was the deplorable conditions for and concerns about children in institutions and almshouses that served to stimulate even more the growth of subsidy arrangements in child welfare. A solution had again become the problem. Many states began to seek alternative forms of child care either by establishing separate state institutions for children or subsidizing the already existing private institutions (Randolph 1976). (Curiously, the early 1980s saw the return of modified almshouses no better than their predecessors for the homeless. They have become the new scandal.)

Despite expressed concerns and arguments, the subsidization of private institutions evolved into a strongly entrenched system for financing social services, reaching its zenith during the early 1930s and then losing ground to the emerging pattern of financing entitled purchase of service (Cruthirds 1972). These financial arrangements were to have long-lasting implications for the nature of the relationship between government and private agencies. Among the effects of the subsidy system were

1. The early and widespread growth of private child agencies through the assurance of continued public support. Rather than supplementing, it often supplanted the government-operated agency system.
2. The assumption of public responsibility, particularly in the field of

20

child welfare. There was little pressure to expand the scope of public institutions since they had extremely low standards and were highly susceptible to partisan politics.

Recurring conceptions of agency character, roles, and relationships were articulated. In a debate over subsidies, the public agency was frequently associated with almshouses, political corruption, and lack of empathy. Voluntary agencies, on the other hand, were seen as undertaking humanitarian efforts and deserving of public funds to help meet social purposes. This positive image of voluntary agencies was reinforced by their self-perceptions as guardians of religious and moral values and vanguards in pioneering new forms of child care (Kramer 1964).

The widespread use of the subsidy system thus encouraged a belief in the primacy of the voluntary agency and residual nature of government as service provider. However, in the 1930s changes in the perceived range of government responsibility to finance and provide social services became evident. Enactment of the Social Security Act of 1935, and the conditions of the economic depression that led to its passage, is generally accepted as the benchmark of direct federal intervention into the nation's social welfare system. The shift from poor relief to the concept of public welfare as a legitimate function of government facilitated the expansion of many public health, welfare, and social service programs. Likewise, government assumed an enhanced role in the gradual extension of state regulation, supervision, and licensing of many not-for-profit and for-profit agencies. The many amendments to the Social Security Act have further articulated and clarified the variety of public roles.

Most pronounced among the changes occurring in the nature and scope of public welfare during the 1930s was the enormous growth in social welfare expenditures, and, for the first time, the amount expended by government exceeded that of voluntary agencies (Wedel 1976). The relative importance of public subsidies to voluntary agencies also declined due to the rapid expansion of functions directly administered by government agencies. The development and implementation of social welfare programs sufficient in size and scope to address the vast demographic and social problems of the 1930s could only be accomplished by government, particularly considering the costs of such a massive undertaking. Some, fearing that voluntarism would be eradicated, urged a sharing of responsibility between the two sectors in the delivery of

21

services, echoing past preferences for role delegation. With the advent of a strengthened public system, the key question concerned the nature of public-private interrelationships: Should there be such a relationship and if so, how and to what degree?

Between 1935 and 1962, several amendments were added to the original Social Security Act, separately and in combination, having the effect of enlarging government's role in the funding and provision of services to a client population increasing in size. One significant trend was the adoption of a "service" philosophy to assist recipients of public welfare, rather than simply the provision of cash or in-kind benefits. In part, this service approach was based on the assumption that the problems associated with poverty went beyond a lack of money and that "rehabilitation" was necessary if the poor were to attain social and financial independence. Significantly, this approach was also seen as integral to diminishing, permanently, the ever-increasing size of the welfare rolls.

In the 1962 amendments to the Social Security Act, Congress initiated a series of programs to strengthen the rehabilitation approach, granting implementation authority to the public sector. Through an open-ended federal appropriation, P.L. 87–543, 75 percent matching funds were provided to states that would establish and implement defined social services under any of the public assistance titles they elected. Another important feature of the 1962 amendments was the official recognition of already prevailing beliefs: services could be used to prevent some vulnerable persons from becoming or remaining dependent on public assistance. Two other features of these amendments are particularly relevant in terms of both precedent and future, unanticipated consequences. The federal financial match was increased to 75 percent from its prior 50 percent level as an incentive for states to undertake or expand services to a more broadly defined population eligible for services. Second, states were, for the first time, authorized to enter into agreements with other public agencies (such as Health and Vocational Rehabilitation) for services that could be "more economically provided by these agencies" (Slack 1979). Thus, purchase of service was introduced into the social services programs. In fact, the inclusion of this provision merely extended purchase of service practices to the social services; heretofore, such related fields as vocational rehabilitation and health had long made significant use of this service delivery mechanism.

By 1967 the political pendulum was swinging back toward a more cautious social services approach. There were those in Washington who were convinced that the "loopholes" in the 1962 amendments were responsible for the spiraling growth in the Aid to Families with Dependent Children (ADC) program. Thus, in response to the growing size of ADC rolls, the 1967s amendments to the Social Security Act were enacted. Although reaffirming the federal commitment to social services, this legislation sought to introduce certain measures that would tie social services more closely to the labor market. Rather than services, preparing people to enter or return to paid employment became the rallying cry. Twenty years later, now called welfare reform, the call was renewed. (The change was in degree, not kind.)

In keeping with the "get people back to work" philosophy, the 1967 amendments expanded available day-care services. Purchase of service provisions were also modified. Under the new law, states were granted authority to purchase services from nonprofit or proprietary agencies, or from individuals or other state or local public agencies. These measures were intended to effectuate the changed conception of public social services. A growing disenchantment with the value of public services, as well as increased skepticism about the efficacy of public service provision, resulted in a new emphasis on work support and private sector linkages.

The use of contracting to purchase work-related services had been a dominant trend in several War on Poverty programs, such as the Job Corps; this established pattern presumably influenced the decision to expand purchase provisions for the newly focused work rather than rehabilitation approach. Accordingly, earlier attitudes of caution about the use of purchase of service were disregarded in favor of using the stronger capabilities and proven expertise of the private sector in this arena (Slack 1979). There had been other recent and successful experiences in the public purchase of voluntary services, fueling the decision to proceed with this type of delivery mechanism. For example, the Vocational Rehabilitation Administration relied heavily and with positive results on purchase, concluding from its studies that this method increased flexibility, improved standards, was cost effective, controlled staff size, and created a network of organizational allies within the purchase of service network.

By 1969 nearly all restrictive language on the use of purchase of service was dropped from regulations, with new rules promulgated to require states to increase their use of contracting. State plans were to "assure progressive development of arrangements with a number and variety of agencies . . . with the aim of providing opportunities for individuals to exercise a choice with regard to the source of purchased service" (Derthick 1975, 20). Subject to the limitations, prescribed by the secretary of the then Department of Health, Education, and Welfare (DHEW), contractual arrangements were to be used for services that, in the judgment of the state agency, could not be as economically or effectively provided by the staff of such state or local agencies and were not otherwise reasonably available to individuals in need of them.

SPIRALING SOCIAL SERVICE COSTS

A combination of features, including broadened statutory authority for purchase of service, federal encouragement to develop such arrangements, states' interest in maximizing federal funds, and the support of the private sector, resulted in rapid increases in the use of public social service dollars by the states. It should be recalled that, under the public assistance titles, there remained no fixed dollar limitation on spending. States sought to maximize the federal contribution through the use of purchase of service. The first goal of the states was very clear. Contrary to legislative intent, they sought to substitute federal expenditures for state expenditures. The quantity of services would likely remain essentially unaltered, certainly an unanticipated outcome. Some states permitted service expansion using voluntary matching dollars as state funds became a smaller component of the total.

As is customary in such matters, expenditures inflated and Congress and the administration reacted. They simultaneously put a ceiling on appropriations, focused the expenditures, and paradoxically granted the states more flexibility within the new set of parameters.

In October 1972 P.L. 92–512, the General Revenue Sharing Act, was enacted, fixing a $2.5 billion ceiling on total federal expenditures for social services under the several Social Security Act public assistance titles. It also restricted 90 percent of the federal funds to expenditures for family planning, child day care, foster care for children, mental retardation, and alcoholism and drug abuse services. This $2.5 billion ceiling, which was carried over into the Title XX amendments (1975) and was later retained with an inflationary index (though cut by 25 percent with the enactment of the Omnibus Budget Reconciliation Act of 1981), applied to states according to a simple, population-based formula, unrelated to the proportion of welfare recipients in the population or other poverty criteria (Slack 1979). Within the dollar and programmatic limits set, the General Revenue Sharing Act, which expired in fiscal year 1986, allowed recipient governments to allocate their funds to almost any governmental service, project, or program. This form of federalism encouraged states and local governments, therefore, to assert choices as to the types of services that would be provided, as well as the means for implementation. Purchase of service was consistent with this newly found power of the states and localities.

On 4 January 1975, additional amendments were enacted. With the passage of P.L. 93–637, the Social Service Amendments of 1974, which constituted Title XX of the Social Security Act, the nature of public social services was fundamentally changed. Henceforth, states would be given responsibility for not only defining services, but for deciding where, how much, and to whom these services should be provided. States now had significantly increased latitude to determine how federal funds would be used. Likewise, the role of the federal administrative arm (then DHEW) in the provision of public social services would be limited largely to technical assistance, with the granting of explicit responsibility for assisting states with their program content and with the administrative requirements newly established.

Title XX was to remain the predominant source of authority and funds for public social services until 1981 when, with the passage of the Omnibus Budget Reconciliation Act (P.L. 97–35), states and localities were given substantially more authority and flexibility to design their human services programs than had existed under the earlier legislation, but with less money. This act authorized a social services block grant program, among other block grants, consisting of the earlier Title XX social services program, the Title XX training program, and day care. To the pleasure of many governors and mayors, a majority of the federal regulations governing the public social services programs were eliminated, but on the negative side, the level of federal funding was reduced by 25 percent. (Inflation also took its toll.) States would no longer have to meet a 25 percent match of the federal contribution, a feature of earlier Social Security Act amendments, but were encouraged by the Reagan administration to make up for this difference in federal funding and finance "real" service costs by promoting private donations and state voluntary contributions.

Among the choices states faced with the enactment of the Omnibus Reconciliation Act of 1981 was the determination of when and how to use the private sector in the financing and delivery of services. The Reagan message was clear: the private sector should have a more expansive role in the planning, financing, and delivery of human services. Partnership building between the public and private sectors was, in the administration's view, an opportunity to overcome many of the perceived weaknesses in the public service system. However, as Salamon comments, the administration misread both the strength of its persuasiveness and the economic realities. "Instead of forging a new coalition in support of a positive program of cooperation between government and the voluntary sector, the administration relied primarily on exhortation and on the expected success of its economic program to suffuse the country with voluntaristic spirit" (Salamon 1984, 271).

Cuts in the federal financing of social services had an immediate and profound impact on voluntary agencies. In FY 1981, it is estimated that federal financial support of nonprofit institutions had reached over $46 billion, 38 percent of the total revenues of nonprofit, charitable service organizations (Salamon and Abramson 1982, 233). In addition to direct funding there are two other primary ways in which voluntary agencies benefit from federal policy. First is tax policy, particularly in regard to charitable-giving provisions. The second means is through purchase of service contracts grants, or third-party payment methods that flow from government to the nonprofit sector. One way in which states could reduce, quickly, their level of social service expenditures was to terminate purchase of service contracts. By so doing, states could redirect the dollars saved to maintain public agency operations. Conversely, states might opt to continue the level of contracting with voluntary agencies, but pass along to them a form of matching funds; e.g., contracted providers could be asked to assume a portion of the costs in a modified version of cost sharing. These two state options, in the face of diminished federal resources, would severely affect the financial status and service-rendering capability of the nonprofit sector. Holding the line on the dollar allotment for contracts was the least likely strategy for states facing a 25 percent reduction in federal funding.

The impact of decreased federal revenues is starkly illuminated by comparing the amount of fiscal support nonprofit organizations receive from government with their other sources of revenue. Private charitable contributions to these organizations from individuals, foundations, and corporations was approximately $22 billion in 1980, 55 percent less than the revenues received from government. For social services, federal support totaled 58 percent of all revenues (Salamon 1984).

For the nonprofit sector to make up the difference caused by decreased federal funding, and holding constant the high probability of cutbacks in the level of contracting, charitable contributions would have to be increased. The issue here, however, is that simultaneous changes were proposed (and finally enacted in 1986) in tax policy, again with a potentially adverse affect on voluntary agencies. The specific issue of concern was a decrease in tax rates. Data indicate that individuals in the higher tax brackets are more willing to give to charities, particularly those who itemize their deductions (Clotfelter and Steuerle 1981). As Salamon (1984) describes it, deductible charitable contributions diminish the "cost" of giving in that the "gift" represents the difference between what the taxpayer contributes and what he or she would have owed in taxes if the gift were not given. People in the higher tax brackets gain the most from charitable contributions. As the individual's tax bracket lowers, the "real cost" of giving rises, thus discouraging giving. Reagan's tax plan, however, benefited most those who, heretofore, contributed the most, with the net effect of reducing incentives to, and likelihood of, such charitable contributions.

Under the best of circumstances, the expected level of charitable giving was of growing concern to the nonprofit sector. One discernible trend in relation to charitable contributions is that the rate of giving has been falling behind increases in overall personal income. Concurrently, more and more taxpayers have been opting to take the standard tax deductions, decreasing the likelihood of their making charitable contributions, because this would no longer count as a tax break (Salamon 1984). The net result of changes in tax law is to decrease even further the likelihood of charitable giving. (See part seven for a more detailed discussion of the impact of the 1986 Tax Reform Act.)

There are at least two other themes of the Reagan administration that concern the use of purchase of service arrangements. This administration made clear its desire to promote stronger linkages between the public and private sectors and, to the extent possible, to shift heretofore public functions and responsibilities to the private sector. This theme, new only in its extreme, comes under the rubric of "privatization." The emphasis

27

on partnership building will be discussed at greater length later in this chapter. Closely associated with the desire to enhance collaboration between the sectors is the emphasis on federalism. Clearly, the current thrust is to reverse the historic and pervasive reliance on centralized decision making, i.e., the federal establishment, favoring, instead, the discharge of public responsibility through state and local governments. It is believed that this decentralization of planning and delivery functions will result in greater responsiveness to the needs of citizens, and more accountability and efficiency. The relevance of Reagan federalism to purchase of service lies in its underlying premise that public responsibilities—no matter the level of government—should be met by delegating functions to the private sector. Ideally, this delegation would include a direct role for the private sector in financing service provision, as well as delivering services.

Several observers hypothesize that President Reagan's social and economic initiatives could be as significant in the long term as the New Deal was fifty years ago. (See Palmer and Sawhill [1982].)

In summary, a number of features of the Reagan domestic agenda tended to favor the use of purchase of service, especially with the for-profit private sector. When viewed separately, the implementation of the principles of federalism, privatization, and public-private partnership building each holds relevance for, and justifies the use of, contractual arrangements across sectors. When viewed collectively, these approaches to the financing and delivering of social services overwhelmingly point to purchase of service as a logical, practical, and proven method of furthering political goals and priorities.

Although there is a tendency in some quarters to view purchase of service as unplanned and an accident of history, this overview of the growth in the use of contractual arrangements indicates their philosophical and ideological consistency with shifts in political priorities and legislative agendas. Particularly in recent years, the evolution from a predominantly federal system of planning, funding, and delivering social services to a system characterized largely by state and local (and increasingly, private sector) responsibility has made purchase of service a significant mechanism by which to accomplish explicit objectives.

ESTABLISHING PRECEDENTS

Purchase of service, as indicated earlier, is not a new or unique invention. George Washington established several precedents. Included was the purchase of goods and services and, conversely, the expression of complaints about several contractors who supplied military hardware (Sharkansky 1980). Wedel (1976) also reminds us that purchase of service has been practiced since colonial days and that purchased services can be traced throughout the history of the American social welfare system. Specific financial modalities have included grants, per capita payments, tax concessions, and lump sum subsidies. He notes that contracting has often been the preferred mode.

Lourie (1979) comments that the increase in subsidized or purchase services in this country in the 1890s and early 1900s was fraught with the same ambivalence and dilemmas as is the case today. The question was asked then, as it is now: Is accountability possible when employees are not your own? He also argues that the civil rights revolution and War on Poverty programs were significant influences on the present popularity of the purchase of social services. Decentralization and community control were advocated, and the community cannot easily control that which is owned, managed, and delivered by a large, distant government. Even local government was distrusted.

One historical example will illustrate the complex history that characterizes purchase of service. Rosner (1980), in describing the Progressive Era (1895–1915) in New York City, tells of the determination of the city comptroller's office to gain control over the locally run small community hospitals receiving partial subsidization from the city. A per capita, per diem reimbursement mechanism was implemented to replace the flat-grant payment procedure. To the comptroller, rationality and cost control were introduced. To the hospital trustees and community representatives, this action constituted political interference. The net result of giving more control to the "good-government" centralized experts was to negatively impact on the small, financially troubled institutions. Some were forced to close. "Adopting as catch words notions of efficiency, bureaucracy and expertise, the reformers assumed power in the central offices of government, industry, and charity services and challenged the rights of communities to make their own social and political decisions" (Rosner 1980, 534).

Thus, by 1899 the system of per capita, per diem reimbursement was inaugurated and "municipal inspection of the financial and moral character of the charity patient began" (ibid., 535).

The tensions generated by those issues were remarkably similar to concerns raised today. The city complained about lack of efficiency. They could make better decisions. Hospitals were concerned both about their financial viability and the city's assertion of authority over their institutions. In the latter part of the nineteenth century, The Charity Organization Society (in some respects, the United Way of its day) feared that a city subsidy system would develop and undermine their authority as leaders of the nonprofit health and social services sector. They responded by setting their own stiff administrative standards. The net result of these several interventions was that some "unworthy" poor previously served were refused medical care and other potential patients failed to participate given the publicity about the the new standards. A 10 percent hospital census reduction occurred. Accounting procedures were improved, especially the hospitals' ability to distinguish prospective patients who could not pay for their care. A change in orientation of the voluntary hospitals was one consequence of this defensive posturing, wherein they no longer felt obliged to treat all of the poor who arrived at their doors.

Over time, two other major shifts occurred. Instead of spending less money, the city's emphasis on efficiency stimulated the identification of many more "worthy poor" eligible for medical care, now defined as a legitimate responsibility of this municipal government. Services funded by the city expanded. Loss of autonomy of the hospital trustees over reimbursement and admissions procedures led to increased city financing. Thus, the city failed to save money, the local community lost significant control of its institutions, and some "unworthy poor" fell between the cracks. There were two positive results. More "worthy poor" were served, as was the bureaucracy.

This turn of the century form of public purchase of private human services was not a uniquely East Coast phenomenon. Levenson (1977) traces Los Angeles County's first service contract to 1907. Massachusetts and Pennsylvania were also early users of this mechanism. In 1961 Coughlin found that 71 percent of the 470 surveyed sectarian agencies in twenty states were involved in some type of financial transactions with units of government. Beck (1971) describes a 1960 survey of twenty-three urban areas. Payments to private agencies accounted for 29 percent of all government expenditures for family services and 100 percent of maternity home care. This was long before the fruits of Title XX, Community Mental Health, Medicare and Medicaid. While Nelson Rockefeller was governor of New York, an integral component of his "creative federalism" was the integration of the private and public sectors by means of contracting (Levenson 1977).

Despite the view of many contemporary authors, the plethora of voluntary programs funded through Title XX, and now, the block grants program, is not unique in this country. In the early 1960s, a series of reports and publications sought to analyze the implications of the purchase of service system; the results probably served as a model for current practices, certainly highlighting the availability of this option. A 1961 Rockefeller Foundation report concluded that the most important source of funds for voluntary agencies would come from increased governmental support (Hamlin 1961). Dissertations by Kramer at Berkeley and Coughlin at Brandeis in the 1960s reviewed the trends and impacts of POS in considerable detail. Key components of their dissertations were published (Coughlin 1961, 1965; Kramer 1964, 1966). Other important articles on this subject published in the 1950s and 1960s include: Burns (1956), Schwartz and Wolins (1958), Johnson (1959), Hilman (1960), Wickenden and Bell (1961), Werner (1961), Berkowitz (1963), Selig (1963), Mintor (1965), Reid (1964), and Geissler (1965). A thorough analysis of the policy issues reflecting the use of public funds by voluntary agencies in the late 1950s and early 1960s can be found in Kramer (1964, 1966).

The justifications for purchase of service and the possible problems relating to its use are remarkably consistent, whether identified at the turn of the century, in the late 1950s, or now. Table 2.1 reflects this historical perspective on the advantages and disadvantages of POS. It should be noted that the number of arguments posed pro or con are less significant than the cogency of each argument. The numbers are not as relevant as the weighting attributed to each factor.

Hoshino's claim that "the drift toward purchase may be mostly unwitting and expedient" (1982, p. 8) appears to be contrary to substantiated history. These cries of despair—and Hoshino is merely an example—may be more a protest against the developments than a rational analysis of historical trends. As Hoshino (1982) himself notes, Benjamin Franklin

Table 2.1. **Advantages and Disadvantages of Purchase of Service**

Advantages	Disadvantages
Cost effectiveness	Difficult to ensure standards and
Accurate cost determinations	adequate coverage
Administrative efficiency	Loss of public control and account-
Greater response to immediate needs	ability
Better service coordination	Abrogates legislative intent
Avoidance of start-up costs required	Undermines role of public agency
to provide services	Increases costs
Avoidance of cumbersome and dys-	Poorer service
functional civil service regulations	Loss of protection for the poor and most
Ease of altering or terminating	needy ("creaming")
programs	Unreliability of contractors
Enhanced quality of services	Loss of autonomy for private agencies
Ease in adjusting program size	Private agencies subject to shifts in
More effective use of talent and human	public policy
resources	Legal mandate to accept low bid
Desirable mix of public and private	Displacement of employees
services	Difficulty in monitoring contracts
Avoidance of political patronage	Reduces experimental voluntary spirit
Ease in measuring/monitoring	Directs private agencies to provide
contractor performance	only publicly funded services
Increased professionalism	
Flexible use of personnel	
Improved program and administrative	
control	
Program flexibility	
Promotion of innovation in policy and	
administration	
Helps retain volunteerism	
Allows for competition in level of wages	
Greater assurance of legal rights for	
clients	
Frees public resources to service other	
important needs	

Sources: Kramer 1964; Wedel 1973; Weinstein 1979; California Tax Foundation 1981; Demone and Gibelman 1983.

secured a public subsidy for the Pennsylvania Hospital, the nation's longest continuing general hospital. The developments, as most in our history, certainly contain elements of expediency, but they are hardly unwitting, as evidenced by the gradual but continuous experience with the purchase of services against sometimes formidable opposition.

32

PUBLIC-PRIVATE RELATIONSHIPS

Purchase of service has been heralded as a means of forging stronger linkages between the public and private sectors, thereby promoting a partnership approach to the design, financing, and delivery of services. This emphasis on the positive benefits to accrue from a mixed service delivery system has been expressed by Presidents Nixon, Ford, and Carter. The Reagan plan is merely an extreme version of a recurrent theme, to which purchase of service, as a means to an end, is philosophically and ideologically consistent.

Under executive leadership, the Office of Management and Budget has, for many years, urged federal and state agencies to rely more on the private sector to meet production and service needs. Hoogland deHoog (1984) points to specific aspects of Reagan's program that promote this private sector reliance within the human services. Under the Economic Recovery Program, for example, comes the expectation that private, nonprofit agencies will increase their services to the needy. Urban enterprise zones have been suggested as the means by which to give businesses the incentives to revitalize economically depressed areas. The U.S. Department of Housing and Urban Development, through its administration of the Government Capacity Sharing Program, has encouraged governments at all levels to increase the use of contractors to deliver a broad range of municipal services.

Typically, the relationship between the public and private sectors is debated on the basis of philosophy or ideology, rather than experience. Empirical evidence is seldom considered, in part because only limited information exists on whether and how auspice impacts on such matters as availability, accessibility, quality, continuity, and cost effectiveness. It is clear, however, that Harry Hopkins's dictum that public money should be spent exclusively by public agencies is increasingly under challenge, with fewer and fewer proponents.

One constant theme has to do with boundary blurring. Public and private organizations are becoming more alike and represent a continuum rather than pure types. The degree to which this tendency to "sameness" is functional is open to question. Data are not offered to support the boundary-blurring hypothesis and, even if found valid, evidence of its dysfunctional aspects is not made clearly explicit. However, the mere suggestion that the distinctive attributes of the private or public sectors

33

may be diminishing and that a more "hybrid" form of organization may be arising in its stead causes considerable consternation and worry among purists.

It is clear that what is public and what is private is now an exceedingly complex question, compounded by the corollary ideological question of what should be public or private. A functional approach to differentiating the two sectors is no longer a helpful exercise, because functions often overlap or are duplicative. To public policymakers, the problem of definition may confuse issues of delegating responsibility and expressing preferences. There is a pervasive inconsistency in describing public and private; similar types of organizations may be under different auspices, or different types may be under the same auspice. For example, community action agencies in some states are within the public sector and in other states they use a nonprofit charter, becoming a quasi-public organization. Community mental health agencies similarly vary. In Massachusetts they may be public or private, but increasingly are of a private nature. In Connecticut they are typically public. New Jersey favors a private sector approach for its community mental health agencies. The range of organizational types is illustrated in table 2.2.

Shepsle (1980) suggests that, if it was ever an accurate description, the public-private dichotomy is no longer valid. He concludes that the public and private sectors today are conceptually indistinct, with two-way penetration. The public sector intrudes through the promulgation and enforcement of regulations; the private, by carrying out public purposes through purchase of service contracts. The regulations, written by lawyers, focus on rights and responsibilities, not role distinctions or performance expectations. We need to forget the old stereotypes about public and private, and instead need to "learn to mobilize research, development, capital investments, and a genuine sense of social participation without regard to the sector that provides the talent, drive, imagination, funds, or direction" (*New York Times,* 19 October 1981).

At a March 1982 partnership conference attended by mayors, nonprofit group representatives, and corporate leaders, the theme was partnership on a larger scale (*New York Times,* 3 April 1982). Now new, but bigger and better was the thrust. In Denver an area under redevelopment has been turned over to a committee of public and private members to regulate such diverse matters as construction design and pollution control. Allstate Insurance Company purchased city bonds in Fort Lauderdale,

Table 2.2. **Types of Health & Human Services Agencies**

Public	Quasi-public	Quasi-private	Private
Classic bureaucratic agencies with civil service staff	Quangos	Privately owned and operated	Privately owned and operated
Legal mandates	Almost exclusive reliance on public funds	Governed by board of directors	Governed by board of directors
Tax supported	Missions consistent with public purposes	Missions may not be consistent with public purposes	Mission established by charter
Public authority	Includes most OEO agencies using private charters and regional health planning	Use private charters but now receive much of their funds from public sources, e.g., Visiting Nurse Associations	Could operate effectively without any public support, but may engage in contracting
Can delegate some responsibilities through POS	May be for-profit or not-for-profit	May be for-profit or not-for-profit	May be for-profit or not-for-profit

Florida, to rebuild a burned-out apartment for the elderly. Loaned executives, as in the United Way, work in many city halls. Mayors from San Francisco and Nashville describe new private-public partnerships. Questions, however, can be raised as to whether the partnerships are not, in fact, built on a public fiscal base, particularly in the case of nonprofit organizations.

Brian O'Connell (1976), president of the Independent Sector, asks "What price independence?" He and others concerned with the consequences of the voluntary sector's reliance on public funds question: "Who will play the visionary role?" "Who will be the critic, the advocate, if they are also the recipients of government funds?" The interests that may be served by accepting government funds must be carefully weighed against the traditional voluntary roles and missions; to what extent are these compromised? Constant vigilance is needed to ensure that organizational purposes are not sacrificed to financial exigencies.

35

DIMENSIONS OF CONTRACTING

Statistics on the scope of purchase of services for all of government are not available. There are, however, a series of reports and studies that provide a perspective on the prevalence of contracting. In fiscal year 1980, the federal government spent $100.1 billion on contracted commercial services, prior to President Reagan's taking office. For 1985 the Office of Management and Budget estimated that the contracting figure would be $173 billion (*New York Times,* 28 April 1985). The OMB remained firmly committed to increasing the use of the private sector for the production of goods and the delivery of routine and specialized services.

In fiscal year 1984, colleges, universities, and nonprofit organizations received $2.1 billion in contract monies from the U.S. Department of Defense for research, development, testing, and evaluation. This sum represented 12 percent of the $18.3 billion in awards made to 2,033 business, educational, nonprofit, and other government organizations receiving contracts over $25,000 (*Washington Post,* 20 August 1985). The total of domestic agency contracts worth more than $10,000 and U.S. Department of Defense contracts valued at more than $25,000 was almost $166 billion (ibid.).

An April 1982 report by the United States comptroller general found, for fiscal year 1980, that for federal civil agencies (excluding the military) engaged in contracting, awards in excess of $10,000 each totaled about $23.3 billion. The comptroller general, at the request of a congressional committee, looked particularly hard at sole source procurements (those contracts let without competitive bids, but through negotiation), finding that about $10.9 billion (47 percent) were so expended.

The comptroller general (1982) also found that of the six federal agencies studied in depth, the U.S. department of Health and Human Services had both the lowest rate of "unwarranted sole source awards and the best record in using the *Business Commerce Daily* to invite competition" (p. 27). Despite this early optimism about the use of bureaucratically responsible procedures in the purchase of human services, charges of favoritism and political bias were leveled against the assistant secretary of the Office of Human Development Services in 1983 and 1984. Although blind reviews of competitive proposals were instituted by OHDS to ensure a fair and open process, allegations suggested that the actual awarding of contracts ignored the highest scored proposals in favor of political friends and philosophically "correct" organizations (*Washington Post*, 28 November 1983; 21 November 1985).

Sharkansky (1980) notes that between 1965 and 1975 government contracting grew by 356 percent, 130 percent faster than total government revenues.

> Social Security and Veterans Benefits aside, a predominate activity of government is letting contracts, grants, and subsidies to corporations for the purpose of performing governmental missions. Although the regulatory functions of government provoke the most publicized outcries, the contracting activity, in sheer dollars and personnel, are vastly greater — 100 times greater in revenue terms alone (Nader 1977, 10).

Purchase of service by state governments is also important, but not all states use this service delivery mechanism to the same degree or for the same purposes. The situation is far from static. With these disclaimers, in 1971 an estimated 25 percent of Title IV-A and Title VI services were purchased (Touche, Ross, and Company 1972). By 1975 about half of all Title XX expenditures were used to purchase service (Office of Human Development Services 1976). With respect to variations among the states, Maine was reported in 1975 to have purchased 82 percent of its Title XX services from private vendors. In Connecticut 81 percent of services were purchased from other public agencies. In North Dakota and California, more than 90 percent of the funds went to direct state provisions of services by the public agency.

Estimates vary on expenditures for the purchase of social services. An Urban Institute study estimated that, exclusive of state administrative costs, about two-thirds of Title XX expenditures nationally were for purchased services, from both other public sources and the private sector (Benton, Feild, and Millar 1978). The U.S. Department of Health and Human Services, Office of Human Development Services reported that for fiscal year 1978, 54 percent of Titles XX, IV-B & IV-A/C expenditures were used for contracting with other social service agencies. Of this amount 33 percent were purchased from private vendors, and 21 percent purchased from other public agencies. In this official report to Congress by the Title XX administrative oversight agency, an important disclaimer is included. These figures may underestimate total POS expenditures from private sources, because public agencies receiving contracts may subsequently subcontract to private vendors. Proportional direct versus purchased services expenditures may also be faulty; the public agency's expenditures for administrative functions are often included in the calculation of direct service costs, resulting in an underestimate of the proportion of service expenditures under POS (Office of the Secretary, DHHS 1980).

Despite outstanding questions about the inclusive nature of POS statistics, possible underrepresentation of the proportion of services purchased to those directly delivered will likely reappear in each separate data collection effort. Comparability by year is still possible. For FY 1980, the nationwide figure for purchase of services under Titles XX, IV-B, and IV-A/C was approximately $2.29 billion, or 53 percent of total expenditures. Nineteen percent of purchased social services were from other public agencies, 34 percent from private sources (Office of the Secretary, DHHS 1981). The proportion of purchased to directly delivered services has remained quite consistent, with a slight increase in the amount obtained from private sources.

Unfortunately, it is not possible to discern changes and trends in POS after FY 1981, at least within the social services. With the passage of the Omnibus Budget Reconciliation Act of 1981, Title XX was amended to become the Social Services Block Grant Program. Many of the requirements under the original Title XX legislation were eliminated, including the mandated annual report. Thus, the 1981 *Report to the Congress* represents the last available compilation and analysis of states' use of purchase of social services.

Another effort to determine the nature and scope of service contracting involved examination of the practices of eighty-nine U.S. municipalities with populations under fifty thousand in four geographic regions (Florestano and Gordon 1980). In one of the four regions, the North Central, municipalities with populations over ten thousand contracted for more than half of their services. Of the total sample, only one-quarter contracted for more than one-third of their governmental services. In order of frequency, professional or housekeeping services ranked first, followed by solid waste collection and street construction. Many of the municipal administrators evaluated contracting positively. They felt they received better quality services at less cost. Exceptions were found by region and size of municipality.

An empirical study of contracting by California's local governments was conducted by Seidman and Seidman, a national accounting firm, on behalf of the California Tax Foundation. Published in May 1981 (thus following enactment of Proposition 13), it surveyed 310 cities, counties, school districts, and special districts regarding experiences with contracting. Eighty-three of the 92 respondents of the 310 surveyed jurisdictions contracted with the private sector. A total of 738 contracts were reported, the majority between local government and private organizations, the latter mostly for-profit. It is not surprising that the different types of local governments in California contract for different types of services.

From the perspective of vendors, prior to the major 1981 federal budget cuts, United Way-supported agencies in the thirty-eight largest metropolitan areas received an average of 46 percent of their annual operating income from federal funds, including those filtered through state and local governments. In New York City the amount reached 71 percent (*New York Times*, 14 November 1983).

Determination of the actual scope of POS is complicated by many variables. One is growth and more recently, decline. According to Bill B. Benton, then deputy secretary of the Maryland Department of Human Services (1981), Maryland's social service program grew from $16 million to more than a half a billion dollars a year from 1972 to 1982. In 1982, $20 million was expended under Title XX purchase arrangements; $1.8 million of it (9 percent) represented contracts with voluntary social service agencies, with the majority of remaining dollars spent on contracts with other state and local government agencies. The total (nearly $20 million) is about 2–1/2 percent of the half billion dollars or so spent on services, a miniscule proportion.

In contrast, in FY 1981, 85 percent of the $194 million budget of the Massachusetts Department of Social Services was expended on the purchase of services, most of which went to the private sector (Hart 1982). Also in Massachusetts, the Division of Alcoholism of the State Public Health Department managed all of its direct services in 1958 through thirteen contracts with hospitals (ten private and three public). By FY 1984 the number of contracts with a variety of providers, almost all private not-for-profits, had reached two hundred (Blacker 1983). In June 1988 the number of vendors had reached about 250, the numbers of contracts exceeded 400. For-profits were still very limited in number (Staff, 1988).

Although measuring the scope of contracting with any great accuracy or reliability is exceedingly difficult, it is clear that the pattern of escalating reliance on this mechanism of service delivery is not likely to abate. Purchase of service, aside from its political popularity, has become a big business. Federal procurement spending nationwide rose from $110 billion in 1980 to $193 billion in 1985 (*Washington Post,* Business, 21 July 1986). In regions such as Los Angeles/Anaheim/Riverside, California, $22.27 million in federal procurement contracts were awarded. Other regions of the country, such as New York and Baltimore-Washington, D.C., rank high as recipients of government contracts. In the Washington, D.C., area, more than ninety-five hundred businesses received contracts in 1985, each averaging $265,000 (Ibid.). These providers of government services have the capacity to wield their own significant influence to ensure continuation of the system. The entrenched interests are strong and, most likely, exceedingly vocal.

EXAMPLES OF PURCHASE OF SERVICES

As already noted, purchase arrangements may take a variety of forms. Government may purchase from other government agencies, quasi-public agencies ("quangos"), private organizations (both for-profit and not-for-profit), and individuals.

Sharkansky (1980), in his overview of governmental contracting between 1965 and 1975, identified examples of the range of purchased goods and services, including those for janitorial, cafeteria and security, design, construction, installation, operation and service of facilities and equipment, personnel selection and training, program monitoring and evaluation, and problem analyses. Hoogland deHoog (1984) cites other prevalent examples of contracting for services, including garbage collection, road maintenance, street lighting, architecture and engineering, and scientific research. Little is inviolate.

The Seidman and Seidman study for the California Tax Foundation (1981) found that a considerable volume of public contracting occurred between public bodies. For cities, trash collection, traffic and signal light service, and building inspections are the most commonly contracted activities. For counties, mental health, drug and alcohol services lead. Other common county contracts include electronic data processing, health services, animal control, and financial services. School districts most frequently contract for computer services, followed, in equal proportion, by maintenance of school plants and equipment, construction and renovation, auditing and laundry. Examples of contracting by local government are trash pick-up, vehicle and fleet maintenance, janitorial and custodial service, garbage removal, computer center operations, paramedical services, hospital administration, sanitation services, operation of waste-water treatment plants, parking meters, window washing, catering lunchrooms, dead animal pick-up, towing and storage of abandoned cars, fire department operations, and building security (*New York Times,* 23 November 1979). The range is large.

A not atypical comment by local officials is one made by mayor Edward Koch of New York City, who suggested to the Public Transit Authority that it hire private companies to provide repair work on buses and subways (*New York Times,* 30 November 1981). His justification was that many transit employees do not give the Authority a full day's work and that Authority officials seem unable to supervise their own employees properly.

The City of St. Paul, Minnesota, terminated its rubbish removal program and assisted neighborhoods in contracting for their own rubbish removal; terminated its youth service program and contracted for the service of a voluntary, nonprofit organization; supplemented its police force with thirty-eight thousand hours of voluntary service; used volunteers to act for the fire department's home inspection service; sold city services to the county; purchased computer services from the county; and developed a public-private partnership for an urban renewal project (Sawyer 1981).

The City of Ventura, California, contracted with Xerox to do their utility billing. Costs decreased and interest income increased because of faster collections (Sawyer 1981).

A four-column newspaper headline read: "City Hoping for Private Operation of Parks" (Goodwin and Guildlen 1980). The City of New York had already ceded its skating rinks and parking lots and hoped to do the same for its golf courses. It sought private contributions and the help of block associations and community groups to maintain neighborhood playgrounds and parks. City consultants designed a ten-year recovery plan, including the creation of a department of managers to oversee and coordinate thousands of projects operated by concessionaires and private groups. The parks commissioner points to the positive results that may accrue: the Central Park skating rink, run by the department, for years was a deficit operation. In private hands the concessionaire increased usage and the department made a profit.

The National Park Service negotiates another type of contractual relationship with its concessionaires. The latter are private organizations operating services (restaurants, motels) in national parks. They pay fees to the Service and may also be responsible for local real estate taxes. Under federal law, a prospectus seeking bids is announced every five years. Current concessionaires have the right of first refusal. They also have the opportunity to match the highest offer before a new contract is awarded. Longer-term contracts can be awarded if the concessionaire does major renovations or makes larger expenditures (Leaning 1983).

During the late 1970s and early 1980s, Medicaid constituted the largest single expenditure for most states. In fiscal 1980 the states paid 44 percent of Medicaid costs, or $12.8 billion. The highest proportion of these expenditures went for reimbursement of hospitals, nursing homes, and physicians, mostly in the private sector (APWA, June 1981).

In FY 1982 New York City let more than $200 million in contracts to child-care agencies, mostly not-for-profit, for foster-care services. The expenditure of these funds was not a routine, bureaucratic venture. A *New York Times* story was headlined: "Politically Tinged Debate on Foster Care Flares On" (19 June 1981). It described the mayor (Edward Koch) as in a "very upset state." The debate was about the conditions of the $200 million in contracts to 72 private not-for-profit child-care agencies for twenty-six thousand youngsters.

The deputy manager of Gainesville, Florida, a city with a population of 85,000, believes that a revolution is occurring in the management of local government. Proposition 13 in California was the signal. Private contracting will be the means to defer or transfer responsibilities. "Local governments are becoming more professional all the time, more business-like, because the financial crunch is mandating it" (*New York Times,* 23 November 1979).

A natural step in the evolution of the purchase of human services was the 1982 proposal of Mayor Gerald McCann of Jersey City, New Jersey, to turn over twenty-five to forty city agencies to the United Way, the Jersey City Medical Center, and other private groups (*New York Times,* 20 June 1982). The mayor viewed this step as a way to achieve several objectives: reduce administrative costs, withdraw the city from the business of offering services that can be better provided by someone else, redefine the role of local government, and reduce the city work force. The mayor and his officials saw a more efficient government in the future.

One year and one reelection later, thirteen social services of the twenty-five to forty municipal services were transferred as planned. Accrued savings were used to increase services. The transfer of nonhuman services—motor vehicle repair, street cleaning, and building maintenance, for example—was to follow if the early transfers were successful (*New York Times*, 12 June 1983). The city will retain police and fire protection, schools, streets, sewers, water supply, public health nursing, and inspection of water, restaurants, and grocery stores. (In many New England communities, however, such services as public health and school nursing traditionally have been purchased from local visiting nurses—now home health associations.) The mayor was defeated in his effort to be reelected.

Troubled by growing deficits and other problems, the State of New York in 1983 signed contracts with a subsidiary of Pan American World Airways to manage two state-owned airports. Modeled after a contract to manage Westchester (N.Y.) Airport, which operates at a profit, the state was seeking "a professional business-like approach." Officials also wanted to avoid adding employees to the state payroll, which would have been necessary if they chose to directly operate the airports. Of the 108 former airport employees, the contractor hired 70; the state redeployed 16 for airport-related jobs. Sixteen people lost their jobs when neither the state nor the contractor hired them (*New York Times*, 2 April 1983).

During FY 1987, the Reagan administration moved to sell or lease many government-owned operations to private companies. Included on the conversion list was Dulles International Airport, National Airport (Washington, D.C.), and even the National Weather Services satellites (*Washington Post*, Business, 21 July 1986). The leasing of the airports to private concerns, although engendering much debate about safety and other implications, was to become an eventuality in 1987 (Sugawara 1985). Within the transportation arena, nothing is sacrosanct. The National Aeronautics and Space Administration (NASA) has been receptive to a plan to replace the Challenger shuttle with a new orbiter that would be paid for and owned by private industry and leased to NASA (*Washington Post*, 30 March 1986). The idea of privately financed orbiters was previously considered by NASA, which is reputed to be "philosophically committed to the goal of commercializing space" (ibid., A5). The privatization of the space industry may receive heightened receptivity now due to the alleged failings of NASA and concerns within that agency that Congress will not appropriate the necessary funds for a Challenger replacement.

A recent occurrence in mass transportation has been the development of special programs for the handicapped and elderly. Studies by the U.S. Department of Transportation suggest the viable development of both publicly operated and publicly contracted, privately operated special transit services (U.S. Department of Transportation 1979). The dual public-private system of delivery allows opportunity for cost and quality comparison studies, but no such data are as yet available. In the 1960s the development and implementation of such programs for special populations would likely have been a public responsibility. More recently, new services for the elderly and handicapped are being operated in many atypical ways.

The Reagan administration's strong preference to turn over functions to the private sector is also being felt in relation to mass transit for the general populace. Private industry is now responsible for the operation of 3 to 5 percent of public mass transit, representing a 2 percent increase over 1981 (*New York Times,* 11 March 1985). Privatization efforts are positively evaluated. "In every case in which the private sector took over a service, it was more efficient and less costly," says Ralph Stanley, administrator of the Urban Mass Transportation Administration (ibid., p. 1).

The Reagan administration is actively encouraging cities to open urban transit systems development and management to private companies. The Dallas Area Rapid Transit Authority, in its attempts to deal with mounting traffic problems, initiated an express bus service that is operated by a private company. The chairman of the Transit Authority, Adlene Harrison, reported, "We were able to start up that service far more quickly than if we tried to do so ourselves" (*New York Times,* 2 February 1986, E5). Washington hopes to see more such endeavors, letting it be known that those cities that demonstrate significant use of competitive bidding for service will be favored for discretionary financing for capital improvements (ibid.).

An Office of Private Sector Initiatives has been opened by the Urban Mass Transportation Administration for the purpose of assisting local agencies to involve private industry in operating transit lines. New federal regulations require recipients of federal transit funds, when expanding existing routes, starting new routes, or taking over privately operated routes, to notify private operators of plans and allow contractor bidding. Periodic review of existing services is also required to determine whether they can be provided more efficiently by private concerns (*New York Times,* 11 March 1985).

Examples of the extending boundaries of purchase of service pervade almost all service arenas. Sager's study of eleven hundred hospitals in fifty-two mid- to large-size cities in the United States from 1937 to 1980, found an almost 25 percent reduction in public hospital beds and an increase of nearly 90 percent in private hospital beds. In the Midwest and Northeast, the decrease reached 40 percent. Although Sager notes many complex reasons for this shift, trends in hospital care from public to private jurisdiction are consistent with patterns throughout all of the human services (Sager 1983).

The 1982 follow-up study of deinstitutionalized clients of New York's Willowbrook State School found that, if managed well, the use of private placement facilities worked. State-operated community residences were found to be more expensive to operate than those operated by the not-for-profit sector and generally provided fewer services (*Washington Post,* 16 April 1982).

Not even the justice system has been excluded from the contracting phenomenon. Publicly held companies have been established in a few northeastern locations to offer alternatives to traditional court room proceedings, which are believed to be expensive, slow, and overburdened. Such corporations include Judicate in Philadelphia, EnDispute in Washington, D.C., and the Center for Public Resources in New York City. These companies are not licensed or regulated, but do follow state laws and procedures on civil cases. The public, however, is excluded from deliberations. Some of these corporations offer hearings, mediation, and arbitration to settle disputes (*New York Times,* 28 May 1985).

The public responsibility to administer incarceration is no longer sacrosanct, as private business is now involved not only in building prisons, but also in running them. Corrections Corporation of America built, paid for, and now operates a jail in Houston, Texas. The corporation receives $25.74 a day for each inmate from the Immigration and Naturalization Service and now detains as many as 350 illegal aliens awaiting deportation hearings (*Washington Post,* 7 May 1985). The district director of the

Houston office of the Immigration and Naturalization Service (INS), Paul O'Neill, claims that the corporation, using its own equity, built the minimum security facility faster than the INS could have, and that its daily fee is lower than costs for the public agency to jail detainees (ibid.). (Typically, in such matters the quality of the program is not discussed.) Contracting for correctional services is merely an extension of a private sector role already established. Private business has for years been contracted to provide food and medical care for prisons and half-way house operations. A U.S. Justice Department study found that thirty-seven adult and twenty-nine juvenile agencies in thirteen states and the District of Columbia purchase some form of service from the private sector for their corrections operations (*Washington Post,* 20 December 1984).

As a part of its privatization strategy, the Reagan administration identified eleven thousand activities it wants private contractors to take over from government. The range is large and includes movie making, health services, geological surveys, and air traffic control towers (*New York Times,* 11 March 1985). Much public attention, through the media, has been focused on this transfer of functions. The *Washington Post* devoted considerable attention in 1985 and 1986 to the proposal that the airports servicing the nation's capital—Baltimore-Washington International, Dulles International, and National—be managed by private concerns. With the approval of Congress, Conrail, the freight rail system, and Landsat, the land-mapping satellite, have been placed on the market for private buyers. All applicants for government loans, grants, and contracts are now screened by Dun and Bradstreet, TRW, and five smaller consumer credit companies (*New York Times,* 28 April 1985). The sale of Amtrak has been proposed, and during the 1985 and 1986 Congressional budget hearings, the curtailment of subsidies for this major rail line was of high priority of the administration. In some cases the goal is to get government out of its funding role, as well as that of manager or provider. In other cases, where the public commitment is more firmly entrenched, the intent is to change delivery auspices. In the latter instance, government maintains its fiscal responsibility for the service but transfers service provision to the private sector.

In the absence of data to contradict prevailing beliefs, the purchase of services is hailed as a means to save money, increase efficiency, and diminish the direct public provider role (thus decreasing the size of the bureaucracy). Questions of quality are less often raised and less easily answered. The quality issue is most often voiced by those opposed to the breadth of contracting in the arena of domestic programs and services. The concern is that inequities in services among population groups may be increased and that the profit-motive serves as a deterrent to quality control and accountability. The debate about cost and quality is likely to continue to reflect ideological and political preferences and beliefs, particularly when little emphasis (or money) is placed on gathering hard data to prove the case either way.

TYPES OF CONTRACTS

For the past several years, the U.S. Office of Personnel Management has offered an array of courses on procurements and contracts. Typically, these courses last from two to five days. One course covered ten different types of contracts (United States Office of Personnel Management 1980). In 1985 the University of Denver College of Law offered its twentieth annual "specially devised high intensity learning and refresher program" on government contracts. The content included contracting techniques and specifications; delays, suspension, and acceleration in the contracting process; cost recovery; terminations; and claims, disputes, and remedies. The program is oriented to the educational needs of procurement professionals (ibid., 1985). Clearly the complexities of the contracting process, including the growing variety in types of contracts, have created a demand and market for skill enhancement opportunities.

Purchase of service is not a unitary concept. The arrangements by which government may purchase services from other public units or the private sector can take several forms. These range from the straightforward purchase on a unit basis of service on the open market to formalized contracts between the public agency and provider that define the type, conditions, and intensity of services to be purchased. The primary issue is the degree of control government will exercise over the services to be delivered, including the selection of clients/patients, the means and frequency of delivery, and the systems instituted for implementation, monitoring, and evaluation. The range of contracting types is suggested in table 2.3.

The most informal pattern of interorganizational relationships is the referral of an individual for services to an agency or individual with

Table 2.3. **Major Types of Contracts**

Firm fixed-price (advertised) contracts	Cost-sharing contracts
Firm fixed-price (negotiated) contracts	Cost-plus-incentive-fee contracts
Fixed-price contracts with escalation	Cost-plus-award-fee contracts
Fixed-price incentive contracts	Cost-plus-fixed-fee contracts
Fixed-price redetermination contracts	Time and material contracts or labor-hour contracts

whom the public agency has no formal agreement and does not reimburse. This type of arrangement is often incorporated into the public agency's information and referral services. The provider agency retains control, or nearly complete autonomy, over the selection of the clients and the content and structure of services. Here, the relationship between the public and private agencies is not formalized or standardized, but instead depends on the initiative of practitioners providing or responsible for the provision of services (Wolock this volume).

A second pattern, more formalized, is the vendor agreement, which encompasses the ten contract types cited in table 2.3. Under vendorship arrangements, funds are allocated by the public agency to purchase specific services for clients. A simple contract may specify the rate of reimbursement for the services rendered. The number of clients to be served may be open-ended or estimated. As characterized in the field of rehabilitation services, purchase orders may also be issued by case managers to obtain products or services on the open market (Gurin and Freidman, this volume). An extension of the purchase order contract is to give the consumer the power and responsibility to secure services for himself or herself. The client is then reimbursed directly at a predetermined rate.

Basically, a contract can be subsumed under two heading: cost contracts or performance contracts. In the former, "the public agency negotiates with contractors for a given number of recipients, service area, or other units of service for a fixed fee or set price based on total or capitation costs agreed to in advance" (Wedel and Hardcastle 1978, 180). In the case of the incentive or performance contract, the focus is on results, not services. (For a discussion of performance contracting, see Gramlich and

Koshel 1975.) Remuneration is based on measurable attributes of service delivery; payments to contractors vary according to the achievement of agreed-upon outcomes. Higher levels of outcome attainment provide greater rewards for the contractors, which are expected to provide incentives for improved performance. "The principle . . . is remuneration based upon performance" (Wedel and Hardcastle 1978, 180). Efficacy is emphasized, which is, of course, risky for the entrepreneur.

The Office of Economic Opportunity, the U.S. Department of Education, and the Job Corps Program, among others, have experimented with performance contracting. That negative results occurred in several instances underlies the complexity of the cost contract but does not necessarily negate the potential of this model. Not all contracts achieve positive outcomes. Performance contracting is one way of delineating the successful from the unsuccessful.

Another purchase model occurs when an agency program is allocated public funds for a general or specific purpose through the public appropriations process. Examples of this model are the programs authorized under the Job Training Partnership Act.

As concerns about accountability have increased, purchase of service contracting has tended to become more formalized. Contracts now often require the delineation of the kinds of service to be delivered and the standards for conducting these services. Specification of the target population, types and levels of service, intake/eligibility procedures, budget and record keeping, personnel assignments and staff qualifications, and various reporting mechanisms may also be mandated. Such requirements may be seen as overwhelming and counterproductive by the provider and may impact on the length and complexity of the negotiating process. The provider agency may be required to submit to the public agency a formal proposal providing the program rationale and detailing its elements. This proposal is then negotiated until a final form, acceptable to both parties, is achieved. Time frames for completion of service activities and evaluation of the services provide a more legitimate basis by which the public agency can monitor performance and assure quality.

It is apparent that there are a wide variety of contractual arrangements that may be used to meet specific circumstances and needs. These vary in the degree of formality and complexity, with a decided trend toward increased specification.

REIMBURSEMENT AND COST STRUCTURE

A major objective of policymakers and administrators is to ensure that services are provided in the most cost-effective manner. Several important matters of policy can be identified in relation to the financing of services, including reimbursement procedures and rate setting for particular services or programs. Equity and incentives, rationality, level and types of payments, responsible record keeping, and assignment of public and private sector roles are all considerations in determining purchase of service cost structure.

Financial issues pervade discussions of purchase of service. Later in this volume, Baumack, Young, and Richardson separately explore matters of cost and reimbursement. As Young and Brandt (1977) note, decisions about reimbursement methods provide an important communication between the buyer (the public agency) and the seller (the contracted private agency). When private agencies are required to match public funds (typically, at a level of 25 to 50 percent), the message communicated is that the products or services to be purchased are of lower priority. There is also some disclaimer of public responsibility. One hundred percent public funding communicates that the service or product is of higher priority and need. If the payment structure for foster-care services is at a 100 percent reimbursement level but adoption services are only partially reimbursed, a clear message about public sector priorities is communicated. If all services are reimbursed at full cost, priorities can be established or identified on bases unrelated to finance.

The private sector is not expected to subsidize a new weapons system for the U.S. Department of Defense, but private human services providers are often expected to contribute, in cash or kind, to the cost of purchased social services. The difference has to do with attitudes about public and private responsibility. Rarely is it argued that the national defense is within the purview of private sector responsibility; even our Constitution allocates powers of defense and war to government. The assignment of responsibility for human services is less clear. The Reagan administration, as noted earlier, favored returning or delegating many service delivery functions to the private sector and saw a public-private partnership as one important means to share responsibility. This partnership may also require a partial service subsidization by the private sector, particularly in cases of purchase of service arrangements. Thus, requiring a financial match of public funds may, this administration believed, prod the private sector's conscience to do what it is expected to do. There is a notable trend, evident in a reading of the request for proposals (RFPs) listed in the *Federal Register,* to require bidders to state in their proposals specific plans to reduce public involvement and maintain the program or service independent of government fiscal support.

The financial components of purchase of service contracts usually reflect more than the dollar value placed on a service or product. Matching requirements are a notable example of the political overtones of such fiscal arrangements; here, prevailing attitudes about role assignments and auspices may be one such factor. Market considerations, more broadly based than one particular contract, also impact on reimbursement rates and cost structures. Lack of competition among private sector providers, a common situation in weapons or aircraft production, places the seller in a much more opportune position to negotiate favorable financial arrangements. Providers of day care, a service for which there is substantial competition, must promise a lot and bid low in order to win a contract and, in fiscal negotiations, are in a far less advantageous position than providers of services for which there are few or no competitors.

Claims that purchasing services are a means to reduce costs are often at the forefront of rationales supporting this form of service delivery. However, such claims are most often made on the basis of assumptions rather than hard data. The few studies that do support the proposition that purchasing services is less expensive than directly providing them seldom measure qualitative differences or account for administrative costs to the public agency to negotiate, monitor, and evaluate contracted programs. Most frequently, cost comparisons focus on the dollar amounts expended by contracted agencies versus the cost to the public agency to provide the same or similar service. When viewed in isolation, contracted services may appear highly cost effective. When the added costs to the public agency for contract oversight functions are calculated as part of the POS overhead expenses, it is less clear that significant savings are realized.

Alternatively, we are unable to locate examples of comprehensive costing of services provided by governmental agencies. Invariably, they exclude many of the overhead charges that permeate government. For example, purchasing, auditing, and personnel services are both centralized and agency-based in state government. Those charges that are agency specific may be identified, but never will appropriate attributions be made to the central agencies. And yet, central purchasing exists to serve operating agencies. Thus, a percentage of its expenses must be allocated to the operating agency providing the service if the rates are to be reliable.

Given the difficulty in controlling the many variables affecting accurate POS cost determination, claims of cost efficiency must thus rely primarily on assumptions and available hard data. The limited information available from expirical studies tends to support the argument that contracted services are less expensive than those provided directly by the public agency. Most such determinations, however, refer to the purchase of concrete services or products, such as fire protection, refuse collection, and municipal services (e.g., water, sewage). These studies are narrow in focus and provide little useful information in relation to the cost of human services, many of which fall into the category of "soft" services—counseling, prevention, and foster care. In these instances the units of measurement are more difficult to identify, and the outcomes often do not lend themselves to easy quantification.

The POS cost effectiveness studies have been criticized on a number of grounds. First, such studies fail to take into account that a large proportion of contracting occurs between government units, rather than between government and private agents. Is this type of contracting less expensive? If not, what is the rationale for its predominant use? Hoogland deHoog (1984) also argues that there is a dearth of hard data on the relative advantages and disadvantages of public versus private delivery, and that comparisons between these two forms are needed in areas in which both types of agencies provide the same service. She further observes that some of the costs associated with contracting out may be underestimated. Before-and-after cost comparisons fail to take into account, according to deHoog, the long-term costs. New contractors, for example, may bid low to get a contract and then negotiate higher rates in succeeding contract years. The costs to the private agency to prepare, negotiate, and administratively operate the contracts are also not always factored into cost studies.

As noted earlier, cost comparison studies of direct versus contracted services have generally been absent in the human services arena. The few cost studies of social services show mixed results. In a mid 1970s study of the contractual arrangements between the Utah State Division of Family Services and fourteen voluntary agencies, Randolph (1976) found that accurate service costing was the most frequently cited problem by private agency executives. Pacific Consultants (Weinstein and Evans 1979), under contract with the U.S. Department of Health, Education, and Welfare, Administration for Public Services, explored the feasibility of comparing the costs between directly delivered and purchased services. They found that states kept more complete and accurate information on purchased services than those provided in-house, thus limiting cost comparison feasibility. Further, cost considerations were not among the most influential factors cited by state managers in their decision to purchase. A methodological difficulty in comparing costs is that the two conditions deemed essential for such studies are often not present: (1) the two methods (direct and POS) must be used to deliver similar types of services and (2) the data needed to estimate the unit cost for each purchased service and each directly provided service must be available.

Many public human services organizations require that the private vendors from whom they contract follow budget-planning guidelines similar to those used within the public sector. An object (line) budget is developed, with each item justified, and all the limitations of, and problems associated with, public budgeting are then replicated in the private sector. In addition, transfers between object items may be severely limited, resulting in the need for frequent contract revisions. At the other end of the continuum are performance contracts, in which payment is based on what is actually produced or delivered. Measures of service outcomes are identified in the contract as the basis of payment, and incentives and disincentives may also be scheduled. The type of contract budget used may have much to do with public agency regulations and style preferences, but may also be affected by the negotiating ability and influence of the private vendor. Examples of variations in contract cost structures are plentiful.

There are several methods of calculating payment rates for services. One method is to relate the number of services to an expenditure base; this base may be expanded or contracted, depending on what is included in it (Copeland 1976). The base almost always includes overhead, depreciation, and other costs of agency operations. Rates of payments may also be negotiated or budget-based. Criteria other than actual costs are used to determine the negotiated rate, whereas budget-based rates are based on actual cost experience, with possible adjustments permitted for inflation and changes in service quality or quantity. Payment rates may also be calculated on the unit cost (the total annual cost of a service divided by the number of treatment/service units) or the proportion of the total cost. Rates may also be variable or fixed. There may be combinations of several types of rate payment methods incorporated into a single contract, e.g., a negotiated, unit-cost rate or a closed-ended (fixed) amount (ibid.).

The rate structure established for a contract has important implications for the service program. If the payment rate is determined on the basis of units of service, the contracted provider must ensure that the hours of treatment, number of home visits, or weeks of day care agreed upon in advance are actually provided and adequate records maintained. Here, payment is not related to the quality of services or to the sophistication of the services provided; reimbursement level will not vary if the services rendered require more highly qualified staff or more extensive preparation. To the extent that rates of payment are fixed, budget-based, and with a constant expenditure base, the vendor may have little incentive to go beyond the minimum contract requirements in either quantity or quality.

Control of line item expenditures may be dysfunctional; when the contracted provider must watch every dollar spent, the goal of POS to provide higher quality services is clearly undermined. The critical variable and appropriate frame of reference should be the client, the services needed, and how best these services might be delivered. The product matters, not the process. However, the specificity with which contracts are written and the often cumbersome financial accounting procedures required may deflect from the product or outcome and focus vendor attention on process. Certainly, contracts for nonhuman services (e.g., garbage collection, fire protection) or goods would not include provisions for the daily management of the provider organization. In the human services, however, there is a tendency to focus as much on how budget procedures are managed and how services are provided as on how well.

The "power of the purse" wielded by public agencies does allow substantial latitude in the type and range of demands made upon vendors. Sometimes role confusion results when the public agency asserts that "state policy should require of these private agencies the same kinds of commitments demanded of public agencies" (Herman 1979, 34). The desire of private organizations to successfully bid on contracts may lead them to permit these demands to be made. The result may be the creation of a quasi-public entity, in which the vendor takes on many of the characteristics of the public agency through contract-mandated procedures and requirements.

Public agencies respond to conflicting and contradictory demands— the public at large, the state legislature and/or Congress, public officials—and accommodation to some or all leads to inefficiency. This is one of the prices of our pluralistic society. It is precisely because of system weaknesses that the public sector has turned to private vendors to provide selected goods and services. Less encumbered by unnecessary baggage, it is believed that the private sector can perform tasks more effectively and efficiently. However, if we now begin to bureaucratize the private sector through the contracting process, the outcome may be to create monolithic structural arrangements, one private and one public, in which costs will continue to rise, competition will decrease, and the standard of goods and services will significantly suffer.

It bears repeating that the product is of utmost concern. Line item budgets are irrelevant, even though budgets and costs sometimes are elevated to the most essential point of negotiations. Rather than replicating government budgeting procedures in private vendor contracts, a more flexible cost determination and fiscal accountability system should be considered. One example of a viable cost structure alternative is deficit financing. Differing from classic purchase of service models, government funds might be more effectively used to finance the deficits incurred by private agencies in the delivery of those services considered to be in the public interest. Sheltered workshops, group homes, and halfway houses, for example, have been shown to be able to generate income usually well in excess of 50 percent of operating costs. Because it is in the public's interest to continue and expand these programs, government could enter into partnership with providers to limit and finance the deficit. This pattern was formerly followed by the United Way and has been used in Israel and Holland with success (Kramer 1979).

A FUTURE AGENDA

There are, as yet, many unresolved issues and questions concerning purchase of services, ranging from the effectiveness of these arrangements to their cost efficiency and how cost structures impact upon vendor performance and service outcomes. Technical as well as policy matters are still in need of resolution, and the public-private partnerships forged through POS are not always successful. There have, however, been some attempts to address the relationship problems that have emerged. One effort to require the government to meet responsible standards in bill payment was the passage of the Federal Prompt Payment Act (P.L. 97–177), signed by President Reagan on 21 May 1982. This law requires federal agencies to pay their bills on time, pay interest penalties when payments are late, and take discounts only when payments are made within the discount period (National Institutes of Health 1982). For the initial period of implementation, 1 October–31 December 1982, the interest penalty for government for late payments of over fifteen days was 15.5 percent.

Unnecessary reporting requirements have also been addressed through the Paperwork Reduction Act of 1980. Following this law's mandate, the U.S. Office of Management and Budget drafted regulations to control excessive demands by government for paperwork. These policies include the following:

Reports can be required no more frequently than quarterly.

Twenty-one days should be given to submit information.

Maximum number of copies to be submitted are one original and two copies.

Records need only be retained, in matters other than health, for seven years maximum.

Separate and simplified requirements are to be developed for small businesses.

Not all of the problems can be addressed through legislation or regulations. The private sector, too, has had to adjust to the realities of the new partnerships forged through purchase of service. In some cases this has involved the need to adapt services to fit the priorities established by government, or to adjust traditional modes of treatment to meet the needs of a different clientele with different problems. From an administrative point of view, changes in record-keeping and reporting systems have had to be instituted.

By the mid 1980s, purchase of service had come under considerable attack and scrutiny, particularly in the defense industry. The human services, however, have not been immune from criticism. Such criticisms range from inadequate accounting procedures to ineffective services. In many circles private contractors are believed to use public funds to support their hard-pressed operations, rather than for intended purposes. Some of these emerging problems in implementing public-private relationships through contracting are explored later in this volume.

That purchase of service arrangements have been found less than ideal is not surprising. Virtually all "solutions" to service delivery problems have been found wanting, to some degree, after implementing experiences have accrued and provided a foundation for evaluation. What is perhaps most instructive in terms of the future of purchase of service is that there is no call to abandon this mechanism. The motivations giving rise to the use of contractual arrangements—a desire to decrease the public sector role and rely on the private sector, a belief in the superiority of private sector services, and the proclaimed notion of cost effectiveness through POS—have, in fact, grown in intensity. Until an alternative to public funding of private services can be realistically identified, the government role of financier will continue to be achieved through purchase of service.

PART TWO

Purchase of Services: Theory and Practice

The government bureaucracy shrinks in the number of civilians it employs, yet is assigned by Congress ever-increasing responsibilities, an apparent contradiction. Who is to carry out these assignments? Some activities are eliminated, some are transferred to other layers of government, others to special authorities, and still others to the private sector. Not exclusively American, the governmental use of private sector contractors, especially for-profits, is nevertheless highly consistent with a strong commitment to free enterprise.

The alternatives to direct government enterprise operate in a gray area on the margins of government, according to Sharkansky. For some, the margins may soon be larger than the core. The continued and expanded use of the private marketplace runs counter to some of the theories of how government should operate, as expounded by political scientists and public administrators, and also raises the question of how public control and accountability are to be maintained. Compared with the rigidities of the civil service and employee unions and the extraordinary complexity of managing a public bureaucracy, almost any alternative is likely to be more responsive to the external environment. It may well be that those theorists who hold that public functions must be carried out by public agents have fallen behind contemporary organizational behavior.

Why the expansion in the purchase of services? Why decreasing confidence in government? Explanations are offered. The causes may well determine ultimate behavior. Kramer outlines the several major causal explanations: We lack sufficient knowledge; managerial skill is poor, planning is inadequate; service is fragmented and poorly coordinated; and resources are inadequate. In the 1980s those supportive of government faulted the inadequate resource base; those with a negative set toward government spoke of flawed administration.

In any case no matter what view one holds about the role of

government and its performance, anger and hostility toward and about the public bureaucracy are very strong. There are few adults lacking in disturbing personal experiences.

To Terrell another important perspective on why purchase of services has evolved into a major option for the delivery of heretofore government services, reiterated throughout this volume, concerns the intermingling of the public and private sectors. Boundary blurring is a common occurrence. Old and long-standing theories about the respective roles of government, the not-for-profit, and the for-profit sectors are obsolete. Needed are new theories about interorganizational behavior that reflect current realities.

The perspective on the need for, uses of, and experiences with the purchase of services on the part of the involved organizations (the government making the purchase, the contractor providing the service, and the client/consumer using the service) vary widely. The limited scholarly and research base about the entire subject of purchase of services largely reflects the lack of concern of public administration, political science, and social work. The most extensive data are derived from the thousands of comparative cost studies engendered because of Office of Management and Budget requirements and the preoccupation throughout governmental agencies with cost containment. The federal agencies are under substantial pressure to compare the costs of direct provision versus purchase of services. Because the results of these studies are frequently not publicized, we know neither how well they are performed nor their aggregate results. We know little about the effects of contracting on the private sector. Opinions abound; it is data we lack. Most notable is the lack of information about the process and outcome of contracting from the perspective of the client.

The gains and losses to the public and private sectors by this expanding interpenetration are most often evaluated on the basis of subjective experience. And even if program monitoring and evaluation were to reach minimal standards, the debate about values has yet to be fully articulated. Is it service availability, accessibility, accountability, cost-effectiveness, quality, or equity that is desired; or is it combinations of these, and in what priority? There is no single answer; much depends on the particular perspective held.

3

Private Alternatives to Public Human Services Administration

Paul Terrell

Since 1970, there has been an upsurge of interest in contracting as a method of delivering human services—especially at the local government level. Once considered quite out of keeping with proper administrative practice, contract alternatives to the direct public operation of tax-financed programs are suddenly being touted as critical resources for government. The League of California Cities, for example, has begun urging municipalities to explore "the potential for *obtaining* services before [moving] towards service *providing*" ("Social element" 1977). Several contributors to the International City Management Association's recent "green book," *Managing Human Services,* warn local officials against narrow-mindedly assuming that public programs can be implemented only through public agencies (Anderson 1977). And a variety of critics of city management as well as "public choice" economists are arguing for the adoption of market-like delivery strategies (including contracts) as a desirable way of countering bureaucratic waste and low productivity (Savas 1977).

The emergence of contracting as a responsible public management option has been significantly facilitated by recent alterations in the character of federal aid. With broadened service responsibilities resulting from revenue sharing and block grant decentralization, cities and counties have had to come to grips, often for the first time, with a number of the most fundamental issues of human services policy and organization. Who is to plan programs? How are problem area priorities to be set? What specific populations are to be served? How can citizens be involved? And, most important for our purposes, how shall services be delivered?

While most of those local jurisdictions involved in human services continue to implement programs directly, a growing number are relying on private organizations, particularly nonprofit agencies. Accumulating evidence, indeed, supports the conclusion that contracting is widespread and apparently increasing, in terms of both dollar expenditures and breadth of use. The Brookings assessment of the Community Development Block Grant program, for example, confirms an important services role for many former Model City nonprofit operators (Nathan 1977). The National Academy of Sciences' analysis of the Comprehensive Employment and Training Act indicates the prevalent utilization of private agencies (Mirengoff 1976). Several revenue-sharing studies show local jurisdictions— especially on the West Coast—contracting out large portions of their allocation for human services (Terrell 1977). And the ICMA volume provides many examples—Dallas, San Diego, Hayward (California)—of localities investing heavily in contract provision (Anderson 1977).

Despite the increasing survey and case evidence, however, the overall dimensions of contracting are difficult to discern. For one thing, the scope of contracting and its importance in terms of total allocations are hardly known. Does contracting comprise a generally accepted alternative to in-house delivery? Does the extent of contracting differ among human service fields? Among regions? Do governments rely on formal request for proposal (RFP) procedures to structure agency applications? Do particular nonprofits capture most of the funds allocated for contracts? Are contracts generally written? Are they monitored? All these questions are basic ones, and without some answers the role of private agencies in public services can hardly be determined or characterized. It is the intent of this paper to begin the process of investigation.

BACKGROUND

Public services in the United States have been traditionally—although far from exclusively—implemented through public instrumentalities. Elected officials enact statutes, provide for their funding, and designate organizations to carry out the services authorized. For the most part, these organizations are public agencies—whether federal, state, or local. Their employees are civil servants—the "bureaucracy" of today's welfare state.

Public programs equal public implementation. The equation is so natural that it hardly needs justification. A taxpaying public is obviously entitled to properly accountable programs, and what could be more in keeping with the public interest than a public administration supervised by popularly elected officials? While a fringe element on the right has always denied the ability of government to do anything well, the idea that public administration ensures the public good has remained the dominant principle underlying the structural organization of services in America.

While dominant, the principle of public administration has hardly been exclusive. Services can be provided in other ways. Government, for example, can promote specific kinds of services through voucher arrangements, or tax deductions or credits. These options have received considerable discussion this past decade (Rivlin 1971). Less discussed, but considerably more feasible in most cases, is government action to facilitate the provision of services by particular private organizations through some type of formal agreement between the parties. Such contract arrangements, indeed, are hardly new. Government has promoted human services by contract for over 150 years.[1]

Until recently, however, such human service contracts were entered into for one primary purpose: to provide care and help for specific populations for whom government had a special responsibility. These populations included wards of the court, veterans, the destitute, the blind and deaf, the "indigent insane," Native Americans, and the like. As early as 1819, for example, the federal government provided direct aid (in the form of a land grant) to a sectarian institution in Hartford, Connecticut, providing care and training for handicapped children, and throughout the nineteenth century, federal land provided major subsidies to a variety of private welfare and educational institutions. States and localities relied even more heavily on charitable organizations to extend help to government wards. Prior to the establishment of formal welfare administrations under public auspices, indeed, governments regularly called on voluntary institutions to raise, train, and protect dependent populations (Elazar 1962; Brown 1929, 1939).

This public/private partnership continues today. Government continues to purchase care on a case basis from nonprofit organizations—especially hospitals, nursing homes, and child welfare facilities—rather than providing it directly. Most of these institutions, indeed, receive a large portion (if not all) of their total support from government.[2]

THE NEW CONTRACTING

In the past fifteen years, contract provision has expanded rapidly as governments at all levels have begun to search for more efficient methods of organizing and administering their vastly enlarged responsibilities to provide for the social welfare. Local governments in particular have come to utilize an expanding number of private organizations for human service purposes. Using a variety of funding sources, city and county policymakers have increasingly entered into arrangements with community agencies to extend a broad variety of services such as job training, individual and family counseling, services for seniors, juvenile diversion, outpatient mental health, primary health care, community development, day care, home help services, and many more.[3]

This new reliance on contracting reflects both the increased public commitment to welfare that began with Great Society legislation and the increased dissatisfaction with the performance of government agencies that started to grow into major proportions soon thereafter. As public social welfare spending shot up (11.8 percent of the GNP in 1965, 20.6 percent in 1976), people's confidence in government's ability to solve social problems plummeted (Skolnik and Dales 1977).

The cynicism about programs that has emerged in the 1970s has focused attention on those various aspects of the policymaking and policy-implementation process that seem to impede the effective translation of resources into positive results. Many schools of thought have arisen to explain such service "failures." Some see the problem arising from faulty intelligence. It's said that we just don't know how to teach children to read, or to prevent drug abuse, or to induce lawful behavior. For others, the issue is inadequate management. Service agencies are faulted for operating on the basis of conjecture rather than planning. Problems are said to be improperly assessed, concise objectives remain unspecified, evaluation is disregarded. A third group of critics sees the performance gap as resulting from fragmented services, from individual agencies going their own ways, unconcerned with coordination, insensitive to the need for "systems."

While these are common explanations for the disappointing results of the Great Society—along with the lament that resources are not (never were) sufficient—a newer thesis is emerging that defines the basic problem in terms of the flawed character of public administration, per se. It is not the effort that is wrong, this thesis goes, but rather that it is carried out governmentally. It is the public nature of service delivery that results in unresponsiveness, inefficiency, and self-serving bureaucracy.

Allegations of governmental ineptitude, of course, are hardly noteworthy. What is noteworthy is that many of today's critics, rather than calling for broad reductions in social welfare spending, are instead proposing a shift in service strategies—a shift, essentially, from public to private provision. Such critics, moreover, encompass an increasingly potent coalition of political forces, a coalition combining "new conservatives," ethnic community-based organizations, traditional social work agencies, and those varied public officials simply seeking more productive ways to squeeze the most from every tax dollar.[4]

RESEARCH APPROACH

To what degree have these developments resulted in local governments coming to rely on contract provision? As a first step toward understanding the character and magnitude of contract delivery, three major sources of federal support for local governments were analyzed: Title I of the Comprehensive Employment and Training Act (CETA) of 1973, which provides support for job-training programs; Title I of the Housing and Community Development Act of 1974, which extends support in the form of community-development block grants; and General Revenue Sharing, first legislated in 1972, which provides "no-strings" aid to all units of state and local government.[5] Together, these statutes provided nearly $10 billion for local governments in fiscal year 1978. Each permits funding for human services, and each allows localities, if they so desire, to contract service provision to nongovernmental bodies.

Questionnaires were mailed to CETA, community-development, and revenue-sharing officials in the 130 largest urban jurisdictions in late 1977 and early 1978. Response rates were 74 percent, 78 percent, and 70 percent, respectively. As far as possible, questionnaire data were supplemented and verified by data from printed sources, principally budgets, program reports, and evaluations.

65

COMPREHENSIVE EMPLOYMENT AND TRAINING ACT

CETA was enacted in 1973. Part of President Richard Nixon's New Federalism, its Title I consolidated over a dozen specific manpower programs into one broad ("block") grant authorizing the provision of "comprehensive manpower services." Within this mandate, recipient units of government—known as "prime sponsors"—were given considerable discretion in setting priorities, establishing an appropriate "mix" among program efforts, and choosing service delivery agents. In FY 1978, Title I provided $1.88 billion nationwide for programs such as outreach, intake, screening, general classroom education, on-the-job training, job counseling, placement, follow-up, and supportive social services.

Service delivery in the employment and training field has always been pluralistic. In the pre-CETA decade, the federal government directly supported an extraordinarily wide assortment of public, nonprofit, and commercial manpower organizations. Under categorical grants-in-aid like the Manpower Development and Training Act (MDTA), the Economic Opportunity Act, and the Emergency Employment Act of 1969, federal departments entered into approximately 10,000 separate narrowly focused contracts with states, counties, cities, school districts, and nongovernmental agencies and institutions.

CETA replaced most of these direct agreements with a far smaller number of consolidated grants to prime sponsors. There are currently 495 such sponsors—445 localities plus the fifty states. Local sponsors must be either cities or counties over 100,000 population or else combinations of local jurisdictions containing at least one unit over 100,000. These local combinations are called "consortia," and there is a financial incentive in the legislation for governments to so group together.[6]

While CETA permits its prime sponsors considerable discretion in organizing programs, it contains a number of standards and requirements to advance national goals. Some of these pertain to citizen participation, others to eligibility, nondiscrimination, planning, and finance. Although the legislation does not require the prime sponsors to use particular kinds of service delivery arrangements (there are no "presumptive providers"), it does draw special attention to the capabilities of what the act calls "community-based organizations."

While there is growing debate concerning just what organizations are and aren't "community based," at the time of CETA's enactment the

66

phrase stood as a surrogate for five organizations that had developed successful employment and training programs for low-income and minority groups in the 1960s: Opportunities Industrialization Centers (OIC), serving inner-city blacks; Service/Employment/Redevelopment (SER, also known as Jobs for Progress), serving Hispanics; the Urban League, serving blacks; Operation Mainstream, serving the elderly; and Community Action Agencies, the local War on Poverty bodies, serving residents of poor neighborhoods. Each of these organizations was locally based and representative of particular at-risk groups. Each encouraged citizen participation in planning and management, and stressed self-help and ethnic identification. And each offered a variety of supportive social services appropriate to the needs of its clients.

These community-based organizations (CBOs) were given special consideration in the CETA legislation to protect them in the change over from categorical to block funding. Prior to CETA, the primary source of support for these agencies had been federal—particularly MDTA and War on Poverty grants. Decentralizing program decision making away from Washington clearly threatened the special relationship such organizations had built up over the years. This concern emerged in congressional discussion. The CBOs all expressed fears that their activities would be cut back or diverted under CETA (Davidson 1972). Along with their congressional allies they were scarcely sanguine about the willingness of local prime sponsors to support "outside" organizations, especially those serving needy but politically weak groups such as the elderly, minorities, migrant workers, and the handicapped. Even a few mayors questioned transferring power out of Washington. According to Mayor Moon Landrieu of New Orleans, for example, decentralization would doom innovative programs by putting "allocative decisions at the local level where the conservative . . . pro status quo groups know they have the greatest say" (U.S.Congress 1972).

Seeking to head off such developments, a coalition of congressional liberals successfully amended the bill to protect already existing community providers. Under the final act, for example, CBOs with "demonstrated effectiveness" in serving the poor and those of limited English-speaking ability are specially recommended for continued funding (CETA, a). Prime sponsors are also required to make "appropriate arrangements" to involve CBOs in program planning (CETA, b). Finally, Title III of the legislation provides for the direct federal funding of "special emphasis programs" serving needy target groups not likely to win support from local government sponsors.

To what extent have local sponsors utilized nonprofit community organizations to provide employment and training services under CETA Title I? Early evidence indicates that, overall, there have not been major shifts from the service delivery patterns established under the previous categorical programs. For the most part, prime sponsors have relied on service arrangements already in place, funneling their Title I dollars through public organizations such as the state employment service, public universities, local school districts (the operators of most skill centers), *and* private bodies such as the CBOs, unions, chambers of commerce, profit-making schools and employment agencies, and social service agencies.

In Chicago, for example, the prime sponsor opted to use Title I to continue the bulk of programs first created and sustained by MDTA and other categorical grants. Under this arrangement, the Woodlawn Organization (TWO), a community organization with considerable experience in manpower programs, was awarded over a quarter of a million dollars in CETA Year I to continue training low-income blacks in upholstery, clerk typing, microfilming, computer keypunch, and offset printing. In FY 1976, TWO operations were funded at nearly $1 million.

In Milwaukee, the prime sponsor used CETA funds to contract with thirteen community agencies in FY 1977, one of which, Big Step, was cooperatively established as a nonprofit corporation with a board of directors chosen from the local Urban League, the Milwaukee OIC, and representatives from construction unions. Big Step's primary objective is to train women and minority-group members for apprenticeship examinations in the building trades. Once individuals qualify for apprenticeship, they are assisted in obtaining and keeping jobs.

In addition to contracting out for employment and training, many CETA sponsors have utilized community agencies to provide "supportive services" such as health and child care, counseling, and transportation. San Francisco, for example, contracted with twenty-six local community organizations in FY 1977, many of which, like Swords to Plowshares, an agency to assist Vietnam veterans, provided counseling and legal services, as well as direct-training assistance.

Tables 3.1 through 3.3 indicate that Milwaukee, Chicago, and San Francisco are not atypical in their reliance on community non-profits.

Table 3.1. **Proportion of Jurisdictions Contracting Out by Funding Source, FY. 1977**

Jurisdiction	Proportion contracting (%)
CETA prime sponsors ($N = 81$)	95.0
CDBG cities and counties ($N = 88$)	67.0
GRS cities and counties ($N = 93$)	33.7
Mean ($N = 262$)	63.7

Table 3.2. **Number of Private Agencies Contracted per Jurisdiction by Funding Source, FY 1977**

Jurisdiction	Mean number of agencies contracted
CETA prime sponsors ($N = 79$)	14.6
CDBG cities and counties ($N = 84$)	5.8
GRS cities and counties ($N = 90$)	7.7
Mean ($N = 253$)	9.2

Table 3.3. **Proportion of Expenditures Contracted Out by Funding Source, FY 1977**

Jurisdiction	Mean proportion of budget contracted (%)
CETA prime sponsors ($N = 80$)	31.8
CDBG cities and counties ($N = 88$)	5.5
GRS cities and counties ($N = 98$)	4.9
Mean ($N = 261$)	13.3

While a small number of prime sponsors have established highly central-ized systems using a single public-sector delivery agent for all employ-ment-related services, most have utilized a number of service-providing organizations, public and private. This, in general, has been the most practical and politically feasible strategy for local government to

69

pursue. Under such arrangements, the CBOs have not been overlooked. Indeed, the preponderance of data indicates that their operations have expanded.[7]

While table 3.1 offers no comparisons with the pre-CETA situation, it clearly indicates the very substantial degree to which prime sponsors rely on local nonprofits. Of the eighty-one prime sponsors reporting, fully 95 percent contract out. Table 3.3, elaborating on the extent to which private deliverers are utilized, indicates 31.8 percent of total Title I expenditures going to directly support nonprofit agencies.[8]

COMMUNITY DEVELOPMENT BLOCK GRANTS

The block grant approach to community development, first proposed by the Nixon administration in 1973, presented quite the same hazards for community agencies as did CETA. In both cases, local nonprofits feared that decentralization would result in independent providers, whatever their merit, being discarded by cities and counties.

In community development, moreover, an additional threat presented itself. Whereas CETA was clearly oriented to the creation of comprehensive employment and training services—a goal shared by SER, OIC, the Urban League, and the other community agencies—Community Development Block Grant legislation (CDBG) offered local governments the chance to select projects aimed at purposes quite different from those sought by local nonprofits. Specifically, CDBG placed few restrictions on the degree to which local governments could stress physical development. By contrast, community agencies (most established under Model Cities) approached community development by stressing human services. Since Model Cities had been created explicitly to direct cities away from their natural emphasis on "bricks and mortar," toward an emphasis on people, the prospect for services under arrangements that gave local government officials wide program discretion was not rosy.

While CDBG meshed together seven formerly separate HUD categorical grants-in-aid, it was Urban Renewal and Model Cities, the two principal community-development programs of the previous years, that were the most vitally affected.[9] Urban Renewal, created in 1949, was primarily a "clear and build" effort, geared to creating new economically viable centers for older metropolitan areas. Because it uprooted a great number of low-income residents in the process, physical rebuilding pro-

70

grams are not frequently viewed as being in the best interests of the urban disadvantaged.

Model Cities, legislated in 1966, was formulated to implement a process of community development that would counter the limitations of physically oriented programs in order to help rather than harm the poor. Funneling resources into approximately 150 poverty neighborhoods around the country, it supported a varied assortment of community-run health, education, employment, and social service programs. Public works were not emphasized; community organization and citizen involvement were.

While both Urban Renewal and Model Cities utilized the contract mechanism, each was concerned with advancing vastly different purposes. Local renewal authorities relied on voluntary sector agencies for one main reason—to assist in the relocation process by inducing cooperation from local residents. Settlement houses, United Way, and other organizations that enjoyed good reputations in the community were frequently hired to persuade local residents of the desirability of renewal and to help in the process of finding new housing for the displaced (Citizen participation 1966).

Model City contracts, on the other hand, were instruments to carry through the entire gamut of human service programs intended by the legislation. Extending the participation tradition of the War on Poverty, Model City operations—while generally managed from within city government—relied on the involvement of outside neighborhood residents and organizations in program planning and service delivery. Nonprofit providers—so-called operating agencies—had the responsibility for establishing and managing a major portion of the funded programs.

Model City contractors operated in much the same fashion as the private "delegate agencies" of the War on Poverty. For the most part they were new organizations, small in size, concerned with developing better approaches to service delivery, and strongly oriented toward advocacy. Most of the contract agencies represented particular ethnic or racial groups, and many had significant participation by the poor in their internal decision making. Staffs, moreover, were often composed of local residents working in paraprofessional roles as social workers, outreach staff, teacher aides, housing counselors, and the like.

Model City advocates were clearly not enthusiastic about the downgrading of community services they perceived in the block grant approach. In testimony before the Congress in 1973 and 1974 they argued that decentralized programs à la the New Federalism would revert community development to its pre-Model Cities pattern. Without a clear emphasis on services for poverty areas, they predicted physical development squeezing out human development, with a concomitant neglect of the acute needs of the cities' neediest residents (Nathan 1977).

In its final form, the CDBG program—very much like CETA—represented something of a compromise between the New Federalism purists favoring minimum controls and block grant critics who demanded protection for existing priorities and programs. Some limited commitment to social welfare concerns is evident in the act. The distribution formula for CDBG funds, for example, is weighted to favor poorer, older communities. Moreover, the 150-odd existing Model Cities communities are somewhat protected by "hold harmless" provisions preventing abrupt reductions in their funding. (Model Cities funding was diminished annually, and phased out altogether by 1983.) There is also a general requirement in the law that recipient cities and counties certify that CDBG programs are "developed so as to give maximum feasible priority to activities which will benefit low or moderate income families, or aid in the prevention or elimination of slums, or blight" (Housing Act, a). Finally, one of the act's seven priority objectives is to promote "the expansion and improvement of the quality and quantity of community services, principally for persons of low and moderate income . . . " (Housing Act, b).

Taken as a whole, however, the legislation provides little support for antipoverty services. Recipient units have broad latitude in defining community development, and the evidence to date indicates that they are investing heavily in physical projects—many related to old urban renewal plans. Even in those cities without any previous involvement in urban renewal, the emphasis is on hardware (Frieden and Kaplan 1976). Overall, only 12.1 percent of the first-year funds and 9.6 percent of the second-year funds have been spent on activities related to the improvement of community services. Removing from this expenditures for police and fire and other services not usually associated with social welfare brings the latter figure down to approximately 4 percent. Almost half of these funds are directed at former model neighborhoods.[10]

Moreover, the legislation itself places a variety of hurdles in front of those communities wishing to emphasize community services. Even if local governments desire to support human services, for example, they are restricted in their ability to do so. While there is no specified limitation in the law itself on the proportion of funds a city or county can spend on social services, the Joint House-Senate Conference Committee Report stated its understanding that no more than 20 percent of any community's funds would be so spent. Generally, HUD has enforced this limit in its oversight of the act. In addition, the law requires that services be supported only when they "support" physical development projects, and even then only in cases where no other source of federal support is available.[11]

Many of the jurisdictions receiving community-development aid, moreover, can hardly be classified as impoverished. The CDBG moneys are distributed by formula and are available to all jurisdictions meeting minimum urban population requirements. Model City funds, by contrast, were project allocated, focusing aid on a limited number of federally selected poverty areas.

Given all of this, it is surprising that CDBG dollars are supporting contract human services to the degree that they are. As table 1 indicates, fully 67 percent of the eighty-eight localities reporting contract out to nonprofits. Most that do are former Model City jurisdictions committed to maintaining support for already functioning community agencies. Overall, as table 2 indicates, 5.5 per-cent of total CDBG spending is channeled through contract providers.

While this figure is low, a good many local jurisdictions are strongly supporting contract human services. San Diego, California, for example, utilized over 12 percent of its CDBG budget in FY 1977 to support community programs having their origins in Model Cities, despite the fact that the city's special "hold harmless" allotment had been terminated in 1976. Committed to a services approach to community development, and unwilling to increase its own payroll, the city council entered into contracts with Travelers Aid, the Salvation Army, United Way, Urban League, and a substantial number of private Model Cities agencies to provide services such as day care, drug diversion programs, and emergency housing. It should be noted that San Diego, in order to secure HUD approval for these services, had to indicate both that they supported physical programs and that other federal funding was not available.

Houston similarly used a significant portion of its CDBG funds to support Model Cities services. When the HUD regional office in Dallas attempted to restrict this spending on the grounds that such services "were not in direct support of eligible physical development activities," Houston appealed to HUD in Washington and won its case. Since then, the city has appropriated approximately $3 million a year—some 20 percent of its total—for the use of neighborhood-based contractors.

Charlotte, N.C., and Cleveland are two other communities strongly emphasizing community social services in their CDBG operations. In FY 1977, for example, Charlotte spent approximately 20 percent of its funds to support forty-four separate projects operated by eighteen independent private agencies. Contract programs included Meals on Wheels, recreation for the handicapped through the YMCA, counseling for homeowners, and a methadone treatment program. Cleveland directed approximately $5 million of its $16 million FY 1977 allocation to contract service—$1 million each to local Model Cities and Community Action agencies and $3 million to other nonprofits. All told, sixty separate agencies (out of 100 applicants) were contract funded.

GENERAL REVENUE SHARING

General Revenue Sharing (GRS), enacted in 1972 and amended in 1976, is the only federal aid program virtually unconditioned with respect to program use. Recipient governments—the fifty states and approximately 38,500 counties, cities, Indian tribal authorities, and Eskimo authorities—receive "entitlements" automatically four times a year which they can spend pretty much as they wish. For all intents and purposes, GRS is a gift from the federal treasury (Rudman 1970).

Unlike CETA and the CDBG legislation, the enactment of GRS provided new federal support for states and localities. Whereas the block grants meshed together narrow categorical grants-in-aid into broader and more flexible aid packages—a notable achievement, but one that did not produce significant additional revenues—GRS has provided approximately $6 billion more to states and localities each year. Moreover, as a fresh invention, a program without any categorical precursors, GRS came free of the interest group baggage that limited localities in refocusing their CETA and CDBG funds. While spending under these programs has been powerfully influenced by historical patterns set in motion by previous federal aid, GRS entered the local policymaking arena with a blank slate.

These distinctive features made GRS a top policy priority of state and local officials in the early 1970s and again in 1975 and 1976 when the original act had to be renewed. While human service interest groups have rarely begrudged the additional moneys for state and local government, they have objected to the unconditional nature of the aid. Revenue sharing, after all, is a marked retreat from federal policymaking and federal standard setting. Making aid available to all states and localities, as GRS does, provides major subsidies to nonneedy jurisdictions. In addition, the absence of federal targeting—the absence of a focus on social problems and needy populations—is tantamount, in the vast majority of situations, to sanctioning expenditure agendas geared toward traditional state and local priorities.

Since GRS is unconditioned with respect to the programs to which it can be applied, it does stand as a rather effective reflection of these priorities. Unpressured by Uncle Sam to utilize the funds in any particular way, recipient units, in fact, have concentrated the bulk of their expenditures on capital improvements, public safety, and tax reduction. Several studies have made it clear that although several local communities (particularly in the West) have strongly supported social welfare programs—often via contracts with voluntary organizations—human services spending for the most part has been exceedingly small.[12]

As table 3.1 indicates, only one-third of the jurisdictions studied reported any contract spending for human services. This is far less than under CETA or the community-development program, and it reflects the lack of social objectives in the revenue-sharing legislation. Among the communities, moreover, just 4.9 percent of total outlays supported contract agencies, again far lower than the comparable figures for the block grants.

While the great majority of the large cities and counties surveyed did not direct any of their GRS dollars to human services—contract or otherwise—several have become heavily involved in contract endeavors. Jurisdictions in the South and West have been especially apt to earmark funds for nonprofit agencies. In FY 1977, for example, eight of the ninety-three communities reporting provided 20 percent or more of their revenue-sharing funds for private human services. Of these, only Columbus, Ohio, was located outside of the "sun belt" states. Among the remaining "high contract" jurisdictions, California counties were especially well represented, with Sacramento and Orange each above the 20 percent mark and San Diego and Alameda each above the 40 percent mark.

These communities, and others, supported a wide range of community-based services. Kansas City, Missouri, for example, contracted with local welfare rights groups, neighborhood centers, and community health clinics, while Alameda County provided tax dollars to the Salvation Army, East Oakland Switchboard, Travelers Aid, San Leandro Girls Club, and more than 100 other local agencies. Wichita, Kansas, as it has for several years, expended approximately 10 percent of its GRS budget for community agencies. In May 1976 the city solicited applications via an RFP process, conducted public hearings, and selected thirteen agencies for funding, including Big Sisters, Planned Parenthood, and the Kansas Elks Training Center. Each agency subsequently entered into a formal contract with the city, with "performance criteria" clearly specified in terms of program goals and objectives and measures of efficiency and effectiveness. The agencies are required to complete quarterly and final reports addressing themselves to these standards.

CONCLUSION

The evidence reported with respect to local contracting with nonprofit agencies warrants a number of conclusions. First, contracting is hardly an anomaly. While the scope and magnitude of its use varies across jurisdictions and funding areas, it stands as a widely used procedure for implementing tax-financed human service programs.

Second, the data suggest that contracting is most likely to occur under the umbrella of those funding sources most clearly focused on human services. CETA, aimed at providing job-related skills to low-income individuals, generated the greatest reliance on non-profit providers. Aid from CDBG, which permits localities either physical or service community-development strategies, funneled far fewer funds through community agencies. GRS, which can scarcely be defined as a social program at all, provided less than 5 percent of its total revenue for private human services.

Third, the findings indicate an increase in contract utilization by local government. Under CETA, CBOs have garnered a major share of the expenditure pie. Contracts under GRS, for the most part, constitute new service undertakings. Only under the CDBG program has the magnitude of contracting diminished. Contracts supported under Model Cities have, in many cases, been terminated. Agencies that have managed to survive are now forced to compete annually for funds against other groups and projects—many not directed to social services at all.

What the expanding use of human service contracting augurs for government and the private sector is not fully certain. It does seem clear, however, that generalizations about government's "loss of sovereignty" or the "jeopardy of private institutions" are considerably overdrawn.[13] The boundaries between public and private have been growing increasingly blurred for many years, and it is unlikely that contracting, any more than tax laws relating to nonprofit organizations and charitable contributions, or state licensing procedures, will unfold in a way that provides all benefits or all liabilities to either sector.

While clearly disturbing to purists in both government and the voluntary sector, therefore, the interpenetration of public and private activities is likely to increase. In the short run this has a variety of consequences. It is clear, for example, that government services can no longer be equated only with public administration, just as private services no longer imply fully voluntary financing. In addition, government will have to increase its capacity to control and manage outside organizations as it increases its reliance on outside provision. This means, at a minimum, that government must be able to define the services it seeks in a tangible way. It also demands greater attention to procedures for selecting contractors, negotiating contracts and controls, monitoring performance, and, in general, ensuring accountability to public purposes.

Private agencies, for their part, will have to accommodate their own operating procedures to the legitimate requirements of government for fairness, efficiency, and equity in service delivery. Public support means, for example, increased paperwork in the form of performance reports. It means restrictions on who can be served and who cannot be. It means increased accountability in the areas of hiring and firing, financial record keeping, internal organization, planning, and citizen participation.

Contracting, in other words, depends for whatever success it might have on an evolution in the character and the behavior of both the public and the private sectors. Contracting necessitates a partnership—one in which each party does what it does best. Contracting, after all, can only be as good as the purpose it seeks and the services it provides. If government fails to set out reasonable and appropriate goals and objectives, then private agencies can hardly be faulted for not advancing the public good. Conversely, faulty agency operations will undercut the best laid out plans and hopes of public policymakers.

The public/private partnership is only in the beginning stages of its development, and considerable evolution in the attitudes and skills of both sectors will be required if contracting is to become a more general alternative to public administration.Nevertheless, development has begun, and there is clearly a growing recognition of mutual need, and mutual dependence, between local governments and local human service agencies. By strengthening voluntary organizations for pluralism and diversity, and by offering government a broader set of choices for organizing the public business, contracting represents an appealing option for the future.

Notes

1. By the 1820s, e.g., most states had entered into agreements with private residential institutions to serve indigent deaf and otherwise handicapped children. For the history of one such institution, the Hartford Asylum for the Deaf and Dumb, founded in 1817, see H. Best, *Deafness and the Deaf in the United States* (New York: Macmillan, 1943).

2. For the character of relationships in the child welfare field, see D. R. Young, and S. J. Finch, *Foster Care and Nonprofit Agencies* (New York: Lexington Books, 1977. Government, of course, also provides a considerable amount of direct and indirect fiscal aid to nonprofit colleges. See C. Kerr, "Higher Education," in J. Bowers and E. Purcell, eds., *Opportunities for Philanthropy—1976* (New York: Josiah Macy, Jr., Foundation, 1977).

3. In addition to the funding sources investigated in this paper—CETA, CDBG, and GRS—localities have also made substantial use of community action, Model Cities, Title XX, and Older American Act funds for contract support.

4. Well-known "new conservative" critics include Peter Drucker, A. E. Savas, and Peter Berger. Drucker's argument for "privatization" can be found in his article, "The Sickness of Government," *Public Interest 14* (Winter 1969): 3–23. Berger's call for an increased reliance on voluntary associations is stated in *To Empower People* (Washington, D.C.: American Enterprise Institute, 1977). Examples of the political clout of community-based and social work agencies in securing contract arrangements at the level of local government can be found in Terrell (1977).

5. Comprehensive Employment and Training Act, 97 *Stat* 839, 28 December 1973; Housing and Community Development Act of 1974, 88 *Stat* 633, 22 August

1974; General Revenue Sharing, 86 *Stat* 919, 20 October 1972 (amended 13 October 1976, 90 *Stat* 2341).

6. An excellent description of CETA's major provisions can be found in the Center for Community Change *(CETA, a Citizen's Action Guide* [Washington, D.C: Center for Community Change, February 1978]).

7. According to Department of Labor figures, approximately $90 million in Title I funds were provided to CBOs through local prime sponsors in FY 1976. These CBOs served 6.4 percent of all Title I recipients. Among the CBOs, OIC, SER, and the Urban League have expanded as a result of CETA, whereas community-action agencies appear to be operating at a somewhat diminished level. However, although the CBOs have not lost ground, there appears to have been some narrowing of their program scope. Prime sponsors, in other words, often utilize the CBOs to provide specialized rather than multi-element services. SER, for example, is frequently called upon to provide outreach services and English language training. Similarly, OICs have been utilized to undertake skill training as a single component within larger prime sponsor systems, despite the fact that OICs have always stressed the comprehensive start-to-finish nature of their operations; see Department of Labor, *Employment and Training Report of the President* (Washington, D.C: Department of Labor, 1977), 54; and Advisory Commission on Intergovernmental Relations, *The Comprehensive Employment and Training Act: Early Readings from a Hybrid Block Grant* (Washington, D.C: ACIR, June 1977), 34–36.

8. This figure does not indicate that the remaining 86.2 percent supports direct in-house employment and training services. First, wages and allowances to Title I trainees are frequently not included in contract totals. Second, approximately 8 percent of Title I expenditures supports prime sponsor central administration, including contract letting and monitoring.

9. The seven programs brought together into the new block grant were: Model Cities, Urban Renewal, water and sewer facilities, neighborhood facilities, open-space land grants, public facilities loans, rehabilitation loans, and code enforcement assistance.

10. The figures include both publicly and privately funded programs; see Department of Housing and Urban Development, *Community Development Block Grant Program, Second Annual Report* (Washington, D.C: HUD, December 1976), 22; Advisory Commission on Intergovernmental Relations, *Community Development: The Workings of a Federal-Local Block Grant* (Washington, D.C: ACIR, March 1977), 50; Nathan et al., 271.

11. For a discussion of the 20 percent proviso, see Nathan et al., 41, 244–246. See also CDBG *Regulations,* sec. 570.200 (9–1976).

12. Revenue sharing has scarcely provided any funds to health or social service programs. In FY 1975, for example, 24 percent of each GRS dollar was directed to public safety, 22 percent to education, 13 percent to environmental protection, 9 percent to general government, and 7 percent to environmental protection. Just 7 percent went to support health programs, and 2 percent was allocated for social services for the poor or aged. See Department of the Treasury, Office of

Revenue Sharing, *Reported Uses of General Revenue Sharing Funds,* 1974–1975 (Washington, D.C.). For examples of communities supporting human services via contract, see Terrell (1977).

13. For an excellent overview of the issues, see B. L. R. Smith, *Accountability and Independence in the Contract State.* In B. L. R. Smith and D. C. Hague (eds.), The Dilemma of Accountability in Modern Government (London: Macmillan, 1971).

4

Policy Making and Service Delivery on the Margins of Government: The Case of Contractors

Ira Sharkansky

Modern government defies definition. It grows, but it also declines. It does more while doing less. It confounds those who would understand it, while adding to the benefits offered the people. Its own officials will not—or cannot—report the true size of the budget or workforce. Because they cannot say exactly what it is, policy makers have problems in controlling it while observers have problems in describing it. Academic specialists in public administration and political science suffer from confusion about the thing that is central to their careers.

Officials do more while they do less by assigning activities to bodies that are not, strictly speaking, part of the government. Just how this happens depends on conditions within each country. The national government of the United States has, in certain respects, actually shrunk in size during the period 1955–1976. Its number of employees declined from 146 per 10,000 population to 134 to 10,000 population. Yet, no one should claim that the national government did less in 1976 than in 1955. It shrunk by hiving off new activities and some old established programs. Washington transferred some activities to state and local governments. It assigned others to special authorities, and to private firms and foundations operating as contractors for government agencies. This essay deals with contractors that operate on the margins of American governments. Yet, central features of this analysis apply to other kinds of bodies that operate on the margins of this and other modern governments.

The inclination to use business firms or other private bodies as contractors is distinctly an American style of conducting public activities on the margins of government. By tradition the United States is a country of free enterprise. It is fitting to use business corporations to design, implement and monitor many of the programs that have turned the United States into one of the most generous of welfare states.

In other countries there is less of a preoccupation with free enterprise and less of a tendency to hive off government activities to private business. The more common pattern is to assign responsibilities to companies that the government owns, or to special authorities that are created by acts of the legislature (Sharkansky 1979). There are also special authorities in the United States and some companies owned by government (Walsh 1978). As in the case of firms operating under contract, these companies or special authorities are distinct from the government even while they are doing the government's business. Typically the employees of government-owned companies or special authorities—like the employees of private firms under contract to governments—are not considered civil servants. The revenues and expenditures of these bodies are not included in the government budget. Usually there is no central listing of government-owned companies, special authorities, or government contractors. Each of these exists in a gray area on the margins of government. Because they are big and important, even though their marginal status makes it difficult to say how big or how important, they create problems for officials, for clients who would receive their services, and for academics who would understand public policy.

One estimate out of Washington is that more people work for private firms under contract to the United States government than work for the government directly. More precise estimates dealing with the Department of Health, Education, and Welfare—one of the most active civilian users of government contractors—is that 750,000 people work under contract to HEW, while only 157,000 are employees of HEW. In 1976, 80,000 federal employees worked to oversee the administration of contracting (Hanrahan 1977). The Department of Defense arranged some 10.4 *million* contracts in one year for a total $46 billion (ibid.) The most recent catalog of United States government contractors seems to have been assembled in 1948—by a contractor. More recently, contractors have conducted courses for federal employees on how to arrange and supervise contracts (U.S. House 1977).

There have long been organizational entities on the margins of government. Now that the margins of some governments may have grown larger than core departments, however, the margins warrant renewed attention. Because they are largely self-governing, bodies on the margin threaten some of political theory with obsolescence. Concerns about elections, legislatures, chief executives, and government departments have limited appeal if governments isolate much of what they do from these devices of political control.

A pessimist could point to the margins of government as disasters in the making. The label "Beltway Bandits" for consulting firms located on the periphery of Washington, Boston, Houston, and Atlanta suggest that contractors are more concerned to help themselves than to help government. Yet the picture is not clear. There are problems of management and accountability, to be sure, but it is not certain that the result of expanding activities on the margins of government is better or worse than expanding activities in the core departments of government. At this time, the disaster is more clearly one of information. Professional observers of the government—journalists, academics, and policy makers—have remained preoccupied with classical topics of elections, legislatures, executives, and the official civil service, when much of the action is elsewhere.

Some years ago Professor Fred Riggs used the term "formalism" with respect to the governmental bodies of developing countries (Riggs 1964). To him, the elections, legislatures, presidents, and prime ministers of Asia, Africa, and Latin America are patterned after the forms observed in Europe and North America, but they do not perform like the originals. Often they mask dictatorships or corruption in the clothing of western democracies. Now we must examine the western democracies with the notion of formalism. How much of their public activities are left to the control of elections and representative government?

WHY CONTRACT?

The manifest functions of government contracts range from the pedestrian to the profound:

janitorial and security service for government buildings;

cafeteria service for government employees;

design, construction, installation, operation, and/or service of equipment, facilities, and supplies (ranging from paper clips to office buildings, rifles to ICBMs);

problem analysis and definition (i.e., to determine just what is wrong and what government may do to fix it);

83

program design (drafting legislation, writing administrative manuals);

service delivery (e.g., operating health clinics, trash collection, halfway houses, counselling services, job training, et al.);

selecting personnel to manage or work in government departments;

program monitoring and evaluation (i.e., determining just what a
government agency—or another contractor—is doing and
whether it is doing a good job.

In short, executive officials contract out virtually any work that the government could do with its own personnel. An exception is the actual approval of public policy. This is reserved, constitutionally, to members of
the executive, legislative, and judicial branches. However, the constitu-
tional branches do contract for the supply of information and advice, with
an eye to decisions they will make.

The *latent functions* of contracting can be more elusive. For the question, "Why should government contract out what it may otherwise do in-
house?", the answer may be:

to abide by requirements to freeze the size of the civil service even
while adding or enlarging the programs that are being offered;

to purchase services more cheaply than they can be had while using
government employees (contractors may pay lower wages
and/or avoid the fringe benefits required for government
employees);

to weaken the power of government employees' unions by giving work
to contractors;

to evade civil service regulations of various sorts (e.g., veterans' preference, maximum salary rules, a prohibition against paying
moving expenses to new employees, or affirmative action procedures) by contracting out a project (the contractor is responsible for staffing, and may be limited only by a total amount
that can be spent on "personnel");

to provide for certain personnel attributes—like specializations or
longevity—not available from regular employees (the Department of Defense contracts for certain persons to maintain scrutiny over complex inventory programs, which is a function not
expected from uniformed personnel who rotate frequently between tasks and places);

84

to reward certain persons for favors rendered in the past by giving
them a contract;

to provide certain programs experimentally, without risking continuation beyond a certain date that can be fixed in a contract;

to save money on the cost of building (government may avoid the need
to pay the entire cost of a building at the time of its construction by contracting for its rent over an extended period of time;
the contractor borrows for the construction of the building and
includes an amount for mortgage payments in the annual
rental fee).

Recent commentators emphasize a growth in contracting. Many attrib-
ute this to the spurt in social programs begun during the Johnson Administration's War on Poverty. A great deal of contracting is prompted
by federal aids, which have climbed sharply. They grew by 356 percent
between 1965 and 1975, 130 percent faster than total government revenues. Because federal money is "soft money" (subject to cuts or curtailment by Washington), states or localities are loath to expand their
permanent staffs for a federally-funded program.

Claims about the newness of contracting must be viewed with caution.
With respect to contractors who supply military hardware, George Washington's complaints preceded those of William Proxmire by almost 200
years. In 1961, the Government Employees Council of the AFL-CIO
noted that it was "gravely concerned over the growing practice in the
Federal service, to contract to private interests, certain governmental
services and functions that have historically been performed by civil service employees (Government Employees Council 1962). At about the
same time, an interagency committee of the U.S. government raised
some basic issues about the control of contractors. In a report to the president, it expressed concern about the capacity of government officials to
oversee contractors adequately and to maintain control over basic policies. In response to this report, a spokesman for contractors raised the issue of excessive control by government agencies over their contractors
(Reagan 1965). Thus, issues of contractor control vs. autonomy have been
well-defined for some years.

85

CONTROVERSIES ABOUT CONTRACTING:
ISSUES OF MANAGEMENT AND ACCOUNTABILITY

Contracting does not proceed quietly. It has warm supporters and intense opponents. There are stories of beautiful successes and horrible failures, each mingled with simple ideology, myth, and personal stakes. On one extreme are right-wing reform mongers who react negatively to symbols of government and politics. They allege creativity, hard work, and efficiency in the private sector. On the other extreme are left-wing reform mongers—like Ralph Nader's Center for the Study of Responsive Laws—and organized civil servants. These groups resist contracting-out to the private sector. Book titles convey their spirit. Nader's Center supported *Shadow Government: The Government's Multi-Billion-Dollar Giveaway of Its Decision-Making Powers to Private Management Consultants, "Experts," and Think Tanks* (Guttman and Willner 1976). The American Federation of State, County, and Municipal Employees published *Government for Sale: Contracting-Out the New Patronage* (Hanrahan 1977).

A report of the Urban Institute sought to assess a series of questions about the benefits and problems associated with contracting by local governments. The document raises several issues relevant to the evaluation of contracting-out vs. the in-house provision of services, such as cost, flexibility, competitiveness, and the quality of management and services. In its conclusions, however, the report concedes the lack of sufficient information to answer its questions in a satisfactory manner (Fisk, Kiesling, and Mueller, 1978).

Despite the hoary character of contracting as a topic, it is appropriate to look again at some issues of relevance to policy makers and academics. Common to each of the issues addressed below are the general topics of managerial control and political accountability. Both control and accountability are strained by the autonomy of contractors. Moreover, there are goods as well as bads in these strains.

Flexibility is a common feature of contracting. Policy makers can select just the kind of contract that seems suitable to their needs and fine-tune details or organizational structure, goals, and personnel. From the consumer's side, especially in large cities, there can be multiple providers of a service within reach (Ostram 1974). Even if the consumer does not have the wide selection that policy makers encounter, some choice is better than none. However, the great variety may be incoherent to all but the expert. The policy maker and the consumer need help to sort through the options. Variety hinders program evaluation according to common or clear standards.

Contractors can innovate in ways not likely to survive in a government office. One State of Wisconsin department contracted for services to high school drop-outs prone to delinquency. The services included counselling, training in basic skills, and work discipline. Among the qualifications that one contractor asked of potential counsellors was:

> in order to facilitate an effective working relationship with ex-offenders, the applicant should have some experience in confinement in a county jail or state correctional institution (although this is not required), (sic) (State of Wisconsin 1977).

The assessment of contracting must compare the opportunities for doing good that result from its inherent flexibility with the opportunities for doing bad with the same flexibility. There are many cases close to the boundaries of good and bad. One state government engaged in a nationwide search for a new division chief. In the early spring it selected a person from another region with a national reputation in the field at issue. The job was to begin on July 1. The candidate wanted the job, but would find it awkward to wait several months to begin work and receive salary. Also, there was the matter of moving expenses. A contract helped to solve these problems. The candidate accepted a consultant's contract until July 1, at a level of compensation sufficient to cover some costs of relocating. In this case, a contract allowed a state government to make its position more attractive to a person who was selected as a result of stiff professional criteria. No personal favors were at stake, although there was a special deal outside the usual procedures and pay scale of civil service.

Flexible procedures for arranging contracts permit great abuse. The General Accounting Office estimates that 85 percent of defense contracts and 71 percent of civilian contracts in sample years were not advertised and bid competitively (Guttman and Willner 1976). Agency personnel identify a contractor they consider appropriate and proceed to negotiate an agreement. There is opportunity for key administrators or elected office holders to steer contracts to friends, family members, party supporters, or to firms allied with organized crime that threaten retribution if contracts do not come their way.

Critics charge that contracting does not offer all the flexibility that its boosters claim. It is seldom easy to shift from one contractor to another. New firms may not want to bid for a community's trask pickup even when the local authorities signal their dissatisfaction with an existing contractor. That business requires a great deal of expensive equipment, plus a site for solid waste disposal. Contractors may use the old gimmick of the "introductory offer" to win a contract. The boost prices when a community has committed itself and closed the door to other options. A critic of contracting reports that residents of Seattle found their charges for contracted trash collection increasing by 98 percent from 1974 to 1976 (Hanrahan 1977).

The quality and efficiency of contracting are not attributes that come automatically. Some claims of reduced costs are simply the product of reduced services. Trash pick-up twice a week by a private contractor will be less expensive than three times a week by the City Department of Sanitation. A memo from the nursing director of a state institution for the retarded complained about a contractor's laundry service in the most homely terms:

> Their work on the whole is almost totally unacceptable. I'm sure most of us as private citizens wouldn't tolerate for one minute sending our laundry out and getting it back like this without complaining and demanding immediate remedial action. . . .
>
> Many of the items sent to the laundry are never returned. . . . Laundry received in the cottage is often not for that cottage and must be resorted. It isn't at all unusual to find laundry from such places as Lake Geneva Bunny Club, Marriot Inn, Holiday Inn, etc. Laundry comes back wet and mildewy-smelly (Southern Wisconsin 1975).

Conflict of interest is a frequent companion of contracting. At times the conflict is blatant and criminal. Vice President Spiro Agnew is the most prominent of many officials who have lost their positions, paid fines, or served time in jail for receiving bribes, kickbacks, or other improper favors from contractors. A high incidence of some 1,000 federal, state, and local officials convicted of felonies during the 1970–76 period dealt with contracts between government agencies and private firms (Hanrahan 1977).

Some contracting is made suspect by cozy dealing. Contractors work both for a government agency and for business firms that are subsidized or regulated by the agency. Peat, Marwick, Mitchell and Co., a large accounting and management consulting firm, was simultaneously a contractor for the U.S. Department of Transportation and Penn Central. DOT asked the contractor to help account for Metroliner costs when the government subsidized Penn Central's operation of the train. Later, Penn Central's bankruptcy was the subject of investigations by the Securities and Exchange Commission and Congress. Part of the inquiries focused on misleading reports about Penn Central's financial condition. According to Wright Patman, Chairman of the House Banking and Currency Committee.

> Information in the Committee's possession shows that this policy of 'doctoring' the financial statements was done at the direction of top Penn Central officials. These documents further indicate that Peat, Marwick, Mitchell and Co. played a substantial role in these successful attempts to misinform the investing public (Guttman and Willner 1976).

At times it is one government that "rips off" another via contracting. State governments have learned to write contracts from one state agency to another in order to make it look like one of them is spending real money for services. This is reported to Washington as the state's contribution to a federal-state program, and draws federal aid on a matching basis. With this gimmick, the State of Illinois boosted its receipts of social service grants by almost twice the national average over the period 1971–73 and caused a bureaucratic furor that reached the president's desk. Illinois also taught New York State how to do it, and New York increased its federal receipts even more than Illinois (Derthick 1975).

Government contracting with voluntary social service agencies raises its own variety of issues. Government expenditures for a group of programs in the child care area grew by 650 percent in the 1950–70 period, while comparable growth in the voluntary sector was only 200 percent (Brilliant 1973). Much of the increase in government spending funnels through voluntary agencies and makes them leading social service contractors in local communities.

Voluntary agencies associated with each of the major denominations have gone heavily into government contracting. One study of Jewish-sponsored social service agencies shows an increase from $27 million to $561 million in government contracts during the 1962–1973 period. Government payments went from 11 to 51 percent of the total income received by these agencies. A study of United Way agencies in the San Francisco area found a doubling in governments' purchase of certain social service over the 1970–75 period (Gilbert 1977). Of the $145 million that New York City spent on daycare, homemakers service, and foster care in 1969, $108 million (75 percent) went to voluntary organizations. Pennsylvania allocated 88 percent of its spending for certain child care programs in 1968 to voluntary agencies (Cole 1970).

Some observers applaud the diversity in social service delivery that is achieved via contracting with voluntary agencies. Clients are freed from dependence on government agencies that monopolize service programs, and the clients may benefit from competition between service providers (Reid 1972). Other observers focus on the dilemmas created by:

problems of coordination among separate agencies that deal in similar services in the same community;

challenges to the autonomy of voluntary agencies via mechanisms of government control;

lack of public control over the programs administered by voluntary agencies;

dilution of the benefits derived from voluntarism in social services, as agencies and their contributors come to rely on government contracts for the bulk of their funds;

problems of church-state separation, felt both by secular interests toward social service agencies having a religious sponsorship, and the religious sponsors who feel the erosion of their traditional social service roles.

CONTROLLING THE MARGINS OF AMERICAN GOVERNMENTS

The large number of diverse contracts and their origin at the working levels of agencies renders them hard to control by legislatures or chief executives. When a Committee of the Wisconsin Legislature sought information on contracting, it was told that:

> it would take 3 to 5 months of searching to obtain the data . . . just for the Department of Natural Resources and Health and Social Services and the University of Wisconsin . . . it would involve searching through 1.5 million documents, and . . . the documents . . . sought . . . not avail-

able by category . . . the data obtained would probably be incomplete, if it could be found at all (State of Wisconsin 1978).

In response to the Legislature's request, administrative departments made some effort to cull information on contracting from 1973 to 1978. The Deputy Secretary of the Wisconsin Department of Health and Social Services sent a memo to his division administrators that reflected something other than a burning desire to cooperate.

> The Legislative Joint Committee on Review of Administrative Rules has requested the Department to provide them with the information listed on the attached. After reviewing this, you will realize, I am certain, that this is an almost impossible task.
>
> In an attempt to reduce this task to more manageable proportions, we are going to provide the Committee with a list of types of contracts we have in the Department, and hopefully convince them that representative samples of the different types would be sufficient. . . . (Wisconsin Dept. of Health and Social Services 1978).

A mixed bag of information came in response to this memo. Two divisions sent in handwritten lists of contracts. One listed a random sample of voucher payments, including only the voucher number and the amount of payment with no reference to the kind of service being purchased or the name of the contractor. Another sent a 10-page list of contractors' names with no indication of the nature of services being purchased.

Federal controls over contractors are also thin. While there is an abundance of control agencies and regulations, weaknesses appear at the working levels. Each of several controllers takes a narrow view of its responsibilities and seems willing to overlook obvious problems that it can define as outside its province. Agencies growing out of the former U.S. Civil Service Commission have a role in certain matters dealing with government employees affected by contracting, but they have not concerned themselves with defining costs or savings due to reducing the government workforce because of contracting. Moreover, they do no systematic checking on contracting by agencies. They wait upon agency requests or upon a complaint filed by an employee who alleges improper treatment (U.S. House 1977).

The Office of Management and Budget has a limited responsibility to check comparative cost figures for contracting-out vs. doing a service in-house, but this only for new activities. When asked about a general program to analyze costs for established programs that are contracted-out, an OMB executive said. "There is no requirement and no desire that any of these actions be reviewed by the Office of Management and Budget (U.S. House 1977).

The General Accounting Office has shown little interest in contracting as a general problem. Its typical treatment deals with contracting along with other issues in program administration. Also, GAO tends to combine contracting with grants in its studies, and thereby blurs the distinctive problems of each (Woodrow 1977).

Contractors help to confound control by seeking to enhance their access to government. The crudest of their techniques can result in disgrace and incarceration for government officials "on the take." Also of interest are subtle payoffs, where the beneficiaries appear to be receiving nothing more than an honor. Some prominent non-profit bodies like United Fund, church, or ethnic welfare agencies choose their boards of directors from government officials who make decisions about contracts. This can look both innocent and prestigious, at least at first glance. Yet, charities and other prestigious bodies have become important contractors. In 1978, the Wisconsin Department of Health and Social Services appointed a citizens' committee to oversee a survey of its contracting. Either through innocence or guile, the foxes were set to count the chickens. Most members of the original committee were officials of non-profit organizations that serve as contractors.

Government contracting has been a live issue in Washington. Circular A-76 of the Office of Management and Budget has put the national government on a pro-contracting course since 1967. The circular was modified in the period 1976–1978, but not in a manner to alter policy in a substantial way. It will "continue to support the policy that the Government should rely on the private sector for goods and services. . . ." (Fettig 1978). Yet, the procedures for costing the advantages of contracting-out vs. in-house activities are to be made more precise, and greater concern is to be shown for government employees who may be affected by contracting-out.

In the details of the 1976–78 review, it is possible to see one of those small points that has crucial impact. The issue was the cost of government retirement programs to be used in assessing in-house vs. contracting-out. The true cost of government retirement is elusive. It depends on unknown future events like inflation and the generosity of Congress to pensioners. Since both factors have been considerable in recent years, the cost of government pensions—and thereby the long-run cost of retaining government employees—can escalate *after* a decision is made to perform a service in-house. *The higher the cost figure assigned to government retirement costs, the more likely that a comparison will favor contracting-out a service.*

Between August 1976 and April 1978, the figure to be used for government retirement costs moved back and forth with all the marks of a pressure contest between contractors on one side and government employees' unions on the other. In August 1976, President Ford's Office of Management and Budget announced that

> New guidance . . . for calculating overhead costs of commercial and industrial activities of the federal government could result in substantially greater use of the private sector, and lower costs (U.S. Office of Management and Budget 1976).

What followed as an increase from 7 to 24.7 per cent in the overhead factor for retirement benefits. This would put an additional 17.7 cents on each federal payroll dollar in comparing prices with private contractors.

The language and the calculations of the Office of Management and Budget shifted with the advent of the Carter Administration. By June 1977, OMB's language showed more awareness of government employees' interests, and its calculations dropped from 24.7 to 14.1 per cent of payroll for retirement costs. In November 1977, OMB's figure moved back to 20.4 per cent of payroll for retirement costs. While the result appears to be a simple compromise, OMB tried to legitimize it with the names of brother agencies.

> This factor was produced by the Civil Service Commission's actuarial model, as modified and validated by the General Accounting Office, using current economic assumptions supplied by the Council of Economic Advisors (Fettig 1976).

PROSPECTS FOR REFORM

The contracting experiences of American governments should not be viewed in isolation. They reflect the general proliferation of activities in modern governments beyond the conventional departments or ministries. Whether the margins of a government are populated with contractors, special authorities, or government-owned companies, the common denominator is autonomy outside the conventional orbit of the legislature and executive or the core departments of government.

Can officers of government put their house in order? The question requires a consideration of the basic reasons for putting activities on the margins. Some of these reasons reveal incapacity. The core departments of the government cannot handle all the activities demanded by citizens and promulgated by politicians. Other reasons for putting programs on the margins of the state reveal some measure of indifference or guile. Politicians respond to some demands out of political necessity, without caring how the programs develop. If there is an available body on the margin of the government, then it may handle the new program without great risk to the politician. If the program goes sour, the autonomy of its administrators allows the government and its political leaders to avoid blame. Politicians also put programs on the margins in order to keep their expenses off the government's budget, or to keep their employees off the civil service list. Politicians can thereby add programs without violating—explicitly—other demands to limit the growth of government. Programs put on the margins are available to patronage demands, from the politicians who create them; to hire a supporter outside the formal controls of the civil service commission, or to provide service to a constituent whose case might not survive the scrutiny of a government office. It is difficult to assign clear or simple motives to any one case of putting a program on the margins of government. More important is to recognize the variety of reasons for putting programs there. Each of these motives would stand in the way of a general reform that brought programs from the margins more clearly into the orbit of governmental control. It may not be a question of the government's inability to put its house in order, as much as a lack of desire to give up the benefits received from having institutions on the margins and performing numerous important functions without close controls from the center.

It is the essence of being a politician to bear contrary pressures; to serve the people *and* to keep taxes low plus minimize government employment; to hire managers who can work quickly *and* to respect all the procedures for clearing major decisions with key government officers; to accept demands that the government hire people according to strict rules that respect traits of competence, ethnicity, sex, or veteran status *and* to allow some bodies to hire who they want. A typical way out of such conflicts is an ambiguous creation. The bodies on the margins of government provide ideal conditions. The margins are *of*, but not *in*, the government. They promise the satisfaction of contrary demands and are essential to the political process.

Is it possible to expect reforms to emerge from *outside of government* if we cannot expect systematic reform from official policy makers? Citizen involvement has been a common theme in efforts to make government more responsive. Political accountability may come not only through the conventional linkages between voters, elected officials, and the heads of administrative hierarchies, but also through the direct involvement of citizens in local service agencies.

Some devices designed with citizens in mind are catching on in many places. Even though they do not aspire to general reform, these devices may render a government more effective and more responsive. The most common example is the ombudsman. This instrument is designed to aid the citizen who feels improperly treated by an agency. The ombudsman inquires into the merits of the claim, and—if justified—will bring the pressure of its recommendations against the errant agency. Depending on the jurisdiction, the ombudsman may deal with bodies on the margins of government, or may be limited to the core departments of government. Generally, the ombudsman has no role in making service decisions, *per se*. Its role is an advisory one, but it is backed up with the prestige and publicity that can be turned against officials who overlook its recommendations.

A weakness of the ombudsman is its being a fixer of bad decisions. Many citizens have problems that are *prior* to being the target of bad decisions. They do not know where to turn in the face of numerous service agencies, especially if their needs do not fit squarely into the orbit of one agency. A client who needs a combination of counselling, job training, medical treatment, and job placement may need to find and visit four separate agencies, and he may not know where to begin. For this kind of problem, a multiple service referral agency (what Australians label "One Stop Shop") is an answer. It should be centrally located, widely advertised, and staffed by personnel who can clarify for clients an incoherent maze of agencies.

It may be that no gimmick incorporated into a large and amorphous government can serve citizens adequately. Perhaps only a private agent

—who works for a fee—will have an incentive to learn the shortest cuts through a service maze and to render advice that truly is in the client's interest. There is an analog in the tax field, where private-sector lawyers or tax advisors sell information that is felt to be more client-serving than the advice purveyed by the tax agency itself. Another analog comes from the travel industry, where travel agents help their clients through a multiplicity of options offered by airlines and resorts that rival the programs of government in their incoherence. In this case, the agents receive fees from the seller of travel services, and not from the client directly.

The models of the travel agent or the private tax advisor may be spread to other sectors of public service. Store-front agencies can specialize in clusters of service that bridge the activities of several agencies in their locales. They would, in a sense, repackage the offerings of different agencies to meet the needs of clients, sell advice as to which agencies a client should visit in which sequence, actually fill out the forms, or accompany the client through the official maze. Payment for such service may come either directly from the clients or via referral chits established by the service agencies.

Academics concerned with policymaking and administration have special opportunities with respect to contracting. Most important is to move contracting from the margins to the focus of our own attention. To round out our comprehension of policy making and service delivery, we can pursue systematic research and teaching about the margins of government—looking at mechanisms that connect bodies on the margins with the conventional mechanisms of government on the one side, as well as with clients on the other side. Crucial is an improvement in basic information. Most writing about government contracting relies on illustration selected according to no systematic scheme. There is no solid information even about the magnitude of government contracting. Academics can join policy makers in urging systematic collection of basic information about government contractors and other kinds of bodies on the margins of governments. Such information would allow systematic comparison of contracting in different jurisdictions, and the knowledgeable selection of specific cases for intensive analyses. At the present time, the lack of systematic attention to contracting—either by academics or government agencies—means that any *crisis* that could be described for contracting is more clearly one of information and analysis than of a breakdown in the activities of policy making or administration.

5

From Voluntarism to Vendorism: An Organizational Perspective on Contracting

Ralph M. Kramer

In this chapter the potential advantages and disadvantages of purchase of service contracting (POSC) in the human services are examined from the perspective of not only government, which is the usual practice, but also from that of the voluntary nonprofit agency as a provider. (Even though profitmaking organizations provide some human services under contract, the dominant suppliers are still nonprofit organizations). Although it would be useful to assess POSC from the standpoint of the consumer—whose interests have generally been considered as synonymous with government—we have virtually no information on what difference it makes to the recipients whether a service is directly provided or contracted. (The few attempts to assess services from the client's perspective include Gibelman 1981; Garrick and Moore 1979; and Miller and Pruger 1978.)

Despite the relative paucity of empirical data and the ubiquitous "softness" of the human services, there is still a reasonable basis for analysis of the relative organizational costs and benefits for both governmental and voluntary agencies (Kramer and Terrell 1982). A series of factors will be suggested that should be taken into account in decisions regarding purchase or direct provision, and some principles of contracting will be proposed. Underlying many of the alleged benefits and dangers of POSC are potential conflicts between the interests of government and its service providers expressed in the strain between accountability and independence. This chapter concludes with a reevaluation of these two key concepts.

THE INTERMINGLING OF PUBLIC AND PRIVATE INTERESTS

One of the most significant trends during the last two decades has been the progressive and pervasive intermingling of public and private funds and functions. The "new political economy," the "contract state," and the "service society" are some of the terms used to describe the simultaneous expansion and blurring of the boundaries between the public and private sectors in the economy and in society. This has resulted in a pluralistic, mixed, and more competitive social service economy, rendering obsolete the conventional conceptions of the role of government and the voluntary sector and their relationship to the profit-making sector.

As a result of these evolutionary modifications, we need new and more appropriate models of interorganizational relationships that will reflect the changing character of the governmental and nongovernmental sectors, help maintain the independence and integrity of voluntary organizations, and lead to better methods of public accountability. For example, although there are theories concerning the private sector and public goods, there is no theory besides pluralism and no rationale beyond expediency for the use of nongovernmental organizations in democratic, postindustrial societies with substantial systems of public social services. The absence of a suitable conceptual framework for the role of nonprofit organizations as providers of public goods has also contributed to the ambiguity and confusion surrounding the functions of voluntarism in the welfare state (Kramer 1981).

In addition to the gradual dissolution of the dichotomy between public and private, there is a backlash of widespread resistance to increased taxes and governmental spending, coupled with a strong animus against bureaucracy. In a context in which many governmental programs shift into low gear, there is growing support for reprivatization and the use of nonprofit voluntary organizations to carry out public purposes. Ideological backing for the voluntary sector comes both from the Left and Right and stems from its perception as a bulwark against further governmental intervention, or at least as an alternative if not a substitute for it. Some even see voluntarism as a means of recovering a lost sense of community. The rationale for the greater use of voluntary organizations, based on the assumption that the expansion of governmental services has ended, marks a 180-degree change in direction from the 1930s when government took responsibility for some social welfare functions because voluntary organizations were no longer able to meet the demands. There is, however, danger that the belief that government has seemingly reached the limits of its capacity and legitimacy can become a premature, self-fulfilling prophecy, too ready to tolerate government failure to continue providing benefits that only the state can insure. *Voluntarism is no substitute for services that can best be delivered by government, particularly if coverage, equity, and entitlements are valued* (Kahn 1973).

Unrealistic expectations about voluntarism are often engendered by its enthusiastic proponents who indiscriminately lump together all forms of nonprofit efforts and regard them all as equally effective in combating governmental bigness and in delivering social services. Yet there are substantial differences in the use of volunteers as unpaid staff and peer self-help, between mutual aid, neighborhood and community-based organizations, and among the various forms of citizen participation (Kramer 1981).

There are many different types of voluntary agencies depending on their health, welfare, or educational functions. Essentially, most of them are bureaucratic in structure; governed by an elected, volunteer board of directors; and employ professional and/or volunteer staff to provide a continuing social service to a clientele in the community. They have also been known at various times as private social agencies, nonprofit organizations, and even as public agencies. Closely related to voluntary agencies are various forms of self-help or mutual aid groups, most of which provide services for their own members. As service providers, voluntary agencies deliver those services they have selected, some of which may be a public responsibility, but where government is unable, unwilling, or prefers not to administer them directly or fully at this time, i.e., the voluntary agency often does what government cannot, should not, or will not do. As a service provider, voluntary agencies may substitute for, influence, extend, and improve the public sector, and/or they may supplement it, offer complementary services different in kind, or they can be a public agent or vendor.

CONTRACTING FOR SERVICE

The vendor role has become more prominent since the 1960s as a result of Great Society legislation such as the Economic Opportunity

Act of 1964, the 1967 Amendments to the Social Security Act, the Model Cities Act, Community Development and Housing, General Revenue Sharing, CETA, and Title XX of the 1974 Amendments to the Social Security Act. The growing availability of matching grants and purchase of service contracting for the social services has changed the character of this service system and altered the distribution of power, resources, and functions between governmental and voluntary agencies. Human services now represent about two-thirds of the expenditures of state and local government, but despite the enormous growth in POSC, there is still little available knowledge to guide policymaking and administration (Wedel, Katz, and Weick 1979).

Contracting has been viewed from three perspectives according to the type of public service, level of government, and extent of reliance on profit-making or nonprofit organizations. One body of literature is focused on the use and relative cost of profit-making organizations providing upwards of forty municipal services, such as refuse collection and disposal, street and traffic lighting, road maintenance, animal shelters, park and recreation services, as well as legal, engineering, and accounting services (Ahlbrandt 1974; Fitch 1974; Fisk, Kiesling, and Muller 1978; Savas 1981).

A broader and more political concern with the "contract state" is found on the national level where there is extensive governmental use of both profit and nonprofit organizations, resulting in diminishing differences between the three sectors. This "new political economy" is characterized by the proliferation of quangos (quasi-nongovernmental organizations), the widespread use of consultants and contractors by federal agencies, and the reliance on universities and think tanks for research and evaluation (Smith 1975; Sharkansky 1979; Guttman and Willner 1976; Hanrahan 1977; Musolf and Seidman 1980; Orlans 1980). Less well known is another body of information about POSC in the social services or, as they are increasingly called, the human services. This experience deserves more attention because of the growing involvement of local government in the field of human services, and because it can also contribute to a better understanding of the policy issues inherent in the use of nongovernmental providers in the production and delivery of public services. These issues take on increased importance because of the cutback environment for social programs in the 1980s that is based on disenchantment with government and public policies favoring decentralization, debureaucratization, and population targeting. Consequently, it is likely that even greater reliance will be placed on the voluntary sector.

POTENTIAL ADVANTAGES OF POSC FOR GOVERNMENT

For government, contracting has generally been an expedient way of extending limited resources, because the cost of the human service is usually less than it would be if it were provided in accordance with civil service and other regulations (Benton, Feild, and Millar 1978; Fisk, Kiesling, and Mueller, 1978). In economic terms the supply of the voluntary agency services and the demand of the governmental agency usually intersect at a price that is below the real cost for both parties. It has usually been easier for a governmental agency to obtain funds for purchase of service than for additional provider staff. Apart from cost factors, government is often in the position of having authority and responsibility for a program, but lacking appropriate or sufficient staff, facilities, expertise, or other resources. The utilization of voluntary agencies and institutions under these circumstances also means that government can offer services such as sheltered workshops or residential care without high, initial fixed costs, as well as without any undesired visibility.

Because human services can be initiated and terminated more rapidly and easily, contracting can give government considerable flexibility, (Sharkansky 1980; Fisk, Kiesling, and Mueller 1978). Contracting is also a means of bypassing rigid administrative and budgetary rules and regulations, such as a freeze on personnel hiring or salary guidelines, as well as a way of getting around political constraints. Unwanted, marginal, or highly specialized services can also be contracted out.

The other advantages of contracting out are related to the specialized competence of the voluntary agency and its capacity to reach certain clientele more easily. Voluntary organizations can also be an effective way of serving small numbers of hard-to-reach or controversial groups, cultural or ethnic minorities, or widely dispersed populations whom government is obligated to serve but where fear or stigma prevent utilization (Rodgers 1976). In addition to improving both geographic and psychological access for clients, voluntary agencies can also be a source of volunteers for service programs and the promotion of self-help (Terrell 1977).

The specialized competence of the voluntary agency may also inhere in the prior existence of its facilities needed by a governmental agency to serve a clientele for whom there is a public responsibility, together with substantial operating experience. In some instances voluntary agencies may almost have a service monopoly as is often the case for day treatment, residential care, sheltered workshops for the mentally handicapped and emotionally disturbed, shelters for the victims of family violence, receiving homes, and other diversionary services for status offenders. Still other voluntary services may be distinctive because they are so recently developed, or are regarded as controversial or inappropriate for government; hence, there are no public counterparts, e.g., "hotline," parental stress and suicide prevention centers, volunteer bureaus, and senior home repair services. There are also some services that depend on being under nongovernmental auspices for their effectiveness, such as anticrime neighborhood organizations, various shelters, and diversionary services.

POTENTIAL DISADVANTAGES OF POSC FOR GOVERNMENT

There are inherent difficulties in maintaining standards and securing adequate accountability from voluntary agencies (Fisk, Keisling, and Mueller 1978; Wedel 1980; Benton 1981). Many are insufficiently bureaucratized, lack suitable information and cost control systems, and, in the case of smaller and newer agencies, have a limited managerial capability. These administrative deficiencies are aggravated by the typically diffuse goals and methods of human service agencies, regardless of auspice, and their inability to produce evidence of effectiveness. This helps explain the widespread substitution of outputs such as the number of interviews instead of substantive outcomes in service reporting and in program evaluations.

The difficulty of specifying outcomes in the human services, as well as the lack of uniform accounting and information systems, also contribute to the complaints of overregulation by government. Because certain processes and activities are easier to count, these indicators become the focus of governmental involvement in the minutiae of agency management (Young and Finch 1977; Katz 1979; Comptroller General, 1979; Massachusetts Taxpayers' Foundation 1980; Sharkansky 1979; Lourie 1979). Yet, evidence suggests that underregulation with little monitoring is much more frequent because governmental agencies rarely have sufficient staff to oversee a contractor's performance adequately. This deficiency is aggravated by the fact that government is often highly dependent on voluntary organizations that may have a monopoly on a particular service. Under these conditions, equity may suffer because of a tendency for a voluntary agency to be highly selective in its intake policy. The result may be that the more difficult and/or poorer clients end up as cases in the governmental agency, whereas the less troublesome and/or middle-class clients are served by voluntary agencies under contract (Beck 1971).

Historically, one of the major objections to the use of nongovernmental providers of public services has been the fear that such relationships would be too easily corrupted by political considerations (Warner 1894). This continues to be a disadvantage because, from the perspective of government, decisions concerning contracting for service delivery can be influenced in undesirable ways by pressures generated by provider agencies and/or their clientele and their supporters in the community. Because of their stake in the outcome, such interest groups often seek to influence the type and amount of the contract, as well as the selection of the provider. To governmental agencies, these pressures represent an undesirable and troublesome intrusion in the decision-making process, often preventing the termination or modification of an existing contract.

The policy of provider pluralism reinforces fragmentation because the dispersed character of the service system lessens the prospects for a more coordinated and coherent pattern. So far it has not been possible to use the fact of 80 percent governmental funding of the human services to bring about a more efficient and rational system. The increasing scope and decentralized complexity of the human services continues to defy a succession of legislative mandates requiring more planning, coordination, and service integration. Other major obstacles are the lack of communication, consistency, and coordination among governmental agencies in a three-tier system (Brilliant 1973; Weick 1979; Young and Finch 1977).

POTENTIAL ADVANTAGES OF POSC FOR THE VOLUNTARY AGENCY

The main benefit of contracting for the voluntary agency is that it can continue to serve its particular clientele and also enlarge the scope of its services, sometimes as much as by a factor of 10. Governmental funds may even be regarded as a more secure source of income than reliance on the uncertainties of fund-raising events and public solicitations, although this is usually an illusion.

The clientele of voluntary organizations may receive a more individualized, less bureaucratized, and specialized service than it might if it were provided by a governmental agency. Funds from other sources, if available, could be released for more sectarian, particularistic, or specialized purposes (Manser 1974).

Other advantages are the enhanced community status, prestige and visibility of the voluntary agency because of its function as a public service provider, together with some increased access to governmental decision making and the opportunity to influence public policy (Kramer 1979; Rosenbaum 1981).

POTENTIAL DISADVANTAGES OF POSC FOR THE VOLUNTARY AGENCY

There is usually a gap between actual costs, assuming these are known, and the rate of governmental reimbursement. Consequently, the voluntary agency has to make up the deficit and, in a sense, ends up by "subsidizing" government. In New York City, where there is the most extensive use of the voluntary sector in the child welfare field, this fiscal gap was estimated at approximately $48 million in 1976 and averaged about 16 percent of an agency's budget (Hartogs and Weber 1978, 1979).

Other rate dilemmas faced by voluntary agencies depend on the size of the difference between their actual costs and the price paid by government. If they undercharge, they incur a deficit; if they overcharge, they can bring into the market competitive, profit-making organizations, and/or they may price themselves out of government's market.

Another hazard of being a nongovernmental provider of human services is the uncertainty of income that is subject to legislative and bureaucratic delays, resulting in recurrent cash flow problems, bargaining over reimbursement rates, and the preemption of organizational resources into a continuing struggle for financing (Rice 1975; Hill 1971; Hewes et al. 1979).

The requirements for fiscal and program accountability for public funds are frequently regarded by voluntary agencies as excessive, onerous, and counterproductive, deflecting resources from the goals of service provision. The demands of these organizational maintenance tasks are a special burden on small agencies because it forces them to become more formalistic, thus vitiating the very qualities desired (Hartogs and Weber 1978). Agencies that sell their services to more than one governmental agency are confronted with multiple, inconsistent, and often conflicting requirements for accountability. Such agencies are caught in a dilemma because the diversity of income that helps mitigate dependency on any single funding source is responsible for these disparate demands for accountability. The latter are also a major obstacle to the coordination of organizations dependent on numerous funding agencies at different levels of government.

Loss of organizational independence is widely believed to be another risk. In addition to compliance with demands for accountability, voluntary agencies receiving public funds are subject to various policy restrictions on who shall be served (client eligibility), by whom (staff restrictions), how (service delivery), and to other unwanted interferences with internal management and operating policies, including requirements for consumer participation. In addition to some loss of control over operations and program policy, there is, in an era of cutbacks, the precarious uncertainty of fiscal dependency on a diminishing governmental source. Finally, by becoming a private, public service provider, a voluntary agency can become a substitute for, rather than an alternative to, government or a means of offering choice. This leads to the last potential disadvantage.

Diminished advocacy, volunteerism, and particularism can be other consequences of a voluntary agency serving as a contractor (Manser 1974; Benton 1979; Lourie 1979). The distinctive advocacy function of a voluntary agency can be constrained through fear of loss of income, or be restricted to the self-interest lobbying of a public contractor constantly seeking higher rates and fewer regulations. Direct service volunteerism can decline because of the possibilities of substituting paid staff for certain types of service volunteers. Active participation of board members can also decrease when the agency becomes more entrepreneurial and relies on government for most of its income. Voluntary agencies may depend less on the fund-raising capabilities of board members and volunteers and more on the ability of professional staff to negotiate governmental contracts and on those board members who have political contacts. Lastly, the distinctive particularism of the voluntary agency, its special religious, sectarian, ethnic, or other minority values may be diluted or lost if it must make its services available to a broader range of clientele as part of the price of receiving public funds (Kramer 1966; Selig 1973).

FUTURE IMPLICATIONS

The preceding summary of the potential values and dangers of POSC to both governmental and voluntary agencies necessarily has a disconcerting equivocal character, not only because of insufficient data, but also because of the inevitable influence of ideologies such as pluralism and the relative values ascribed to accountability, access, autonomy, choice, cost efficiency, equity, or effectiveness. There is very little evidence that would help identify the conditions under which any one of the costs and benefits of POSC are likely to occur. It is obvious that we need much more research on such topics as the comparative costs between POSC and direct provision; the impact of different modes of service delivery and auspices on clientele; and more objective ways of measuring service quality apart from various forms of professionalism.

Benton (1981) has noted, "Contract technology in the human services is still relatively primitive compared to other areas of public enterprise." Among other unanswered questions regarding different components of the contracting process are: Should bidding be competitive in the human services? Should low bidders always be accepted? If so, how can we insure quality considerations? How can the driving out of the small, less bureaucratic agencies who may be unable to compete in the bidding process be avoided? How can costs be determined that are fair in the light of so many complexities, e.g., eight different potential payment mechanisms and eleven variables to take into account in pricing (Lourie 1979)? What monitoring and evaluation systems are desirable and feasible? What role is there for citizens in the contract management process?

The future of contracting is surrounded by great uncertainties because of the new fiscal and interorganizational conditions confronting state and local governments. One can only speculate whether the backlash against government spending will result in more functions being privatized. It is not assured that voluntary agencies will benefit from the backlash against government because they may seem to be less costly and ideologically more acceptable. Although lower costs are usually cited as the primary advantage of contracting, it is uncertain whether this value will override a tendency to keep as many functions within government in order to preserve budgeted staff positions. The advantage of specialized competence or greater access to clientele offered by voluntary agencies may be of less importance to government in the face of substantial cutbacks in the human services. Community and political pressures may also be insufficient to overcome the fiscal pressures of austerity, particularly if the voluntary agency services are not mandatory. Apart from appropriations, legislative requirements and preferences will also influence the prospects for contracting.

Consequently, it is even more important for both governmental and voluntary organizations to assess the previously cited advantages and disadvantages involved in the choice between direct provision or contracting. In addition, perhaps better decisions might be made if the following questions were also considered:

1. To what extent is there public acceptance of this service as a governmental or voluntary responsibility? How is the service viewed by legislators, public officials, and clientele?
2. What is there in the nature of the service that seems to require governmental or voluntary auspices? Would contracting contribute further to the erosion of governmental responsibility? Are there any sectarian or voluntaristic aspects of the service that are not within the province of, or that are inappropriate for, a governmental agency?
3. Where will the needed service best be integrated? What is the best way to avoid fragmentation and encourage coordination?
4. To what extent is the voluntary agency qualified and prepared to provide the service in accordance with the required conditions at least as economically and effectively as government? How would acceptance of public funds affect or displace other aspects of the voluntary agency's program?
5. How ready is the governmental agency to delegate responsibility and provide the voluntary agency with the necessary standards and technical assistance? To what extent can government specify the service product and pay the full cost of the service?

AUTONOMY AND ACCOUNTABILITY

Whether these questions are answered or even posed, the future interorganizational environment will be one of greater scarcity, interdependence, competition and entrepreneurism, and a sharper politicalization of the mixed economy in the human services. Under these circumstances, issues pertaining to accountability and autonomy will loom large, reflecting the different and often competing organizational interests and values. For example, the much-vaunted independence of a voluntary agency may be viewed by outsiders as arbitrary, idiosyncratic, or self-serving behavior, just as pluralism is frequently regarded by others as duplication, fragmentation, or even "organizational anarchy." Independence is naturally prized by the supporters of a voluntary agency, but others, less partisan, may value equity and entitlements more than provider autonomy and pluralism and be more concerned about the consequences of governmental domination by private interests.

From the point of view of government or an underserved population-at-risk, a reduction in the autonomy of a voluntary agency would not be considered a calamity if it meant that the agency would function with a broader conception of the public interest, i.e., if it were operated more in accordance with the wishes of certain groups of clientele and less that of staff and board. Conversely, governmental demands for service and fiscal accountability may be perceived as administrative busywork and an illusion of "business-like" accountability. This illustrates the adage that one person's accountability is another's harassment. Voluntary organizations may also challenge the belief that there is more accountability in the public services on the grounds that governmental agencies are usually reluctant to disclose information regarding their operations, and they often fail to respect the client's entitlement to service and redress of grievance.

The conventional dualism between autonomy and accountability, on the other hand, may be more artificial than real, and they may be much less opposed than many people believe (Mansfield 1971). For example, a strong, independent, voluntary agency can be more accountable because government can pinpoint responsibility. Furthermore, some accountability requirements can be beneficial to a voluntary agency as it seeks to improve the efficiency and effectiveness of its performance. Contracts can be a tool to structure and guide program operations. When a program description is broken down into mutually exclusive, sequential, functionally interrelated components, it can be used as a monitoring guide, an administrative focus, a planning tool, a basis for evaluation, and for contract renewal (Gundersdorg 1977).

Both terms are, however, ambiguous, value laden, and require analysis. For example, how autonomous should or can a voluntary organization be, and regarding what aspects of its functioning? To whom should a voluntary agency be accountable, for what, when, and how? How much accountability should government require and in what forms?

To begin with autonomy, it is obvious that no organization can be completely independent, because all policy decisions are subject to many external and internal constraints. Autonomy, being a matter of degree, is relative and conditional. Autonomy is also not an end in itself, but a necessary means for the accomplishment of the organization's task and maintenance goals, justified pragmatically by its contribution to more effective performance. The distinctive nature of organizations is that they are not self-sufficient or wholly self-determining but are, instead, inescapably dependent on their environment for their essential resources. The prevailing natural state of organizational life is one of interdependence in which organizations "use" each other via trade-offs in which resources are exchanged for a measure of control (Jacobs 1974; Mindlin and Aldrich 1975). Furthermore, voluntary agencies are not private, freewheeling enterprises; rather, they are, strictly speaking, public agencies because they require sanction from the state in the form of a charter or legal recognition of their nonprofit, charitable, tax-exempt, corporate status, and they must often be licensed. The community in which they function is the source of their legitimization, service mandate and domain, good will, and more tangible resources such as funds, clientele, staff, and information.

In actual practice the little evidence available suggests that there is much less encroachment on the independence of voluntary organizations than is commonly believed. In a study of voluntary agencies in the United States, England, the Netherlands, and Israel, it was found that dependency was significantly mitigated by the payment-for-service form of most government funding, the diversity of income sources, the countervailing power of a voluntary agency service monopoly and political influence, and the minimal accountability due to the trade-offs of a mutual dependency relationship (Kramer 1979; Massachusetts Taxpayer's Association 1980; Carter 1979; Perlmutter 1971; Burian 1970).

The concept of accountability is particularly difficult to grapple with, because its popularity in the human services is exceeded only by the lack of agreement about its meaning. It has been viewed as both an end and a means; it has been defined in terms of procedures, results, disclosure of information, recourse, compliance with regulations, and it is often indistinguishable from such concepts as evaluation, efficiency, effectiveness, control, and responsibility (Etzioni 1975; Newman and Turem 1974; Gates 1980). At a minimum, accountability means having to answer to those who control a necessary scarce resource (Marmor and Morone 1980). It therefore involves an obligation to report how the organization is discharging its service and fiscal responsibilities in appropriate detail so that evaluative and other decisions can be made. Although disclosure requirements of "public accounting" and red tape may be costly nuisances and may even deflect agency resources, they do not necessarily impair an agency's freedom. Indeed, there is considerable evidence that government has a severely limited capacity to assure accountability via effective contract monitoring and performance evaluation. Because of this, there should be more concern with the implications of the shift in the major governmental role from service provider to case manager, middle man and broker, as well as to the possible erosion of governmental responsibility by contracting.

Perhaps the issue can be rephrased as to how to make public service providers more accountable without restricting the very qualities of flexibility and individualization that may make voluntary agencies desirable. At the same time, to prevent the regulated from regulating the regulators, we need to discover an appropriate organizational distance between governmental and voluntary agencies; a midpoint that is not so close to produce excessive restrictions, overenforcement of rules, or cooptation, or so distant that it is not possible to protect the public interest and to assure compliance with stated objectives. The search would be for that golden mean where government could, at arm's length, hold its contractors accountable without interfering with or constraining the distinctive features of voluntary agencies (Young and Finch 1977; Litwak and Meyer 1966). In the process each will have to acquire new or improved organizational competencies. Government will have to increase its capacity for more effective contract management and to improve its bidding and review procedure, product specification, monitoring and accountability requirements. It will have to learn how to cope more effectively with provider coalitions and how to use such structures for the development and enforcement of standards. On the other hand, voluntary organizations under contract as public agents will have to strive for greater equity and efficiency in service delivery, improved managerial capability, and to accept a greater measure of paperwork, citizen participation, and some program restrictions when they become private, public service providers (Terrell 1979).

The quest for the principles to bring about a better balance between provider autonomy and accountability in contracting will be elusive and demanding, but it is essential for the future of a pluralistic social welfare economy.

PART THREE

The Technology of Contracting

Not surprisingly, the increasing use of purchase of service arrangements has been accompanied by a growth in technology, complexity, and bureaucracy. The focus of this section is on these emerging technologies to implement the purchasing of services. The topics covered include procurement rules and regulations; marketing; human services; negotiating contracts; transferring fiscal resources; rate setting; and unit cost contracting. Although the focus is on technology, appropriate content is included on the growing complexity of contracting arrangements and the emerging bureaucratic contracting industry.

Given the volume of contracting in which the federal, state, and local governments engage, attention to process inevitably became a focus of concern. The process by which contracts are arranged is an essential component of the subject of purchase of service, because it sets the stage for how, when, and under what circumstances and conditions the purchase of services will occur. Cognizant of the need to develop procedures in this emerging contracting era, the American Bar Association Consortium, after five years of effort, produced a Model Procurement Code for state and local governments, which has been widely adopted by the public sector. Its adoption by all levels of government suggests that this code is having considerable influence on the procedures used by the public sector to purchase goods and services. Interested readers are encouraged to secure copies of the complete ABA text and to become familiar with the codes of their state and local jurisdictions. Where adopted, it sets the boundaries for all governmental contractors. A brief overview of the Model Procurement Code appears in this section.

Negotiation is the process by which government and a vendor come to terms on the substance and scope of the contract. There are two elements to negotiations: programmatic and fiscal. The two may be combined or undertaken as separate steps in the process. Gibelman and Demone review the principles of negotiating purchase of service agreements, emphasizing its dimensions and how it is done.

Given that a major motivation for government to contract out goods or services is to obtain these at lesser costs, fiscal negotiations may be the key element to securing a final agreement. The Fines review theoretical marketing concepts as they apply to human services as products. They examine the parallels between the processes of dispensing human services and the marketing of ordinary goods. Young views purchase of service as the transfer of fiscal resources, concluding that buyers of human services get what they pay for. He identifies three major dimensions: service, clients, and a competitive structure. An appropriate fit of these characteristics should be the objective of the buyer. Young describes means by which to achieve this fit.

Rate-setting procedures may serve to include or exclude providers, and provide the rationale and basis for controlling contract costs. The method by which rates and fees are calculated are determined by government. Developmental costs, interest, costs of facilities, and inflation are all variabîes of note. Also to be established are matters of income, fixed and variable costs, procedures for billing and payment, and fines for late payment. Other matters of concern include prepayment, invoice processing, and pre-auditing.

Richardson places purchase of service arrangements in a cash transfer context. He begins by analyzing control strategies that result in the promulgation of regulations. Next he moves to matters of rate setting by explicating provider costs, differentiating between those that are reasonable and unreasonable. He outlines means by which rate structures, accounting, cost funding procedures, and actual rate decision-making strategies can be improved.

Baumunk walks the reader through the details of unit-cost contracting as used by government for the purchase of social services. Basic to unit-cost contracting procedures is the designation of service and its method of measurement. She also identifies the limits of the procedure. Knowing when to use unit-cost contracting is essential if it is to be applied effectively.

Formal standards and procedures, elements of contemporary managerial technology, are viewed as essential for realizing an enforceable, programmatically and fiscally sound contract. Even the most elementary procedure would include use of requests for proposals (RFP), including clear content and unambiguous language; widespread public notice; a clear-cut timetable; formal and clearly understood contract approval mechanisms; specific role delegations to legal, fiscal, and program officials; formal logs of the contract processes; and a final contractual procedure. Program consultation during the contract, contract monitoring, program evaluation, and uniform accounting all need explication. Matters of client confidentiality need similar review and concern (Human Services Provider Council 1975).

The technology developed and applied to purchase of service arrangements encompasses all that is currently operative in public administration, except for one important feature: personnel policies and practices are the responsibility of the vendor. To the degree that the contractor (the governmental agency) establishes detailed conditions regarding personnel, they will merely recreate the public agency, but under private auspices. Logical areas for the public expression of concern about personnel are in respect to matters of quality and equal opportunity. Without anticipating the details of personnel practices, the public regulator could establish standards requiring that personnel hired meet experiential and educational criteria equivalent to those providing other services within the same agency or in line with civil service requirements. Just as affirmative action requirements can be imposed upon contracted agencies, matters of personnel quality can also be set forth in general terms. Operating details are unnecessary, if not inappropriate.

In light of the many issues and questions that have emerged in relation to efficacy, effectiveness, and efficiency from an outcome perspective, it is perhaps understandable that government agencies have sought to exert controls on the contracting process. It can reasonably be assumed that the public sector, as the contractor, will continue to develop more elaborate control mechanisms, using contemporary managerial and fiscal technologies. It is incumbent on the contracted vendor to master quickly the new ground rules and technology.

A Model Procurement Code
for State and Local Governments

Harold W. Demone, Jr.

The American Bar Association's (ABA) Model procurement Code project, completed and published in 1979 following five years of effort, has had a significant influence on public contract procedures, including those used in the purchase of human services. Interested readers are urged to secure full copies of the seventy-five-page model code from the American Bar Association in Washington, D.C. Basically, it provides "(1) the statutory principles and policy guidance for managing and controlling the procurement of supplies, services, and construction for public purposes; (2) administrative and judicial remedies for the resolution of controversies relating to public contracts; and (3) a set of ethical standards governing public and private participants in the procurement process" (p. vi).

O. S. Hiestand, a member of the ABA Coordinating Committee to Develop a Model Procurement Code, summarized the salient features of the code in a 1979 article in *Contract Management*. Following is an excerpt from that summary.

Coverage. Although the code covers all public expenditures of funds for the procurement of supplies, services and construction, waivers are provided in respect to gifts, bequests or cooperative projects where terms may require otherwise. For example, a donor may provide support for the library to be used to purchase books specific to one publisher.

Procurement Organization. The code creates a State Procurement Policy Office and Chief Procurement Officer. Respectively they would be granted the authority to (1) promulgate, audit and monitor the appropriate regulations and (2) procure supplies, services or construction.

117

Delegated procurement responsibility to operating agencies subject to Code and Policy Office regulations is integrated into the Code. Thus, for example, a Department of Public Health would remain responsible for its own purchasing under the general provision of the Code.

Source Selection and Contract Termination. Competitive sealed bidding ("formal advertising" is the federal equivalent) is identified as the preferred method of bidding. An invitation for bids (IFB) is promulgated, bids are publicly opened at a previously announced time and place, and the award is made to the lowest, responsible bidder whose bid meets the requirements and criteria set forth in the IFB (for federal agencies the term "RFP", request for proposals, is used). The criteria for evaluation of the bids can include relative judgements (e.g., quality, workmanship and suitability) but such criteria must be objectively measurable.

Competitive Sealed Proposal. This method is used when competitive sealed bidding is not practical or advantageous. In federal terms it is equivalent to "competitive negotiations." It requires both the issuance of a request for a proposal and the awarding of the contract to the bidder whose proposal is seen as most advantageous to the public agency, given price and the evaluation factors set forth in the Request for Proposal. If discussions are conducted, bidders are to be afforded equal treatment.

Small Purchase Procedures are authorized and procedures recommended. The ABA recognizes that the costs of bidding small purchases will likely exceed their costs.

Both *Sole Source Procurements* and *Emergency Procedures* are provided for in accordance with recommended standards.

Special Competitive Selection Procedure for designated *Professional Services.* A special competitive selection procedure is designated for professional services, examples of which include those of accountants, clergy, physicians, lawyers, and dentists. The specific determination of what constitutes a professional service would be at the discretion of the state or local legislative body when and if it enacts the Code.

118

The selection procedure requires public notice, issuance of an RFP, and selection of the most qualified offeror based on the criteria in the RFP.

Cost Data. The Code requires the submission and certification of cost or pricing data for contracts awarded by the competitive sealed proposal method, and similarly for contract modifications and change orders. Any type of contract, except a cost contract, may be used. Cost reimbursement contracts are permitted if they are likely to be less costly or if it is not practicable to use another type of contract.

Contract Modifications are authorized in the code, including changes, stop work, variations in quantity, and price adjustment. *Legal and Contractual Remedies* are established covering bid and award protests, performance and other breach of contract disputes, and suspension and debarment actions.

An absolute right is established for bidders and contractors to have their grievances heard in court. An administrative appeals board could also be established to decide on protests, performances and breach of contract disputes, as well as suspension and debarment actions.

Cooperative Purchasing among several public agencies would be explicitly authorized. For example, several health agencies could establish a single RFP for pharmaceuticals or computers.

Small and Disadvantaged Businesses are covered in a policy that establishes a procedure to assist them in learning how to do business with the public sector. Special provisions for progress payment and adjusted bonding requirements are included.

Ethical Standards and sanctions are provided and shall be applicable to all participants in the public procurement process. The standards cover conflicts of interest, gratuities and kickbacks; contingency fees, and misuse of confidential information.

Conclusion. Although this Model Code is a proposal and not obligatory in whole or part for the several thousand state and local jurisdictions, its five years of development, extensive use of process and involvement, positive sanctions, important sponsors and general level of responsibility will likely see widespread adoption of it in most of the larger jurisdictions. As of September 1, 1981, only 13 months following its completion, 18 states had adopted the Code and 27 others had some sort of identified effort. In only 15 states was there no evidence of action (American Bar Association 1981). Thus providers may want to participate in legislative debates about the Code and certainly, after the fact, familiarize themselves with its detail.

Its principle weakness is the assumption that objective measurable criteria can be developed for all services. We know of no such acceptable criteria for legal services. The helping professions operate in equally complex environments with equally complex offerings.

7

Interagency Cooperation for the Delivery of Human Services: A Marketing Perspective

Adell P. Fine and Seymour H. Fine

Increasingly, human service institutions are adopting a marketing philosophy as they realize that family counseling, substance control, and child abuse prevention can be considered as products—social products. Therefore, their abilities to dispense these products must benefit from a business approach. It is not a very new concept. The idea that a service may be seen as a product is rooted in a remark by a psychologist, G. D. Wiebe (1951), "Why can't we sell brotherhood like we sell soap?"

In the health field, for example, interest in marketing can only be described as phenomenal. Hospitals are clamoring for marketing directors, and a huge literature on health-care marketing has emerged, even with its own journal by that name. The trend has caught social workers lagging somewhat behind, but they are catching up. Jack Rothman, senior author of a new book on marketing human services refers to the dispensing of human services as social marketing, which, strictly defined, implies the marketing of ideas. However, Rothman's usage is semantically correct because social products usually contain significant ideational components. Further, the social marketing rubric has lately come to subsume the more popular subject of nonprofit marketing and, of course, most social service agencies are public or nonprofit organizations.

A general view of social marketing may be obtained from the works of Fine (1981). This chapter mentions only briefly some of marketing's tenets as applied to social work, and concentrates on one of them—distribution channels, chosen because cooperation between social agencies resembles the use of middlemen by commercial firms. To place the channel topic into context, the reader is directed to Figure 7.1, which

Figure 7.1. **Elements of the Marketing Definition**

Marketing is a process by which a supplier (marketer) plans the distribution of goods, services or ideas to consumers.

Price	Promotion	Place	Product	The Market
Cash Time Effort Psyche	Advertising Word of mouth Public relations Special events	Distribution channels (parties to the process) Delivery	The offering that fills clients' needs and wants Packaging	People with needs, wants, motivation Segmentation research

illustrates a definitional scheme of marketing wherein the distribution channel is seen as one particular element.

SOCIAL MARKETING IN SOCIAL SERVICES

The figure lists the "four P's" of marketing—product, price, promotion, and place—and the markets to be served. Marketing is a transactional process in which the marketer (agency) designs a *product* (service) in such a way as to fill needs and wants of the consumer (client). These needs are ascertained in advance through marketing research, which is one type of social research. A *price* is paid, usually in money, and/or in such "social prices" as time, effort, anguish, or risk. The marketer is assumed to have *promoted* the product (as well as the image of the agency) to a target market (audience, constituency) after segmenting (grouping) it according to some relevant criterion such as age, family status, or socioeconomic factor. This is done whether the product is an automobile or divorce counseling. The *place* concerns the delivery system by which the product is made available to the market. No matter how well the product or service is designed, priced, and promoted, the process fails if the offering is not readily accessible to the client at a convenient time and place. In the marketing sense, place is synonomous with the goal of accessibility.

To achieve that goal, the social service planner must view the agency as but one in a network of community organizations. There is increasing awareness among social workers that it is frequently difficult for one agency to perform all of the required functions in the overall service process. Service delivery is facilitated significantly when the agency cooperates with other organizations in a system wherein each member performs those functions it is best able to perform. That reality is completely parallel to the situation in the marketing of commercial commodities where various intermediary middlemen are employed. The system or network of firms so consitituted is known as a channel of distribution.

The corporation is often faced with the "make-or-buy" decision: Should a component of a product be manufactured in-house or should it be obtained through subcontracting out to a firm specializing in that product? Similarly, should a school social worker serve as a leader with a group of children or should the system contract with a social agency to send a group worker to perform that function? Decisions of this nature are always based on whether the subcontractor can supply the product in better quality, more quickly, and/or at lower cost. Not only can two or more agencies cooperate on cases, but on programs as well. For example, a family service agency and a nearby university can pool talents to stage a workshop on some topic of mutual concern. Both insititutions gain obvious publicity benefits, and other advantages as well. The university becomes more aware of the agency's services and might later refer troubled employees for counseling. In turn, the agency learns of course offerings germane to social work and can utilize academic expertise for training in such areas as management, law, or medicine.

INTERAGENCY COOPERATION

The significance of interagency cooperation in social work may be seen in the light of recent directions toward specialization in social work training and practice. As with high-tech society in general, the field of social work has become increasingly varied and complex. These changes have created a need for people and institutions who are capable of performing specialized functions. Changing forms of service delivery and of professional roles for social workers are already impacting upon social work education where the system appears to be opening up to include ancillary subjects in the curriculum (Bassoff and Ludwig 1979). Bracht and Briar (1979) have raised the question whether social work and legal education can somehow be blended. Indeed, a degree combining law and social work is currently offered at George Warren Brown

University in St. Louis, and Columbia University awards a master's degree in social work and business, to cite just two evidences of the trend.

At the practitioner level, recent articles advocate cooperation between the social agency and sociologist (Bromley and Weed 1978), cultural anthropologist (Green 1978), lawyer (Bernstein 1980), school (Phillips 1978), dentist (Levy, Lambert and Davis 1979) and police officer (Carr 1979). Bloom and Parad (1976) investigated empirically some of the obstacles to such interaction, as did Lowe and Herranen (1978), who focused on channel conflict between nurse and social worker. An even larger literature stresses teamwork between social workers and health-care professionals (Williams et al. 1978; Forman 1976; Lurie 1977). These are but a few of a plethora of papers, all of which clearly indicate that social service professionals and organizations do not feel they can go it alone in an environment growing increasingly complex. The formation of a distribution channel structure broadens the scope of service delivery capabilities. That point was stressed by Reichert (1982) as he commended "efforts by social workers to compensate (for fragmentation in service delivery) through referral systems, coordination, networking, multiagency case conferences, case advocacy, and other devices."

Within the social services sector, cooperative networks can be classed into three forms: collaboration, referral, and subcontracting (Table 7.1).

Collaboration is the simplest and most common form of cooperative network. Two or more organizations work informally together on a case, pooling opinions and diagnoses, and even coordination services—such as the joint venture in business. Yet, virtually no management or control is transferred, and each party performs its own roles and functions. For example, a caseworker in a welfare agency providing monetary support to a family might meet with a caseworker of a family agency where all or part of the family is receiving counseling or therapy. Functional collaboration can optimize service efficacy in resolving difficulties facing the client. For an extreme example, a welfare check might be withheld until a parent enrolls in an Alcoholics Anonymous program.

Referral results from collaboration and implies actual transfer of all or most management and control responsibilities from the primary to a collateral agency. The choice of agency is not based on contractual agreement but stems from the primary worker's knowledge of, and experience with community organizations and their areas of expertise.

In subcontracting, an agency ordinarily expected to perform a service

124

Table 7.1. **Interagency Cooperation in Social Work**

	Collaboration	Referral	Subcontracting
Formality of network structure	low	medium	high
Transfer of functional control	nil	high	medium
Transfer of management	nil	high	low
Accountability of collateral to primary agencies	nil	medium	high

contracts to have that service performed instead by another source. The clear implication is that the other source is able to perform more efficiently (by some standards) than the contractee or granting agency. This is the most formal of the three network structures (see Table 7.1). The management role and certain other functions are usually retained by the primary agency. In its most simple form, a primary agency delegates just one function, as in the case of a prison that contracts out the function of psychological testing to a testing service. At another extreme, the agency can contract out all of its functions and become a case manager, or what in marketing is called a "desk jobber," similar to the role of a builder who invites subcontractors to carry out the tasks of masonry, plumbing, and electricity.

In Bergen County, New Jersey, the State Division of Youth and Family Services (DYFS) is legally mandated to deal with cases involving the legal protection of children. Clients are referred to DYFS by physicians, schools, the police, and other community sources (C. Venti, personal communication, no date). The agency has direct responsibility for about half of its operational functions, including group counseling sessions and foster day-care services. On the other hand, it contracts out the other half—virtually all treatment and direct services—to private medical practitioners and such community-based organizations as mental health clinics and residential treatment facilities, (see Figure 7.2).

DYFS assigns cases involving protective services (such as child abuse, emotional neglect, sexual molestation, incest) to the Family Life Center (FLC), a hospital-sponsored therapeutic agency. The FLC is thus a treatment arm for DYFS, which compensates FLC on a per-case basis according to terms set down in a contract, even though FLC is also supported by

Figure 7.2. **A Channel of Distribution for Protective Services**

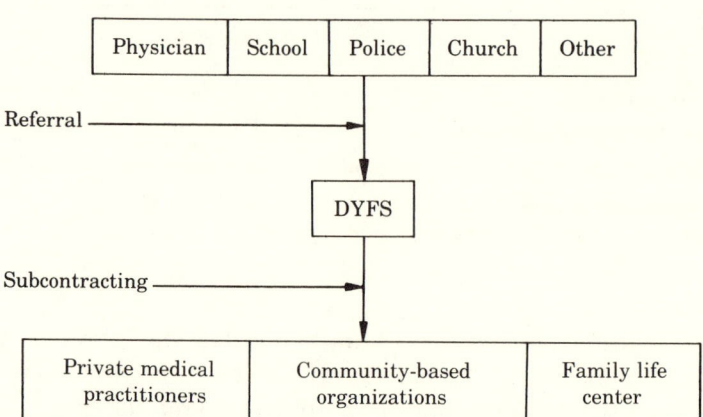

federal and county funds. Under the contract, and with its legal responsibility, DYFS retains case management functions, whereas control of operations is transferred to FLC as the collateral agency (see Table 7.1). For example, FLC has final word on matters relating to treatment modality (whether individual, family, or group approach). DYFS usually assigns a staff person to maintain liasion relationships and to attend FLC case conferences; client progress is discussed at least quarterly. The primary agency decides whether and when to terminate a case, usually on the advice of the FLC therapist. The FLC maintains a maximum caseload of ninety cases so that it can accept a new case only when it terminates an earlier one (J. N. Kessler, personal communication, no date).

This relationship illustrates the subcontracting structure as formalized by an agreement. Of course, it need not be bound by a written instrument; copies of communications between the parties can also serve as a contract. Verbal agreements are legal too, although fraught with potential for conflict. In any case, a key feature is the primary agency's capacity to monitor the case and to see that cases are followed through by the collateral agency.

Typically, the agency will simultaneously employ more than one of these three cooperative formats for delivery of a particular service or different forms for different services. The objective is to most efficiently, effectively, and equitably reach and serve the desired target clienteles.

126

CHANNEL LEADERSHIP AND CONTROL

Whether the system is formed through collaboration, referral, or subcontracting, its members should agree upon a "channel captain." Unless one institution or individual assumes that role, leadership is unspecified and fragmented, and no one, least of all the client, can be certain about whom to turn to for substantive decisions. Still worse, any institution may invite additional and sometimes extraneous agencies to join a case, whereas another might decide to drop out.

In the commercial sector, the channel captain often emerges in some natural manner. Motivated by profit, businesspeople find little difficulty in agreeing upon a leader. But with public and private nonprofit organizations, leadership is more likely to be left to chance, and hence often overlooked completely. This is a serious matter for the referring or primary agency to consider, if for no other reason than the client's feeling of security as the treatment process progresses.

As with the business marketing channel, the social services network is susceptible to disagreement. Indeed, the same points of contention arise between channel members—who will do what, and for how much money. The wholesaler complains about retailer's high markup and reluctance to carry large inventory, and retailers bewail wholesalers' infrequent sales calls. Collateral agencies cry for higher salaries for their professional workers than those received by primary personnel: "We do all the work, have more training, and bear the risks." Primary staffers would like to dispense with required client visitations: "Let them (collaterals) do it; they're paid enough, have smaller caseloads than we do, and are more familiar with the family."

SOME OBSTACLES IN IMPLEMENTATION

Implementation of the channel concept in social services also has its unique obstacles. One concerns a lack of clarity concerning roles and functions within the typical agency. If I go to a bank and ask the bank to sell me stocks and bonds, they will refuse and refer me to a stockbroker. However, if I go to a mental health clinic with a pain in my back, the clinic staff is often uncertain as to whether to treat me or refer me to a physician. A prerequisite for the existence of channel relationships is that the parties to the process define and agree on the assignment of roles, functions, and activities both within and between agencies.

Another obstacle stems from the social worker's temperament. There is a tendency among agencies to perceive themselves as self-sufficient, complete entities capable of performing virtually the entire spectrum of services required by their clients. Social workers tend to prefer to work directly with the client. When treatment is subcontracted away, the primary worker is left with only the managerial function. This might violate the original purpose of her training as a social worker; she has lost the direct service role and contact with the client. The change of role from client treatment to case management can be inconsistent with the social worker's choice of career. Is an MSW necessary to prepare a person for performing case management functions? Why cannot an MBA or an MPA do the administering and leave MSW's to do the social work? How removed is the manager from active involvement in ethical and humanistic principles? Does the philosophical base of the social work profession become diluted when the agency engages mostly in case management and less in direct services?

A third obstacle facing channel proponents is feedback and accountability. General systems theory has taught us the importance of information feedback in the operation of such systems as distribution channels. In that regard, it is instructive to compare channel structure via the two devices of subcontracting and referral. In both instances, the collateral agency has an obligation to keep the primary agency informed about case progress. But there is a large difference in motivation. Under subcontracting, the feedback mechanism is built into the contract. In the case of referral, if the collateral agency wishes to obtain continued referrals, personnel may be motivated to maintain satisfactory relations with the primary agency and to report back even if only to maintain good will. So in subcontracting, accountability is forced by the terms of the contract, whereas in referral, accountability just makes good business sense. In any event, some social agencies do not recognize the need to be accountable to a referring agency and will neglect to report back on client progress. This is poor business practice; in fact, it is poor social work practice as well.

Because of that neglect, primary agencies may perceive collaterals as doing a poor job. As a result, they refrain from referring and instead attempt to carry out all case functions by themselves. It is quite possible that this decision has resulted in the recent proliferation of social workers and psychologists engaging in private practice in competition with collateral agencies. What has resulted is a "short channel" of generalists performing a wide variety of functions, instead of the more efficient "long channel" of several specialists or, ideally, a combination of generalists who are comfortable using specialists where necessary and indicated. The latter practice is used in medicine. Some social work educators have proposed differentiation in training, with the B.S.W. being required for generalists and master's level programs reserved for specialists (Turner ed. 1977). For example, with respect to the two agencies mentioned earlier, DYFS workers are often B.S.W.s, whereas the FLC is staffed primarily with M.S.W.s.

Finally, the suggestion earlier in this chapter that social services adopt marketing does not imply that business philosophy should unduly influence social workers' thinking (Rosenberg and Weissmon 1981). Indeed, the profession of social work must guard against the possibility of venturing too far afield lest it dilute and confuse its legitimate roles. In that regard, Bartlett (1970, p. 208) has cautioned that the identity of social workers should not be lost by overemphasis on borrowing from other professions. She points to the example of "treatment," which social workers borrowed from medicine, and used it to devise a clinical approach that tended to supplant concern with groups and communities.

One must decide which concepts are appropriate to social work and which are not and, further, how to fit new ideas into the social work knowledge and values system. The notion of enhanced service delivery through a distribution channel is suggested as one such idea.

SUMMARY

Social services institutions naturally seek ways to increase visibility and utilization. They are beginning to look to marketing as one model from which they can borrow techniques for the improvement of service delivery to target audiences. Some have had strategic marketing plans drawn up to serve their special needs. Many organizations in the human services industry are middlemen in the sense that they perform certain specific functions so well that they deserve to have those functions farmed out to them by other agencies. The situation is comparable to that of wholesalers of tangible commodities who perform the marketing functions of warehousing, credit, delivery, and so forth. In both circumstances, suppliers as well as consumers benefit from the inclusion of these intermediary institutions within a network or channel of distribution. Contracting by public agencies not only fits the mercantile model, it is often quite advisable.

By considering services as though they are objects, the social worker is able to borrow concepts from the business world. One examines familiar processes through a different lens and gains new insights while enhancing one's understanding of established perceptions.

Negotiating a Contract:
Practical Considerations

Margaret Gibelman and Harold W. Demone, Jr.

Negotiations occur all the time, everywhere: nations negotiate; management and labor negotiate; community groups negotiate; spouses negotiate with each other and their children. In purchase of service contracting, negotiation is often a key process in securing a final agreement between the contractor (usually a government agency) and the service provider (another public, voluntary, or proprietary agency or individual).

With the enormous growth in purchase of service contracting between public and private organizations and the increasing numbers of interorganizational exchanges and mergers, both public and private sector employees are now commonly involved in negotiations for a variety of essential and legitimate objectives. Negotiations can commence anywhere along the contracting continuum: at the preproposal stage, negotiations can be initiated to map out the nature and scope of a service program and establish budgets; at the postcontract stage, negotiations may focus on modifications to the original agreement.

Nierenburg (1973, 4) describes negotiations thus: ". . .whenever people exchange ideas with the intention of changing relationships. Whenever they confer for agreement, they are negotiating." Cohen (1980, 15) talks about negotiations as "a field of knowledge and endeavor that focuses on gaining the favor of people from whom we want things." In his view negotiation also involves the elements of information, time, and power. These elements are especially pertinent to the contract negotiation process, where the presumed goal is to reach agreement on contract components, including scope of program and cost, personnel and time, in order to operationalize or continue one or more services.

None of the definitions limit negotiations to two individuals or even to two sides. Many may participate in the negotiating process, representing a variety of viewpoints. Sometimes two or more service providers may seek a contract from a public body, in which case all parties to the potential contract will participate in negotiations. Similarly, one contract may transcend the jurisdictional boundaries of any one government agency, involving several public agency representatives in the negotiating process. Generally, all parties enter negotiations willingly or at least the pressure is not stimulated by a court of law. The negotiators usually serve as representatives of larger systems, such as health or human services organizations. Occasionally, however, an individual consultant may submit a proposal for funding by a public agency and enter into negotiations about its terms independent of organizational sponsorship.

ELEMENTS OF THE NEGOTIATION PROCESS

Explanation, clarification, and compromise are essential elements of negotiating. These reconciliatory characteristics, however, do not negate the power struggles that may permeate the process. Depending on the past and current relationship between the government and service-providing agencies, the negotiating atmosphere may be more or less cooperative or adversarial.

The government agency, serving as contractor, brings to the negotiations the power inherent in an authoritative position. The funding body, after all, holds the power of the purse and can deny or ultimately approve the end product of negotiations: a contract. The provider, on the other hand, may be a "sole source," i.e., the only vendor with whom negotiations are being held. The sole source status may be bestowed when the service provider is the most logical, capable, or only source able to offer the service. In such instances its bargaining power is greatly enhanced, and it enters into negotiations with the government agency on a more equal basis.

In situations in which negotiations concern a contract renewal, the provider agency may also be in a relatively secure position, particularly if it maintains a positive track record. Even if the program or service to be renewed is put out for competitive bid, the agency that has already provided the service is at an advantage, assuming that the contractual relationship has proved positive for both parties. If a lower budget or political factors are on the side of a new competitor, however, the competitive advantage of the agency currently holding the contract may be diminished. It is not uncommon for political factors to enter into the negotiations, at least in terms of affecting the attitude of the public agency or the pressures put upon it. An individual may, for example, be a large financial contributor to the campaign chests of key elected officials (no matter what the level of government), inevitably creating covert pressure for the public agency to adopt a more cooperative negotiating stance.

In the interactional dynamics, the funding body usually holds the advantage of time, except possibly at the close of a fiscal year. Cohen (1980, 14) notes, "The other side doesn't seem to be under the same kind of organizational pressure, time constraints and restrictive deadline" as is the applicant. In the case of renewal contracts, for example, the government agency may have little to lose by delaying or stalling negotiations, even if it means that a final agreement is not reached until after the expiration of the initial funding period. For the service provider, however, such delays may entail staff layoffs, curtailing services to the detriment of the clients, or compensating for the cut-off of funds through the use of internal resources. Negotiating delays are not uncommon and are a frequent topic of complaint from provider agencies who consider themselves to be at the mercy of bureaucrats' whimsical timetable.

The flow of information, or, conversely, the withholding of information, is another essential element in negotiations. Information can be a shared commodity. Negotiations that take place at the preproposal stage include information sharing by government about the goals to be addressed and budget parameters and information seeking about the ability of the agency to undertake the proposed service program. After a proposal has been prepared, the information flow in negotiations may focus on such activities as performance expectations, line item cost constraints, affirmative action requirements and plans. The provider agency, however, may not be an equal partner; more information is likely to be given than received. Cohen, (ibid, 19) notes, "The other side seems to know more about you and your needs than you know about them and their needs." The information-seeking powers of the public agency are likely to be more sophisticated and broadbased than that of an agency, which may rely on intuition, rumor, and past experience to interpret the wishes and intent of government.

The elements of the negotiating process may, to varying degrees, be absent. In the case of information sharing, for example, government may know what it wants from a provider, but not adequately convey such. The result may be a breakdown in communication, probably originating with the request for proposal (RFP) stage, where what is wanted may be vaguely worded or open to interpretation. Lack of clarity on the part of the government agency may also reflect uncertainty about the best approach to offering a service and the desire to allow discretion in negotiating and finalizing a contract. Requests for proposals may also be poorly written, necessitating that bidders contact federal or state officials for clarification. The questions posed may range from, "Is Office of Management and Budget clearance needed" to "How many projects will be funded and at what dollar value?" Service providers may also want to know to what extent a particular approach is viable and whether contracts will be spread among many vendors or concentrated among a few. Government is at the information advantage; vendors may even be unsure as to whether they stand a chance in the competitive process.

Negotiating a competitive contract can be significantly simplified if the RFP is written clearly and expectations of government are clearly communicated. Much time can be saved if the pre- and post-proposal negotiations can avoid clarification of intent and review of vendor suitability. The straightforward declaration of eligibility criteria for vendors and the detailing of the services to be rendered (where, to whom, and under what conditions) can aid the provider agency in preparing a proposal and entering negotiations with an accurate understanding of government's position. The more accurate, detailed, and clear the information contained in the RFP, the more likely it is that applicants will provide the necessary information for proposal evaluation and contract negotiations.

Information, time, and power may be among the elements of negotiating over which government exercises the upper hand. Government also can control the negotiating environment, ranging from such factors as degree of formality, cooperation, clarity, and specificity. However, there are instances in which the applicant can enter negotiations as a more equal partner. Government may be under pressure to begin a project or program. The fiscal year may be drawing to a close, with pressures to expend appropriated funds or risk cutbacks in the next fiscal year. An applicant and/or its program may be politically attractive. There may be only one logical service provider. Their competence may be clearly evident.

An external factor impacting upon the equality of the negotiating team is the amount of money available for contracting. In the 1960s successfully negotiating a contract was a far more likely prospect than in the 1980s, even if the merit of the proposals was identical. Higher appropriations and/or the designation of a higher proportion of the budget for contracting out increases resources and reduces competition. Historical factors also enter into the negotiating environment. The past relationship between the provider and funding agency will impact upon the attitudes of the negotiating parties and likely result in greater informality and less specificity. The skill of the applicant in negotiating is another essential element equalizing the process.

KNOWING HOW TO NEGOTIATE

As purchase of service has grown into a billion dollar industry, the formalization of the contracting process has quickly followed suit. Potential providers of public services are expected to be able to negotiate an acceptable service package that meets the needs and specifications of the funder. The justification of a proposed program is now demanded, whether the applicant be sole source or engaged in competition with other providers. It will also have to document its capability to deliver a service and prove that its plan of action is the most responsive to the goals and objectives set forth by the funder. If, after a contract has been successfully negotiated and implemented, modifications are needed in the plan, the provider must reenter the negotiating arena to convince the government on the appropriateness and need for change in program scope, design, or cost. Thus, the ability to negotiate on behalf of oneself and/or one's organization is critical; the successful applicant will have to demonstrate its bargaining skills from the initial application stage through the conclusion of the contracted program.

When contracting for services was first being applied to the health and human services on a broad scale, negotiations followed a fairly standardized format, based on a relatively simple contract proposal document. Access of the applicant to government agents for information and clarification was, generally, available. But similar to any growing enterprise, the sheer volume of contracting resulted in the perceived need to formalize the process, in part to ensure objectivity and adherence to affirmative action guidelines. The identification of implementation problems—discrepancies between what was promised by providers and what was delivered—also led to requirements for a detailed proposal, assurances of provider capability, and accountability.

Negotiations may be more routine and simple with a new contract. In the case of renewals, both the government agency and provider may seek clarifications and protections in the light of implementation experience. The negotiations may consequently be longer and more detailed for second applications or renewals. As Copeland (1976, 4) states:

> . . . As controversies arise in the administration of the contract, each party will want various kinds of protections for itself, or specific obligations which it wants the other to undertake, written into the contract. The more of this detailing of each party's obligations and responsibilities thought to be necessary, the more onerous the contracting process will become to both parties—and the more negotiation time will eat into service performance time . . . and into service monitoring and technical assistance time for the state agency.

The formalization of contracting procedures is evident in the types of information requested by the government agency in the RFP, all of which are subject to discussion, analysis, and negotiation. The information requests range from extensive descriptions of the program, methods of delivery, administrative procedures, and fiscal monitoring and control. Copeland (1976) provides an exhaustive list of the items for inclusion in the proposal, which serves as the negotiation base. Items include

Line item budget
Staff assignments, qualifications, and supervision mechanisms
Narrative explanation and budget justification
Relationship of the budget to specific program elements
Unit of service definition
Accounting systems and procedures
Client eligibility criteria
The process and outcome of the services to be given
Program need
Monitoring and evaluation procedures
Affirmative Action/Equal Opportunity policy statements
Organizational description, including governance, history, service providing capability
Licensing and accreditation verification
Management plan

It is not unusual for a proposal to be fifty or more pages in length (although sometimes a page limitation is imposed). It is also not unusual for government to request, during the negotiating process, revisions in the document. From the authors' personal experience in negotiating contracts with a state agency, four rewrites of a proposal were required. In many instances this need may arise less from the quality of the original proposal than from the changing or unclear requirements of the funding agency. From the perspective of the applicant agency, patience and fortitude may be among the key criteria for successful negotiations. Motivation must also be high.

The need for negotiating skills is reflected in, and recognized by, the increasing number of universities and private training enterprises that offer workshops, seminars, and short-term courses focused on the subject of negotiation. Until recently, formal training in negotiation has been lacking among degree-granting programs in business, management, and the human services. Heretofore, most knowledge development and skill application related to negotiating had been acquired on the job through trial and error or under the mentorship of supervisors or administrators who have some experience as negotiators.

Negotiating involves a keen understanding of organizational dynamics, role clarification, problem identification, conflict resolution, and consensus building. AMR International, Inc. (Advanced Management Research), has, for several years, sponsored two-day seminars on "Successful Negotiations: Strategies, Executions and Pitfalls" across the country. Several major themes are identified: (1) negotiating in today's external environment; (2) what makes an effective negotiator; (3) assessing needs and setting objectives; (4) preparing for negotiations; (5) negotiating for mutual gain; (6) behavior in negotiations; and (7) follow-up after negotiations. These teaching areas imply that, with proper training, certain techniques may be acquired that will enhance the bargaining position of an organization or individual. The Wharton School, University of Pennsylvania, initiated in late 1985 a series of two-day seminars in several cities for "all people involved in the negotiation of real estate transactions." (The tuition and fees for the two days were $1,190!)

Negotiations are willingly entered. The bidder on a contract wants to win the award and thus is (or should be) prepared to justify the proposed program and associated costs, explain and clarify points of information, make modifications as requested to accommodate to the requirements of the funding body, and compromise on points of program or budget that, if done, will increase the successful outcome of negotiations. Government enters into negotiations to ensure that (1) the proposed program accurately reflects the priorities and goals set forth by government; (2) the applicant is capable of providing the program or service; (3) missing or ill-defined components of the proposal are clarified; (4) costs are justified and reasonable; (5) staffing is appropriate; and (6) all substantiating documentation has been made available.

Despite the shared goals of negotiation by all participating parties (government wants a program implemented; the applicant[s] wants to receive the contract and offer the service), there are still times when the process may engender anxieties. As previously noted, the applicant agency is frequently in a subordinate position, because it is dependent upon government to approve or reject the proposal. Thus, the applicant must prepare for negotiations, including anticipating issues and questions that may arise. The applicant must also review and decide upon, in advance, the points on which compromise is possible or desirable and, conversely, what requirements may be seen as violating the integrity of the program. The issue of when to say no is important and involves a high degree of self-assessment about one's own organization and its proposed program.

It is essential that the agency or individual entering contract negotiations know both itself and its partner (government). Is there internal organizational agreement about the program elements and what can be "bartered"? The applicant must know what it wants of and from its proposed program within the context of its overall agency services and clearly perceive the compatibility (or lack of) between proposed program goals and agency goals and missions. The costs in money, prestige, and influence of the proposed program must be understood. Applicant negotiators must also be aware of the programmatic implications of potential compromises and decide, *before* entering negotiations, their "bottom line," i.e., a standard or point of reference to guide deliberations. Later, if these standards appear to be at risk in negotiations, decisions can and should be made about the desirability of compromise or even continuing the negotiating process.

WHO NEGOTIATES?

Frequently, several people participate in negotiations, representing each side. A team, an individual, or a team with a clearly designated leader are all legitimate choices. Ordinarily, a team without a leader may find itself at a disadvantage. Whatever option is selected by a side to the negotiations, the presentation of a unified, collective front is important. If a team approach is used, each member should be assigned a specific responsibility or area of expertise, such as the budget, staffing, or program format. The chief negotiator for both groups should be someone who is respected and who carries some weight within the respective organization.

The issue of who should participate in negotiations will have an obvious and profound effect on both the process and outcome. If a government agency assigns its chief contracting officer to head its negotiating team, it is appropriate for the applicant agency to designate its director or associate director as representative. If a program officer is assigned to negotiate on behalf of the funding agency, the designated project director would be a logical choice as chief negotiator for the applicant agency. The negotiator's position in the hierarchy should be matched by the other party. When negotiations take place among "unequals" in power or position, the less influential partner may have to consult with organizational superiors for sanction or approval of decision-making issues. The higher-ranking negotiator may also try to manipulate or control discussions or circumvent decisions by directly contacting the other negotiator's superior.

When there are complicated issues to be negotiated, or when the parties are meeting in negotiations for the first time, the participation of senior staff in the deliberations is advisable. The authority associated with high position may facilitate discussion and enhance the process of consensus building and agreement. In negotiations that are likely to be straightforward and the issues known in advance, the power to speak on behalf of the organization may more easily be delegated to those of lower rank. For example, when it is known that government will fund a group home for the retarded, but the budget line items must be justified by activity, program staff can appropriately represent the applicant organization. In fact, in such instances they may be better able to respond to questions than their superiors.

The negotiators from each side should determine in advance the style of negotiating, timetables, and logistical arrangements. Each side, of course, should also assess the extent of power and influence held by the other side. Evaluating the bargaining position of the other is a significant preparatory step; as much as possible should be known about the other organization, including its leadership and decision-making processes and its history in past contract negotiations or contract performance. What strategies will the other side likely employ? How tough are the negotiators? How strong is their position? Potential roadblocks and obstacles to the resolution of issues should be anticipated.

The task of setting the agenda is particularly important in guiding the process and outcome of deliberations. To Schelling (1963, 68), the ability "to set the stage in such a way to give prominence to some particular outcome that would be favorable" is significant. What is known about the other party will help to define the ordering of the agenda. In some instances it is most appropriate to begin with items on which there is ready consensus, tackling the more difficult issues later. This approach allows the building of a positive, cooperative environment. On the other hand, if the outcome of negotiations is in real question, addressing the consensus items first may only obscure the real issues and potentially waste the time of both parties should agreement not be reached on contention matters.

Which side will carry this responsibility is a major question in agenda setting. Most frequently, it is the funding agency that raises the issues and questions about the proposed program and therefore identifies the agenda items. However, this does not negate the possiblity that the applicant may influence the ordering of the agenda. Depending on the experience of the negotiators, government may not sufficiently prepare; the applicant should always be ready to suggest the topics for discussion and items on which agreement must be reached. Limits should always be set on the scope and number of areas to be covered in negotiations.

THE PHYSICAL ENVIRONMENT

There are three choices in selecting the site for negotiations: their place, your place, or a neutral location. Most often, the applicant will be asked to come to the offices of the funding agency. Should the applicant be able to persuade government representatives to meet on their turf, psychological advantages may accrue to the former. If a neutral site can be arranged, neither party is at a disadvantage. One option is to alternate the place of negotiations, meeting first in the offices of one party and next at the offices of the other party.

The logistical arrangements are important, as they influence the negotiating environment. Are there rooms for separate, small-group meetings? Is there a convenient place to eat or have catering arrangements been made? How many should sit at the table, and in what place? How many people should be seated in rows behind the table? Attention to such details must not be overlooked.

BUILDING A STRATEGY

There are a number of procedural, logistical, and planning questions that must be addressed prior to and during negotiations. Ground rules must be established. The meeting must be called by one party or the other. When and where the meetings are to be held must be addressed. Spokespersons must be identified.

All internal differences should be resolved before formal negotiations take place. Any public display of disharmony can impair the position of a negotiating party. For example, if the negotiators for the applicant agency disagree about the need to hold firm on certain program components or budget lines, the funding agency may well press its views all the harder. Arguments presented by the applicants must be grounded in a position of strength, entailing unanimity of purpose and consensus on the means by which the desired outcomes may be achieved.

One negotiator from each side should be assigned the task of analyzing the various positions held internally and the degree of agreement and disagreement. To the extent possible, the negotiating team should also assess the degree of consensus held by the other party. Negotiation strategies are built on such information.

141

NEGOTIATING

Negotiating is a give and take process. It is also a straightforward business conversation. Negotiators are well advised to write down the names and identifying data of those participating and to be cognizant throughout the process of the information that has been gathered on the other party.

If negotiations are held to finalize a contract on which there is already general agreement, confrontation is unlikely. When there are identified issues on which clarification is sought, some compromise may be requested and granted. There will be discussion, but it will still be peaceful. When an applicant agency is asked to meet for the purpose of presenting a "best and final" offer, discussions are often of these two types. The funder may well question at least some component of the proposal, be it staffing, budget, or program. When the provider capabilities are already established, discussions might center on justifying the proposed approach or elaborating on the statement of the problem; e.g., an informational session on noncontroversial issues.

Negotiation of issues on which there are clear differences of opinion takes the process one step further. Here, the transactions between the parties are more formalized and compromise is expected and sought. The potential for increasing or decreasing tensions exists. The methodology of a research proposal may be considered to be inadequately explained or too complicated for the intended purposes. Adaptations in the original proposal are likely to be requested and, on the basis of changes made by the applicant, negotiations will be continued.

Negotiations may contain some difficult moments, highlighting the need to keep discussions and agenda as flexible as possible. As the situation changes, adjustments in process will be required. Using a fallback position may become necessary, but counterproposals are often effective.

In flyers promoting their training programs, AMR suggests that negotiators table uncertain assumptions. They also advocate using hypothetical situations before dealing with specific issues. Nierenberg (1973) advocates asking questions and listening well. He urges that attention be paid to nonverbal communications ranging from sounds and silence, gestures, posture, and facial expressions. Personal bickering should, of course, be avoided; personalities are unimportant and diversionary. It is the issues that are important and that require a businesslike approach.

Developing and implementing strategies and tactics is a complex task, because they must be sufficiently diverse to address negotiators who are ready to compromise, those who are not ready, and those who are not ready but will be if the terms suit them. Cohen (1980) suggests that many negotiating tactics should be applied, including admitting that one does not have all the answers (humanizing oneself) to bring about more receptivity on the part of others.

Impasses

When and if an impasse is reached, informal talks may be appropriate. The use of coffee breaks or meals may be crucial for promoting informal discussion and should be extended if progress can be made in this manner.

At times, it is appropriate and necessary for one side or the other to say no to a particular request. For example, if the government agency asks that a more complex evaluation procedure of a service program be instituted but is not willing to increase the budget for this component of the project, the applicant must decide the impact on the overall program and the financial liabilities that may accrue to the organization. Turf issues may also arise, threatening the process and outcome of negotiations. Who will monitor what? Does the funding agency have the right to review the process by which the program is implemented, rather than just its outcomes?

The authors experienced a negotiating crisis when a state agency, as a component of a large training program, requested that a course be implemented on recently promulgated rules and operating procedures specific to that agency. The funder, under the assumption that only an insider would have the appropriate knowledge to teach this content, made known its expectation that it would have the deciding vote in selecting the instructor. However, the university had its own criteria for hiring instructors, including standards of education and experience. The university's bottom-line position, developed in past negotiations, was that the selection of instructors was solely within the purview of the educational institution. The university thus did not agree to offer the course under the outlined conditions but instead suggested that the agency offer it on an in-service basis.

This example points to several risks in negotiating and how discussions may break down on the matter of a single point. The funding

143

agency may decide that without resolution on the point of contention, there will be no contract. Although the university may not wish to compromise, it may have to decide between forfeiting the entire program or backing down on its position. Or, the university may offer a different solution: a joint selection process for the instructor. The university's decision may in part rest on the extent to which contract funds are needed or the program is perceived to be of value. There may also be forces within the university urging compromise. On the other hand, the funding agency may be under pressure to successfully negotiate the contract; there may not be any other educational institution with the ability to offer the program. In this circumstance compromise may be more likely on the part of government.

Ultimatums enter negotiations when one party informs the other that without compromise or acceptance on a particular point, the entire contract is in jeopardy. When choosing to offer an ultimatum, four criteria are useful to test the potential effectiveness of this strategy: (1) The other side has no choice; if the ultimatum is rejected, it stands to lose a substantial investment. (This implies that ultimatums may be most effectively employed toward the conclusion of negotiations rather than at the beginning. (2) The ultimatum must be palatable and communicated in a manner that does not belittle or threaten the other party. (3) In offering an ultimatum, its rationale should be documented and legitimated. (4) If possible, the opposing side should not be left without alternatives; the exchange should be structured to allow the other party to make a choice even though the alternatives are considerably less desirable (Cohen 1980).

NEGOTIATING STYLES

Demands can be extreme or within realistic, established limits. In the extreme one party may adopt a "win at all costs" attitude. For Cohen (1980), there are six steps in negotiating this competitive win-lose approach:

1. Extreme initial positions, which start with tough demands or ridiculous offers that affect the other party's expectation level.
2. Limited negotiating ability, where negotiators themselves have little or no authority to make any concessions.

3. Emotional tactics whereby a party or parties to the negotiations raise their voices, act exasperated, and convey that they are being exploited. Occasionally they will stalk out of the meeting in a huff.
4. Adversarial concessions, which are viewed as weakness. Should one side concede on a point, it is unlikely to be reciprocated.
5. Stingy concessions which, after a period of delay, reflect only a minuscule change in position.
6. Ignoring deadlines and acting as though time is of no significance.

When confronted with a win-lose style of negotiating, it should be remembered that this is a tactic. If the other party was not serious about a contract, they would not be in negotiations. Once a tactic is identified as such, its effective potential is reduced. The negotiators faced with any or all of the behavioral manifestations of this approach may opt to (1) curtail, for the short or long run, discussions; (2) fight fire with fire; or (3) attempt to change the relationship from the competitive win-lose variety to a more collaborative exchange that can meet the needs of both parties.

Another style of negotiating is the mutual satisfaction approach, characterized by warmth and friendliness. Here, the parties are moderate in tone, admit of occasional error, indicate when help is needed to understand or clarify a point, speak with tact, and show concern for the other side. There are efforts made to see the problem from the perspective of the other parties and to harmonize and reconcile needs. Absolutes are avoided. This approach characterizes negotiations between parties that have worked well together in the past; established mutual satisfaction of past performance and trust; and know each other on a first name, friendly basis.

When negotiating from this mutual satisfaction perspective, it may still not be possible to avoid all conflict. However, every attempt is made to determine the cause of the conflict and to understand the other's point of view. As Cohen (1980, 161) notes: "Successful collaborative negotiations lie in finding out what the other side really wants and showing them a way to get it, while you get what you want."

A third negotiating strategy is win-win, in which an effort is made to have both sides gain as a result of bargaining. This is accomplished by building trust, gaining commitment, and managing the opposition (Cohen 1980). The process of building trust occurs over considerable time and may be motivated by purposeful decision. Trust, in this strategy, makes it easier to obtain needed information from the other party and helps to build mutual respect for ideas and positions. Relationships of trust lead to collaboration, in which moderate risk-taking is possible and both sides are willing to assist in problem solving.

A case example of the win-win strategy occurs when government enters negotiations with a leading nonprofit firm with whom it has done business over the last ten years for a research program. Both sides are committed to quality, know what resources and activities are needed to accomplish the project's goals, and have individually and collectively decided to negotiate as smoothly and rapidly as possible. Both sides are willing to be honest about presenting their needs and demands, and each knows and respects the limits and circumstances of the other. They work together.

Fisher and Ury (1983) urge a more generic negotiating strategy that they entitle principle negotiation. This approach is both hard and soft, with the focus on the merit of the issues. Mutual gains are sought, but when interests are still opposed, the results should be based on fair standards independent of either party.

We have stressed interorganizational negotiation, but intraorganizational negotiating also takes place, especially in complex systems. Ginsburg (1981, 89) describes the budget process as "Games People Play." "Ask any ordinary, mild-mannered, middle manager to tell you how much money he needs for the coming year, and suddenly you're face to face with a character you barely recognize, an actor who plays his role with passion and eloquence in the hopes or wringing a few more dollars out of his thick-skinned boss."

The strategies used in intraorganizational negotiations are similar to those used between organizations. These may range from threats of resignation to following precisely and without complaint the policies handed down. In between are the full gamut of maneuvers designed to provide gains for one party (an employee, unit, or program within an organization), or at least secure its position, while extracting these gains from those within the system who hold the power to deny, grant, or withhold the sought-after item.

TOWARD SMOOTH NEGOTIATIONS

As mentioned earlier, negotiations are usually a give and take process. No matter what negotiating style is adopted, there are certain principles that should be followed by both parties. These include

Maintaining control of the meeting, including its tone, content, and the behavior of participants;

Maintaining open lines of communication with superiors and involved staff about the progress of negotiations;

Maintaining patience; when faced with a frustrating situation or impasse, approach it with tact and aim toward meeting one specific need;

Avoiding demands for the impossible;

Avoiding bluffs, unless there is certainty of your position and a willingness to follow through; and

Setting realistic time frames for negotiating and adhering to them.

In addition to these process considerations, the success of negotiations will be significantly enhanced if each party has clear authority to negotiate on behalf of his organization. Each side will do well to clarify points of congruence and divergence in their respective organizational environments, include mandates, philosophy, mode of operation, and general and specific program goals. The desired outcome of negotiating should be understood and verbalized and internal and external constraints recognized. One party or the other (perhaps both) may have to be content with achieving less than its desired aims.

Agreements reached during negotiations tend to develop incrementally. When complete, the terms should be written and subject to review and approval by both parties. There should be clarity about dates and the agreement should be signed, which avoids later disagreement about the terms reached.

Much of the writing about negotiating focuses on what to avoid. This is because negotiations are not always successful. The process can break down or the outcomes be far from that desired by either side. To increase the likelihood of a positive outcome

Do not avoid doing your homework.
Do not talk too much.

Do not become involved in personalities.
Do not get locked into a single, unyielding position.
Do not ignore the importance of setting forth alternative strategies.
Do not be impatient.
Do not be impetuous.
Do not forget the desired outcome; the goal should always be in sight.

The Transfer of Fiscal Resources in Purchase of Service Settings

David W. Young

In this chapter, the focus of attention is on transfer of fiscal resources within the context of purchasing—not selling—human services. Although the discussion centers on the purchaser, the principles drawn are of equal importance to both purchasers and vendors of human services. To the extent that both parties recognize the degree of the complexity of the issues and can thus communicate in a more informed way about the transfer of fiscal resources, it may be possible for them to develop more rational and cost-effective transfer processes.

Several biases underlie the content of this chapter. For example, a principal operating premise is that purchasers get what they pay for. As a rule, vendors do not cheat, steal, and plunder from purchasers. Indeed, most vendors—be they private social service agencies, hospitals, nursing homes, community action programs, halfway houses for drug dependents or alcoholics, free-standing mental health facilities, and so on—are motivated to deliver high-quality services at reasonable cost. They are also motivated to stay in business. Thus, to the extent that the payment mechanism for the transfer of fiscal resources—what hereinafter will be called the transfer price—motivates them to deliver services other than what the purchaser had in mind, or at a higher cost than was envisioned by the purchaser, the responsibility lies with the purchaser, not the vendor.

To be more concrete, over the past decade the human service field has witnessed a variety of what might be labeled "unintended consequences" in purchase of service situations. The following examples illustrate the problem in three human service fields: health care, mental health, and social services (Young 1978; Young 1981; Young and Allen 1977).

In health care we have seen hospital stays of excessive lengths for Medicare and other patients; overutilization of ancillary services; transfer of very sick, but not acutely ill, patients from nursing homes to acute care hospitals; and less than optimal reliance on outpatient care or home health services in favor of more inpatient care. In the mental health field, we have seen minimal efforts to move patients from institutional care to free-standing—deinstitutionalized—facilities, and treatment modes that are more custodial than therapeutic. In the social services, we find children spending a good portion of their youth and adolescence in foster care rather than being returned to their natural families or placed in adoptive homes. We also have seen a continuation of child abuse in families where the child has been removed, treated, and returned. And so on.

The reason for these allegedly unintended consequences is really quite simple: we get what we pay for. Unfortunately, although the reason is simple, the solution is not. The establishment of a good transfer-pricing structure is an inherently difficult task. A good structure is defined as one that communicates the proper set of signals to vendors and that, if not motivating vendors properly, is at least neutral, i.e., it doesn't motivate vendors *improperly*. (A particularly interesting article that addresses these issues is Frost, 1978.) The remainder of this chapter will be devoted to a discussion of the elements that make up a well-designed transfer-pricing structure in the human services.

PURCHASERS, VENDORS, AND DELIVERY PATTERNS

As a first step in developing a sound transfer-pricing structure, it may be useful to focus on purchasers and vendors and the ways in which they interact. Purchase of services can take place at three levels: federal, state, and local (cities, towns, counties) government, and can involve three levels of vendors: state government, local government, and private agencies (both for-profit and not-for-profit). The result, depending on the initiator of the purchase decision, is nine different purchase options, as depicted in figure 9.1.

Several points should be stressed with respect to figure 9.1. First, the options do not necessarily depict situations in which the next step is delivery of service by the vendor to the client. For example, in situation F1, where the federal government (FG) purchases services from a state government (SG), the SG may, in addition to delivering services directly to

Figure 9.1. **Purchase Options: Relationships between Purchasers and Vendors**

Option	Federal Government	State Governments	Local Governments*	Private Agencies	Clients
F1	FG purchases from SG Ex.: Medicaid				
F2	FG purchases from LG Ex.: Community action programs, model cities				
F3	FG purchases from PA Ex.: Medicare, federally funded community health centers				
F4	FG delivers care directly to C Ex.: Veterans Administration				
S1		SG purchases from LG Ex.: Chapter 766[1]			
S2		SG purchases from PA Ex.: Community mental health agencies			
S3		SG delivers care directly to C Ex.: State schools for the retarded[2]			
L1			LG purchases from PA Ex.: New York City child care[3]		
L2			LG delivers care directly to C Ex.: L.A. county adoption service		

[1]A state-funded program in Massachusetts for serving children with special needs in the regular school system of the town in which the child lives

[2]State-run institutions in Massachusetts that care for the mentally retarded and physically handicapped

[3]New York City system in which the city purchases child-care services (foster care, adoption, institutional care) from some eighty voluntary (private) agencies

*A variety of intralocal governmental activities can take place within this category in which, say, a county government purchases services from cities and towns, or vice versa. For purposes of simplicity, this level of detail has been excluded, as have all other purchase of service arrangements within a single category, e.g., between two private agencies or two state governments.

clients, purchase some services from either local governments or private agencies. This is the case with the Medicaid program, for example, where a state may deliver services directly to Medicaid patients (through state hospitals, for instance), but may also purchase health care services from private agencies (e.g., hospitals or community health centers). Thus, option F1 may result in either S1, S2 or S3. And S1 may result in L1 or L2. Similarly, F2 may result in either L1 or L2. The result is that, depending on the initial purchaser of care, fourteen potential service delivery pathways exist from a purchaser to a client. These are shown in figure 9.2.

A second point concerns the strategy that leads a local government to opt for L1 rather than L2, or a state government to opt for S1 or S2 rather than S3, or the federal government to opt for F1, F2, or F3 rather than F4. Although the issue is beyond the scope of this chapter, it is a crucial one in the general area of purchase of service contracting, since it represents, for each level of government, the fundamental purchase of service decision: direct delivery vs. contracting out. This decision has been discussed in detail in Young (1978) and involves a wide variety of interrelated concerns: cost comparisons, economies of scale, flexibility in the face of increased or reduced demand for services, risk, performance evaluation, and others. In each situation the interaction of these several factors is unique, requiring sound managerial judgment if the most cost-effective course of action is to be taken.

The final point of importance is that, although the transfer-pricing structure that is used between any two of the actors in figure 9.1 is important, this chapter focuses only on those relationships that involve a contract between a governmental entity and a private agency. The three relationships in figure 9.1 that describe this situation are F3, S2, and L1.

There are three reasons for choosing this limited focus. First, it represents one of the most common and problematic purchase of service arrangements. Second, it has received fairly widespread attention in the literature on purchase of service contracting (Bowers and Bowers 1976; Dowling 1974; Hill 1971; Schorr 1970; Young 1978; Young 1981; Young and Allen 1977), but no clear conclusions have emerged. Third, the principles developed in this somewhat concrete set of situations can be applied with little additional effort to the remaining options in figure 9.1. That is, if we can develop some valid principles for private vendors, i.e., vendors who are not a priori obligated by statute to deliver services, we

Figure 9.2. **Potential Service Delivery Pathways**

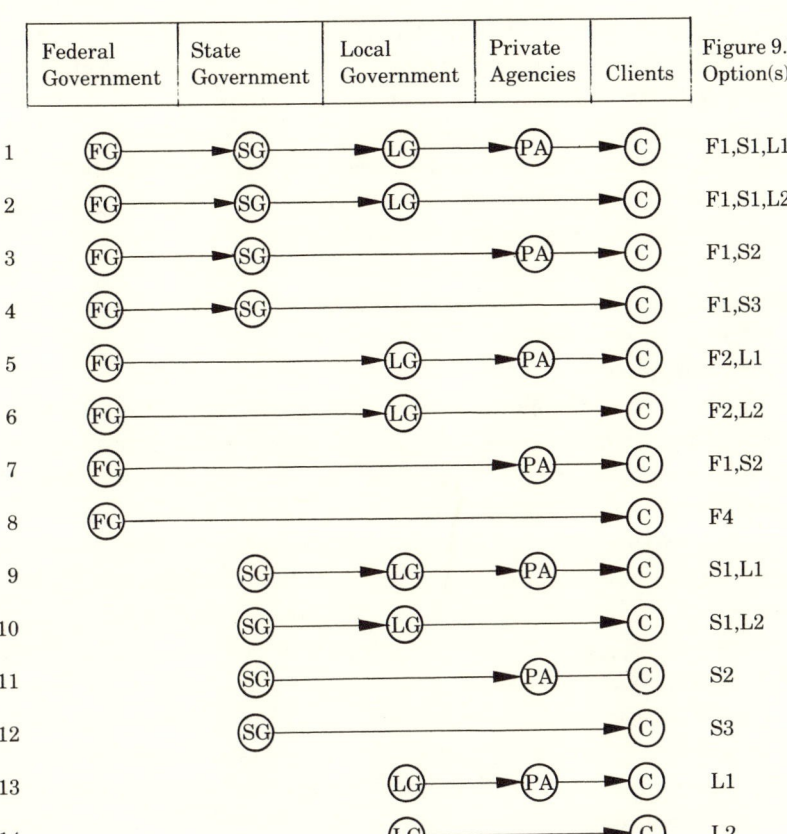

	Federal Government	State Government	Local Government	Private Agencies	Clients	Figure 9.1 Option(s)
1	FG	SG	LG	PA	C	F1,S1,L1
2	FG	SG	LG		C	F1,S1,L2
3	FG	SG		PA	C	F1,S2
4	FG	SG			C	F1,S3
5	FG		LG	PA	C	F2,L1
6	FG		LG		C	F2,L2
7	FG			PA	C	F1,S2
8	FG				C	F4
9		SG	LG	PA	C	S1,L1
10		SG	LG		C	S1,L2
11		SG		PA	C	S2
12		SG			C	S3
13			LG	PA	C	L1
14			LG		C	L2

should have a relatively easy time applying those principles to organizations that do have statutory obligations, e.g., governments.

THE TRANSFER-PRICING ENVIRONMENT

In order to develop methodologies for establishing a transfer-pricing structure, we must first examine the environment in which the structure is to be established, since clearly a transfer-pricing methodology that is appropriate for one setting may be quite inappropriate for another. An appropriate methodology for establishing an adoption reimbursement fee to a private agency, for example, almost certainly will be of little use in establishing the fee paid to a halfway house for a six-month community outreach program. What, then, are the important elements of the transfer-pricing environment that constrain, and sometimes govern, the formulation of an appropriate transfer-pricing methodology?

Although a wide variety of environmental factors can interact to influence the development of an appropriate transfer price, there are three that would appear to have somewhat universal applicability: service context, client characteristics, and the competitive structure. These are shown schematically in figure 9.3 and explained below.

Service Context

The service context refers to the overall type of organizational activity for which the purchaser wishes to contract. In some instances the purchaser will only wish to see an operating entity in place and thus will provide start-up assistance. Federal support of demonstration programs is one example of this type of contract. During the start-up period, the organization may or may not serve clients. In other situations the purchaser may wish to have the vendor engage in an outreach effort to contact potential clients and determine their needs. In still others the purchaser may wish to have an organization ready to serve clients even if it does not do so during a given period of time. Finally, the purchaser may wish to reimburse a vendor only for its ongoing activities with clients.

In many instances a combination of service options exists. One of the most frequent combinations is the situation in which a purchaser may wish to have a vendor both be ready to serve a certain number of clients and to actually serve some as well. The most obvious example is a hospital, but others also exist. Mental health facilities, social service agencies, group homes, and halfway houses are all situations in which the purchaser typically wants an agency to provide services to some clients in an ongoing manner and be ready to serve others should the need arise.

Client Characteristics

Clients can be described in terms of both their demographic attributes (age, sex, race, religion, income levels) and their service characteristics. Of these two, the latter generally is the most important in purchase of service settings. From the purchase of service perspective,

154

Figure 9.3. **The Transfer Pricing Environment**

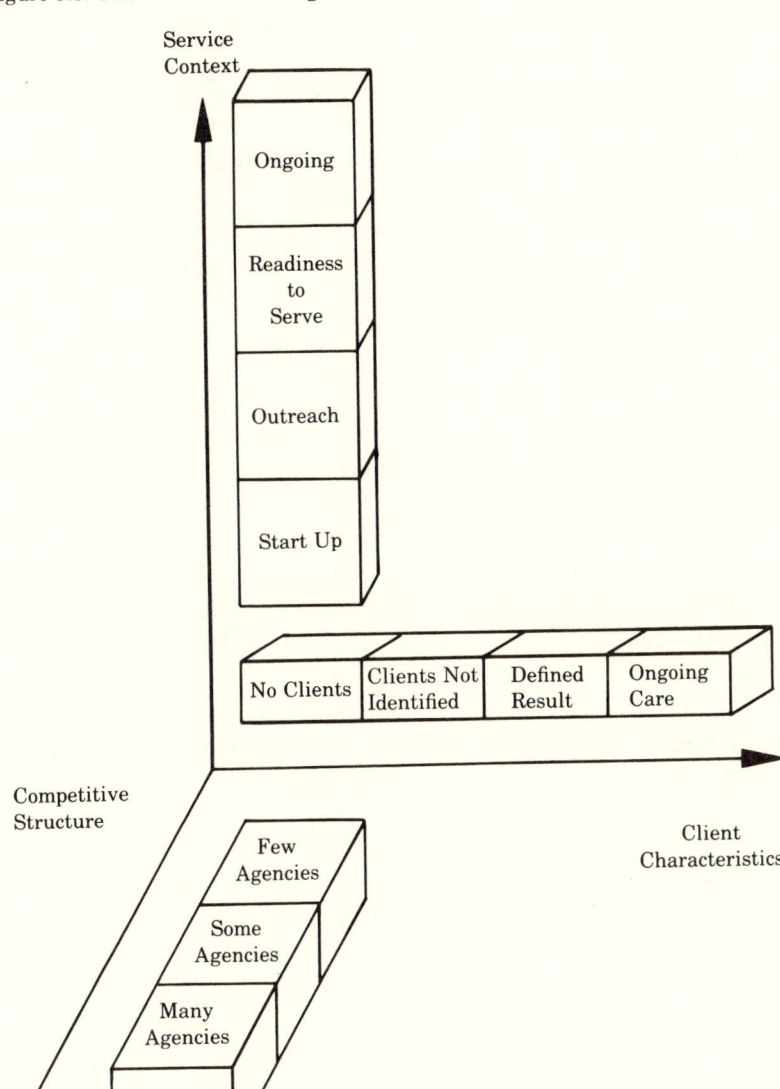

The 3-dimensional idea was adapted from Abell (1980).

relevant client characteristics can be classified into four situational categories, depending on the services delivered: (1) no clients directly involved; (2) many clients are served but none is identified individually; (3)

clients are identified directly, services are delivered, and each client is discharged with some defined result accomplished; and (4) clients receive ongoing care of some sort with no particular objective intended other than the care process itself. Some examples may help to clarify these categories.

The first, where no clients are involved, generally occurs in the context of start-up activities, where a purchaser provides funding to assist an organization in establishing a readiness-to-serve capacity. It also could exist in the rare circumstance of a vendor who has a readiness-to-serve capacity but delivers no client care.

The second situation is one in which clients receive short-term or intermittent care, such as a meals-on-wheels program, a senior drop-in center, an emergency shelter, or a pregnancy counseling agency. In many of these situations, clients receive the service offered on a one-time or infrequent basis, but are not identified in such a way as to permit follow-up efforts or tracking of any sort.

The third situation is one of the most common in a human service context: that in which an identified client receives services over some period of time with the ultimate objective of completing a defined task. Hospitalization for an acute illness is one example, adoption is another.

The fourth situation is also quite common. Again, the client receives services, but now with no particular defined end result. Examples are chronic care hospitalizations, foster-home care, mental hospital institutionalization, and so on.

Clearly, in some instances a client or group of clients may be classified into more than one of the above categories. The fact that some human service settings serve clients with several different kinds of characteristics is not a limitation of this classification scheme, however, but a strength. It is precisely because of this fact that the scheme can be useful to purchasers in developing transfer-pricing structures that attempt to match the payment process to the desired service package. In many instances the need will arise for a series of transfer prices rather than just one. This matter will be discussed more fully following a description of the third environmental factor.

Competitive Structure

As figure 9.3 indicates, a description of the competitive structure is deliberately soft, using the terms *few, some,* and *many* to characterize the nature of competition among the agencies offering their services to purchasers. The terms are used only to illustrate the need for the purchaser to assess the marketplace in which services are being bought and sold. If there are many agencies offering similar services, the purchaser generally will have more power to negotiate prices than if there are only a few agencies offering very different services. Indeed, in some cases the purchaser may stimulate the development of new competitive services. The situation encountered by New York City in purchasing foster care services—in which some eighty agencies all offer similar services—is considerably more enviable, for example, than that of Blue Cross purchasing an emergency appendectomy for one of its insured patients in a one-hospital town.

NEGOTIATING THE TRANSFER-PRICING STRUCTURE

It is within the framework of a particular transfer-pricing environment—a given mix of service context, client characteristics, and competitive structure—that the transfer-picture structure is established. An emphasis on the word *structure* is quite appropriate because a purchaser frequently is not purchasing a single service but a mix of services delivered to a mix of clients. And just as Solomons (1965) stipulates that different multidivisional corporate situations call for different transfer-pricing structures, so it is in the human services as well. What then are these human service scenarios, and what do they imply for the mechanism by which fiscal resources are transferred from the public to the private sector? In order to answer this question, we must return to the three-dimensional framework described in the last section.

The first point of importance to note is that although there are forty-eight (4x4x3) possible combinations of a service context, client characteristics, and competitive structure, we need not discuss each one individually. This is true not only because there are some invalid combinations (e.g., start-up service context with perpetual care client characteristics), but also because some elements can be discussed independently of others. The competitive structure, for example, can be looked at by itself relatively independent of each particular service context-client characteristic combination.

The second important point is that there are certain prototypical combinations, the discussion of which can be illuminating for the more unusual situations. Consequently, instead of looking at each valid combination, two prototypes will be discussed with the hope that the discussion will both clarify why certain purchase of service arrangements have produced alleged unintended consequences and describe how these consequences might have been corrected with a more appropriate transfer-pricing structure. I use the term *alleged* because in my opinion the consequences were quite predictable at the outset with only a cursory analysis of the transfer-pricing structure and the signals it sent out.

Prototype 1: Foster Care versus Adoption

Young and Allen (1977) have argued that adoptions in the New York City child-care system remained at low levels because of the imbalance between the one-time fee paid to agencies for adoptions and the daily fee paid to the same agencies for foster care. The imbalance was such that the agencies, although desirous of placing children out for adoption when necessary, could not afford to do so. What went wrong?

First, as indicated above the competitive structure was characterized by many agencies offering similar services; thus, it should have been possible to set the adoptions payment at "cost." This did not happen, however, because cost was never appropriately analyzed. From all indications the analysis was inhibited by a complex relationship that existed between service context, with both readiness to serve and ongoing operations, and client characteristics, which included a combination of defined result and ongoing care. In effect, agencies, because of their readiness to serve, had certain fixed costs that were covered by per diem payments for foster care. An adoption, which was reimbursed by a one-time fee, resulted in the elimination of the ongoing foster-care payment and hence in a failure to recover fixed costs adequately.

The solution to a situation such as this is threefold. First, if readiness to serve is desired, it must be paid for. This may be accomplished by reimbursing fixed costs on a periodical basis (e.g., monthly) rather than on the basis of volume. Fixed costs by definition occur with the passage of time, not with volume, and readiness to serve implies that some level of fixed costs will exist associated with that readiness. Second, the variable and semivariable costs of the defined result (adoption in this instance) must be assessed carefully. In the above example, because fixed costs should have been covered by period payments, variable and semivariable

158

costs were the only relevant costs. Finally, in the context of a defined result, it is important to recognize that the payment for each result must include the cost of failed attempts, since not all attempts generally are successful. As Young and Allen (1977) indicate, a transfer-pricing structure of this sort was not utilized, and hence adoptions remained low while some twenty-eight thousand children resided in foster care. (Editor's Note: A more successful experience in San Mateo County, California, using a different pricing mechanism is described by Elsa Ten Broeck elsewhere in this volume.)

In this context one additional point must be stressed. In those situations in which the purchaser incurs a one-time cost that serves to eliminate an ongoing cost, a reasonable level for the one-time cost can be determined rather simply by means of discounting the cash flows from ongoing cost savings to determine their present value. This is a standard procedure used in many for-profit capital investment decisions and would seem quite appropriate in human service settings as well. (See Young and Allen 1977; Anthony and Welsch 1981, chap. 9, for additional details.)

In sum, the answer to why New York City has some twenty-eight thousand children in foster care is simple: it gets what it pays for. In this situation by not reimbursing an agency's full cost for adoption and by not reimbursing on a period basis those fixed costs associated with a readiness to serve, New York City is paying agencies to "keep the beds full," i.e., to maintain children in foster care.

Prototype 2: Excessive Inpatient Stays in Hospitals

A variety of substitutes exists for inpatient hospital care and, in particular, for long hospital stays. Ambulatory surgery, nursing home convalescence, and home health care are three of the better-known options. Why, given these options, do hospitals admit patients who could be treated in an ambulatory mode, or keep patients needing inpatient care in the hospital rather than utilizing more cost-effective modalities? Once again, as described below, the answer lies in a misfit between the service context-client characteristic combination and the payment mode chosen.

Similar to social service agencies, hospitals have fixed costs associated with their readiness to serve, but for which they are reimbursed on a per diem (i.e., volume) basis in accordance with a patient's stay. (Outpatient care, including ambulatory surgery, constitutes a minor part of most hospitals' revenue.) Additionally, there are certain one-time costs associated with a patient's entry into and exit from a hospital (Wood 1982). These, too, must be recovered via the daily per diem.

In this instance there are two problems. First, once again the fixed costs associated with a hospital's readiness to serve are not being reimbursed on a period basis. Additionally, however, we have a situation in which we are reimbursing for a defined result on an ongoing care basis (see figure 9.3), i.e., a misfit between what we want—a cured patient—and what we pay for—a day in a bed. Because the per diem does not cover a variety of large one-time costs incurred early in a patient's stay, hospitals are motivated to extend a patient's time in care in order to make up the deficit during the convalescent portion of the stay. This is because during convalescent days, when the variable costs of care are low, the per diem rate remains at the same level. The hospital thus earns a surplus of these patient days and attempts to use it to recover the deficit incurred during the early days.

Again, what is happening is that we are getting what we pay for—days in beds. Although regulatory measures such as utilization review procedures, administratively necessary days, and the like may be necessary, purchasers of care should also examine their transfer-pricing structure; in this instance it does not fit with what they wish to purchase.

Although the examples could continue, they would serve only to repeat the theme: purchasers of services must first analyze what they want, and then structure transfer prices in such a way as to avoid penalizing vendors for giving appropriate services. In many respects the Diagnostic Related Group is an attempt to do this, i.e., to obtain a better fit between the transfer-pricing structure and the kinds of services desired. Although the DRG system has a number of limitations (see Young and Saltman 1982), it nevertheless has been designed in recognition of the fact that the desired result of a hospital stay is a cured patient and not a given number of days of hospital care. In the terminology of figure 9.3, the DRG system is paying vendors for a defined result rather than ongoing care.

Lessons and Implications

Other examples of appropriate or reasonably appropriate transfer-pricing structures could be found, but the fact is that the human service field is replete with purchase of service settings in which misfits exist between what purchasers wish and what vendors provide. Although not all of these misfits result from inappropriate transfer-pricing structures, many do, and for many more the transfer-pricing structure is a major contributing factor.

Although this chapter has focused most of its attention on purchase of service contracts between a governmental entity and a private agency, it also has attempted to put these particular arrangements in their broader context, as only one of a variety of relationships between purchasers and vendors. Although the details of some of these other relationships will no doubt differ, there nevertheless are lessons and principles that apply to all purchase of service situations. Two such lessons emerge from the discussion in this chapter. First, in terms of service context, the most problematic situation occurs with the juxtaposition of ongoing care and readiness to serve. Readiness to serve requires that a vendor commit itself to a base of fixed costs. These must be negotiated and reimbursed on a period basis if readiness to serve is to be clearly separated from ongoing operations.

The second lesson emerges in the context of ongoing operations, namely, that if we wish a defined result, we must carefully analyze its cost and pay for it on a lump sum basis. If we wish ongoing operations, we should pay for them on an ongoing basis. If we wish some combination, we cannot reward agencies for doing one and not the other, because invariably they will do what we reward them for. Stated simply once again: we get what we pay for.

10

Purchase of Services, Third-Party Payment, Market Conditions, and Rate-Setting

David Richardson

The goal of human services programs is to improve client status through the provision of services. In their efforts to reach this goal, policymakers can choose from three alternative human services program models: direct service provision, cash transfer, and purchase of service (POS). Each of these models relies upon a different strategy for obtaining the desired quantity, quality, and cost relationship. The models can be differentiated by how they organize and deliver services and by how they operate as a control mechanism. This second component will be emphasized here.

The decision to employ the POS model creates the need for regulation and thus rate-setting. The necessary causes for rate-setting are found in the goal of the human services program coupled with the selection of the purchase of service model as the vehicle for obtaining this goal.

PURCHASE OF SERVICE MODEL

Form

The purchase of service model is best described by comparing it with a cash transfer approach. For both models the major role of the human service program is funding, not direct service delivery. Moreoever, the role of the POS funding source is similar to that of the consumer in a cash transfer model, except that the POS model cannot rely upon the competitive market control of individual consumer behavior.

In the cash transfer model, the client, in his or her consumer role, is

THIS ARTICLE is based on Project Share's *Rate-Setting in the Human Services: A Guide for Administrators* 24 (September 1981).

Free to buy or not buy services according to needs and preferences,
Responsible for locating providers, and
Responsible for deciding upon the quality of service required and the
price to pay for such services.

In the POS model, the funding source itself takes on the consumer role.
Specifically, it defines the services required by the target population,
locates providers of such services, and enters into a contractual relationship with them. Although the conditions and extent of such contracts may vary widely by program, their common elements include the
following:

Definition of the service to be provided, including components of quality standards
Rules defining the funding source's responsibility and method of payment for services rendered

Typical of services "purchased" were those listed in the Title XX
amendments to the Social Security Act and the new Social Services Block
Grant program. For example, a state department of social services may
identify a need for residential treatment programs for emotionally
disturbed youths. The state agency may also ascertain that voluntary
or proprietary providers of such services already exist. Rather than
constructing and staffing such facilities itself, the state agency would
contract with providers to make residential placements available for its
clients. Other examples of services often purchased by state or local social service agencies include group day care, family foster care, home-
maker/chore, and counseling or family services.

The term *purchased service* is not typically used in health-related programs, though for chronic diseases and substance abuse they may follow
this model. For acute conditions, programs such as Medicaid and Medicare are defined as third-party payment mechanisms. A distinction
sometimes noted between third-party payment programs and the social
service POS model is the level of agency versus client control over service
authorization. In many social service POS programs, the human service
agency is totally responsible for the decision to initiate or terminate the
service. For instance, an agency, not the client, would be responsible for
authorizing the placement of a child in a residential treatment program.
Conversely, in Medicaid and other third-party programs, the decision to

163

utilize a particular service is made by the recipient, although termination is customarily the responsibility of the provider.

To whatever extent differences exist between POS and third-party payment approaches, they do not alter the basic relationship between the funding source, the client, and the provider. It remains the responsibility of the funding source initially to define service requirements, locate providers, determine their eligibility, contract for service delivery, and assume responsibility for payment. This funding source versus client responsibility for consumer and payment decisions dramatically affects the control methods that must be used in the POS and the third-party program.

Control Strategies

The control strategy relied upon in the POS model is the regulation of providers by the funding source. Regulation is an extremely problematic task. It is often viewed by classical economists as an inferior control mechanism to direct management or competitive market forces. However, factors exist that preclude the use of management and market controls in POS programs.

The inapplicability of direct management controls to the POS program should be readily apparent. In the direct service model, the human service agency owns the resources for service delivery. In the POS model, the service providers control the resources. Thus, the human service agency that funds a POS program does not have direct management control over staff hiring or decisions on whether to incur certain costs.

The reason market controls are not effective in the POS model are less apparent. Nor does the market model work for the public agency providing the service directly. It possesses the same limits as the POS agency. Because the role of the human service funding source is that of a consumer agency seeking to identify and purchase services, it might be anticipated that potential service providers would compete for POS arrangements.

To be sure, some market behavior can be observed in certain POS program areas. To the extent that real competition exists, the analogy between controls in the cash transfer model and the POS model is accurate. However, circumstances exist in most POS arrangements that preclude the effective functioning of a competitive market, hence its controls. The primary impediments to applying a market situation to the POS model are:

Displacement of the client as a true consumer,

Greater purchasing power by the funding source consumer than by private consumers,

Preponderance of not-for-profit firms in certain human service program areas,

Barriers to free entry into and exit from the human services market by firms, and

Monopoly or market control by a few providers.

The first impediment to true market conditions in a POS situation is the POS model's negative impact on consumerism. This occurs in two related ways. First, the individual client served in a POS model is not responsible for paying for the service. POS models may require copayment or cost sharing by higher income clients. However, in many programs, the impact of such arrangements is minimal due to the concern to keep the client's costs to the lowest possible level. Rather, the costs of services are the responsibility of the funding source. Because services are essentially free to the client, he or she has no incentive to play a typical consumer role. The consumer has no incentive to use services only in the amount required and thus may overutilize them. Similarly, the consumer will not be required to make cost-quality tradeoffs or to consider accepting lower quality services to reduce costs.

The number of clients served in the POS program may be small compared with the number of private pay clients using the same services. If so, the economic impact of the POS clients' "nonconsumer" behavior will be felt only by the funding source. However, if program clients constitute a large percentage of all clients, their service decisions have a society-wide impact. These clients (or the funding sources that purchase services for them) become the predominant force in the market. Unless the human service funding source applies controls (i.e., sets rates), program clients can price private pay clients out of the market.

As an example of these dynamics, many authors cite the impact of the health-financing programs, particularly Medicaid, on rising nursing home costs. The argument is that because nursing home placements are essentially free to Medicaid eligibles, certain proprietors initially raised rates to such high levels that self-paying clients could not afford their services.

The second limitation to a true market economy in human service POS settings relates to the characteristics of the service providers. One key characteristic is that not-for-profit providers predominate in many human services programs. Not-for-profit providers may not be induced to voluntarily control costs because they do not need to earn a profit. Indeed, voluntary providers may have objectives that are contrary to cost control, such as the expansion of service, scope, and quality, or enhanced prestige in the community. A more fundamental problem created by a voluntary service system is that not-for-profit institutions have great difficulty in attracting capital from profit-seeking investors. They must rely upon costly and uncertain methods, such as fund raising, for resource acquisition.

The difficulties in capitalizing voluntary agencies may create an effective barrier to the entrance of new, or competing, institutions to a service area. This situation results in a quasi-monopoly for the preexisting voluntary institution, or at least a market within which only a handful of potential providers exist. Obviously, such an arrangement reduces competition. When, simultaneously, the real consumers of services are also a limited set of third-party (POS) funding sources, no effective traditional market can exist.

REGULATION: THE NECESSARY CONSEQUENCE OF THE POS MODEL

Given the absence of effective market and management controls, the funding source for human services POS program is put in a difficult position. Clients may have little regard for the prices paid for services, permitting providers to raise charges ad infinitum. Since the clients are not responsible for payment, the providers' concern for quality may become secondary. These factors suggest continual pressures for price increases without corresponding improvements in quality. Unless dollars available to the funding source increase in direct proportion, the quality of service that can be purchased will continually decline.

To grapple with this problem, the human service funding source regulates providers to obtain defined levels of service quantity, quality, and price. Two components of regulation exist: (1) program standards and controls and (2) rate-setting. Program standards and controls are used to establish and obtain the desired quality of service.

Examples of programmatic standards are federal and state licensing and POS contract requirements, which dictate conditions such as the size and amenities of the POS providers' physical plant, necessary components of a service program, and client-staff ratios. Controls used to obtain compliance with standards include program monitoring, evaluation studies, and subsequent corrective actions (e.g., technical assistance, fiscal penalties).

The form and nature of these program standards dictate the resources and activities of the POS program. In turn, the provider must purchase such resources, hire staff, acquire supplies. For each of these program elements, the POS agency pays a price. Together, these prices yield the provider's costs for providing the requisite services. Rate-setting defines the conditions and amount of reimbursement to providers for the costs of service delivery.

Rate-setting, a regulatory activity undertaken by the POS program funding source in lieu of competitive market or direct management control over POS providers, has the following goals:

To determine the provider's costs of service delivery
To differentiate unreasonable from reasonable costs
To establish payment rates and/or reimbursement policies that keep providers and program costs at reasonable levels

In the remainder of this chapter, some observations on the state of the art of human services rate-setting will be made, including a summary of just what the rate setter can and cannot expect to accomplish vis-à-vis the goals underlying rate-setting. Next, a set of recommendations will be presented to improve the state of the art and finally, conversion of POS to cash transfer or direct operation will be discussed.

RATE-SETTING CAPABILITY AND PERFORMANCE
VERSUS BASIC RATE-SETTING GOALS

Goal 1: Defining Provider Costs

Only price-based rate-setting models avoid the requirement of defining provider costs for service delivery. The priced-based approach is applicable only if competitive market conditions exist. The absence of these conditions in almost all human services POS programs dictates the use of cost-related models. Hence, the requirement to define provider costs is the first step for the majority of rate-setting programs.

The techniques available for this cost definition step include traditional expense accounting, cost finding, and cost models. (Cost models are typically used as analytical aids to discriminate against reasonable/unreasonable costs. The conclusions on cost definition, therefore, apply only to the first two accounting methods.)

The basic accounting techniques, which have been developed over centuries, theoretically provide a more than adequate state of the art for POS cost definition. These techniques, do, however rely upon considerable professional judgment for appropriate application. The precise methods selected will depend upon general or extremely specific objectives over which the providers and funding source may be at odds. The administrative costs of cost definition may be high or extreme if a detailed knowledge of provider expenses is sought.

Although the necessary technology for cost definition exists, it cannot be taken for granted by the rate setter. Extreme care and a high level of skill must be employed if the first objective in rate setting, cost definition, is to be obtained.

Goal 2: Differentiating Between Reasonable and Unreasonable Provider Costs

This is the most fundamental goal underlying rate-setting. With such a discrimination, the funding source has the basis for deciding what costs it will or will not reimburse providers for. Without it, there is no rationale for accepting or rejecting provider costs, other than the exhaustion of the funding source's budget resources.

There are two basic requirements for this goal to be fulfilled: first, a clear definition of human service output and second, knowledge of the best and most efficient combination possible and use of the provider's resources (inputs) and other factors that affect the costs of producing this output.

The need for a definition of output is self-evident. The rate setter's concern is to decide the amount he or she is willing to pay for a service delivered by multiple providers. Until this service is precisely defined, the rate

168

setter accepts a range of costs from providers, each of which may be delivering a different (unknown) good.

Assuming that output is defined, the definition of "reasonable costs" is the lowest cost for which a provider can deliver the specified output. This lowest cost will be obtained to the extent the provider:

Identifies, acquires, and uses the best possible combination of inputs to service production (e.g., facilities, staff, equipment linked in the most efficient service process possible);

Pays the lowest possible price for each of these inputs;

Adopts management practices that obtain the highest level of productivity and efficiency from the inputs selected; and

Takes advantage of the quantity of service-cost relationship, including economies of scale.

To exemplify these requirements, assume that the rate setter is attempting to set prices for automobiles. With respect to output, he or she has available a tangible and functional set of specifications: namely, the output must have wheels, an engine, and an interior, and must start, turn, drive at a specified range of miles per hour, and stop.

This tangible output, a car, is produced by a defined automobile manufacturing technology. The rate setter also can directly investigate the factors (inputs and prices) affecting manufacturing costs. Again, we are dealing in the realm of tangible, physical, and known commodities. Inputs are assembly line machines, raw materials, warehouses, and specialized workers with predefined tasks. The extent to which each of these factors of production can deliver necessary components of the automobile can be measured and the best possible combination of them can be defined.

The automobile rate setter could, with sufficient time and analytical resources, conduct studies to identify reasonable automobile production costs versus unreasonable expenses due to imprudent or inefficient manufacturing processes.

Conversely, the human services administrator-rate setter possesses none of these advantages. The intended output of human services is alleviation of client problems or improvement in social, economic, or status dimensions. To date, the complexity of human needs and service systems is greater than the ability to measure or understand them. We have no unambiguous measures of quality of human service output.

These limitations preclude the administrator-rate setter from knowing what combination of inputs would best yield the (undefined) output. For instance, in rehabilitation of juvenile offenders, is multidiscipline team group counseling preferable to individual counseling? Is counseling preferable to basic life skill development (e.g., education, job training)? Are facilities best located away from the pressures of urban areas, or should clients contend with such pressures as part of the rehabilitative process?

These variations in service design abound in POS programs and, perhaps more than differences in prices or other cost factors, underlie differences in provider costs. Our inability to define and measure output and to ascertain the best combination of inputs is the fundamental constraint underlying all techniques of human services rate-setting. We lack a technology that yields a science of "reasonable cost" discrimination.

In lieu of this capability, all rate-setting methods address the reasonable cost problem via comparison of providers' historical and/or current practices and costs. Namely, reasonable costs are defined in relation to the range of costs that exist across the POS programs in question. This is nominally the case in comparison group prospective rate-setting. It is no less the case for specifications of limits in retrospective models or in techniques such as budget review. In all these procedures, the administrator-rate setter draws (systematically or intuitively) on a knowledge of costs across providers.

Since reasonable costs are operationally defined in terms of distribution of provider costs from lowest to highest, the explicit assumption is that low-cost providers are efficient whereas high-cost providers are not. In view of the history of human services POS programs and prior regulatory methods, this approach to defining efficiency may be extremely misleading.

We know that human service regulation did not, until recently, contain strong incentives for provider cost control. One might suspect that not only are the costs of some individual providers high but also that the entire current cost range of providers is higher than necessary. For example, we might ascertain that the current per diem cost for residential child-care providers ranges from $100 to $250. We do not know if this cost should in fact range from $50 to $200 or even be lower.

We also recognize that current costs are a reflection of past expenditure decisions, many of which cannot be easily undone, for example, a provider's fixed costs for prior plant and equipment purchases. We cannot relocate providers with "excessive" facility costs or replace their services in short order, even given the capital financing and political will to do so. Hence, as limited as our knowledge of truly reasonable costs is, we may have difficulty implementing cost controlling rate decisions.

Goal 3: Establishing Payment Rates That Keep Provider and Program Costs at Reasonable Levels

The lack of scientific basis for determining reasonable cost, coupled with the provider's historical resource commitments, detract from the setting of "ideal" rates, however they are derived. Rate-setting is, moreover, a highly politically-charged undertaking and one in which providers frequently have a great deal of power. It is their program that is regulated, and they are often the only source of information crucial to making rate decisions. This is true of "hard" cost data that can be obtained in an ongoing cost-reporting system. It is equally true of the knowledge of day-to-day program and fiscal operations necessary to evalute the reasonableness of costs. Hence, whenever rate setters seek to control payments, providers can be expected to utilize their monopoly on information to explain why costs are different than they appear and why they cannot be easily controlled. These arguments may well extend to claims of higher service quality, which are politically appealing yet difficult to evaluate empirically.

Finally, individually and in the aggregate, providers hold the ultimate trump card: total or selective withdrawal from the POS program. Rate decisions that appear eminently desirable from a cost perspective take on an impossible light if this card is played.

RECOMMENDATIONS

Despite these severe limitations to the foundations of rate-setting, steps can be taken both to further the state of the art and to better work within current constraints.

Strategies for Improving the State of the Art

In the current political climate, recommendations for increased federal involvement and funding are problematic. Despite the intent to limit human services spending and deregulate federal program involvement, the federal role of technology development and transfer may continue to be seen as valid.

Given this expectation and recognition of fiscal constraints, federal support should be given for a social service rate-setting evaluation and research and development (R & D) program. The most immediate need is for an inventory and a straightforward evaluation of state rate-setting practices in major social service categories (e.g., day care, institutional foster care). Currently, there is no central (i.e., federal) repository of sample rate-setting practices, let alone a comprehensive inventory. This condition forces each state to mount its own independent rate-setting development effort, often at high cost and without the benefit of other states' learning experiences.

To be most useful, such an inventory of rate-setting practices should include a pragmatic and technical description of the rate-setting models as well as an evaluative component. Technical description should define the mechanics of the rate-setting methods, including rate structures, accounting/cost-finding procedures, and actual rate decision making strategies. The evaluation component should assess the administrative burden of the methods; the extent of provider technical compliance with reporting requirements; and a basic (not unnecessarily sophisticated) assessment of the impact of the rate-setting models on cost controls, service quality, and service availability goals.

The benefits of such an inventory would be threefold. First, a repository of current practices would be created that could be used in a technology transfer mode. Second, the extent to which current practices approach the state of the art would be identified. Third, fruitful directions for research and development would be identified.

We would anticipate that the proposed initial evaluation would identify R & D needs in areas such as

Model accounting and cost-reporting systems linking POS providers and the funding source,
Analytical methods for analysis of POS program costs factors, and
Analytical models for interprovider comparisons.

One particularly fruitful approach would be for the funding source to offer providers computerized accounting packages in a service bureau mode. For instance, a state department of social services would develop a model accounting system for residential treatment programs. Providers would utilize these data for storage and analysis of basic accounting data. This would, in turn, provide the state agency with a flexible cost data file with which to meet its analytical rate-setting needs. Obviously, the philosophy underlying such an effort would have to recognize that fiscal management is the internal responsibility of each provider. Hence, the funding source should not serve as the providers' accountant. The funding source would simply act as a vendor making an accounting system available to providers.

Improvements to the State of the Art

Administrators who must deal with rate-setting obviously cannot suspend their efforts until a research program unfolds. In the interim they must attempt to operate within the state of the art. First, the administrator-rate setter must strive to put rate setting in a proper and supported context vis-à-vis other regulatory and management efforts. It is especially important to acknowledge that rate-setting decisions cannot be made without adequate planning and program evaluation.

The planning information required to support rate setting is a reasonably accurate estimate of client demands for POS services and POS provider capacity to meet such demands. The requirement for these data is that efforts to control rates (program costs) may well be contrary to provider recruitment (service availability goals). Specifically, the approach most often taken with rate-setting cost control is to limit rates to some level less than the higher range of provider costs. This approach places high-cost providers in the position of withdrawing from program participation. It may also reduce the incentive for potential providers to enter the service market.

The criterion for setting rate limits may thus be the impact of those limits on service availability versus client demand. Limitations in basic planning data, often found in social service programs, deprive the administrator-rate setter of this key criterion.

The funding source should take seriously the issue of the financial management skills of POS providers. It is one thing to set incentives for cost control behavior via limitation of rate increases. It is quite a separate problem for POS providers to analyze their cost experience and identify methods for increasing efficiency. Research in health care rate-setting has shown that providers (e.g., hospital administrators) often do not possess such an orientation or skill. This may be due to the limited cost control requirements placed on providers in previous years (e.g., program development era).

The same problem can be expected in social service voluntary agencies such as residential treatment, family services, and day care. Historically, such programs have operated without the level of cost containment that exists today. Furthermore, the managers of many of these programs have been selected because of program knowledge rather than financial control skills.

The rate-setting funding source can address this potential problem both directly and indirectly. The development of improved cost reporting, particularly in prospective rate-setting models, can force providers to question costs in a serious manner and can provide the data necessary for answering initial cost questions. Beyond these indirect benefits of rate-setting, the funding source can, and probably should, consider programs of technical assistance to providers.

Finally, the rate-setting agency must adopt a pragmatic approach to defining and monitoring program quality standards that directly affect provider costs. Given the lack of acceptable outcome standards, the trend has been toward ever-increasing specification of component and process standard definitions. When these standards take on inflexible forms (e.g., staff-client ratios, required hours of programming), providers are deprived of the ability to combine inputs in an attempt to control costs. The funding source that continually promulgates such standards is itself defining mandatory increases in program costs for which POS providers should not be held accountable.

It is true that much of the responsibility for unnecessary or badly researched quality regulation lies at the federal level. The current interest in federal deregulation should, however, give state funding sources the latitude to reduce regulatory burdens on providers.

Conversion of POS Programs to Cash Transfer or Direct Service Programs

The best way to deal with the intractable problems of regulation and rate-setting is to avoid them entirely. This can be done to the extent that POS programs are converted to the alternative basic models of human service delivery.

The conversion of purchased social services to cash or voucher transfers is a distinct possibility. Day-care, homemaker, and family services are all programs for which a competitive market exists, or would exist in the absence of contractual regulation by public human services programs. They also are programs for which service costs can be readily calculated, hence, for which the value of a cash transfer sufficient for service purchase can be set.

The political climate for such converisons exists. The "cashing out" of social services has been a long-time interest of fiscal conservatives. In the past disadvantaged populations have opposed such actions as being merely budget control devices. However, representatives of social service beneficiaries are increasingly supportive of service deregulation. Their argument is that public purchase inevitably creates a maze of rules that is inflexible, unrelated to individual needs, and dehumanizing.

The conversion of POS programs to those directly managed and delivered by public funding sources is a less easily evaluated option. In general, society does not support such models, which are viewed as "socialized" forms of human services delivery. Yet, as the proportion of funding for such services increases, so too does the level of public regulation. Hence, regulation serves as management in absentia, and bad management at that.

The conservative drift in social program philosophy will meet a real anomaly in considering conversion of POS programs to direct management. On the one hand, it seeks to reduce government intervention and regulation. On the other hand, it seeks to apply modern management principles derived from the private sector.

Reliance on purchased human services avoids public ownership of such programs, but it deprives the only funding source of the basics of management control, substituting a web of ineffectual regulations.

Ideal social philosophy may have to bend to pragmatic operational realities. There are many social service programs in which government is not a sole or key purchaser. For these, reliance upon the POS model, if not a cash-out strategy, seems logical. However, there are a number of services for which government is the only funding source and in which POS models predominate, for example, most residential treatment programs. For these programs government may wish to acknowledge that it has acquired a responsibility from which it cannot divorce itself. Direct management and control of such programs by the public funding source would thus seem an option worthy of consideration.

175

11

Unit-Cost Contracting for Health and Social Services

Earlene Baumunk

U nit-cost contracting is essentially an agreement to pay a provider a fixed rate for each delivered unit of a standard defined service. It can range from full cost to a rate less than the cost of a provider delivering a service. It is sometimes called unit-price contracting and fee for service. Payments rendered to provider agencies under the terms of these contracts are made upon receipt of verification of service delivery on a service unit basis and only for actual units of service delivered.

Unit-cost contracting for human services has been utilized by governmental bodies on a limited scale for a number of years, but the complex myriad of federal regulations and guidelines has prevented widespread use. However, with the current national trend to deregulate, this form of contracting is assuming greater popularity and increasing importance.

Under a unit-cost contract system, cost determination is based upon the rate paid for a delivered unit of service rather than budgetary line items or functional categories. Such information regarding program operational costs is critical to planning, resource allocation, and rate-setting. At a time when those in human services are faced with crucial decisions regarding who receives what and how much, the unit-cost system can help make administrative cost decisions more objective. Since diversity in the process itself is possible, unit-cost contracts can also be implemented and administered in a variety of ways.

THE UNIT-COST PROCESS

The basic unit-cost process is characterized by the simplicity of the contracting procedure, a stress on performance and adaptability to changing circumstances.

176

The first step in any service procurement system is the initial decision as to which service(s) to purchase and what quantity to purchase. This procedure involves assessing service objectives and needs, defining a unit of service, determining the rate necessary to obtain the service, and ascertaining the number of units desired and/or obtainable under available funding.

The definition of services, their units of measure, and the mechanisms for rate-setting are essential to the unit-cost contracting process. Each party to the agreement needs to know precisely its expected responsibilities under the obligation. Specifically delineating the services to be delivered or the task to be accomplished at an agreed-upon rate of payment could have a direct influence on the quality of the contractor's performance and the nature of the results obtained. This forms the criteria upon which the evaluation of the service provided will be made.

The designation of a specified unit of service and a fair and reasonable rate under a unit-cost system may also encourage the entrance of new providers into the vendor network. By purchasing desired services from among the largest number of potential provider agencies, reputable agencies can be selected and the quality of services improved. The unit-cost concept emphasizes a review of agency capabilities prior to formal contracting. Final selection of a provider agency can be based on an evaluation of the agency's ability to provide the service(s) as well as insuring an adequate financial and management system.

With the institution of uniform rates, the establishment of program standards and a standard defined unit of service, the need for lengthy contract negotiations can be reduced. A unit-cost boilerplate need not be lengthy or detailed, specifying only those rights and obligations necessary under state and federal laws and for the protection of both the governmental agency and the contractor. Annexes may be attached to the primary document to detail those mutual obligations agreed upon during the negotiation stage. The relationship between the contracting parties during this stage is of a legal nature. The contract is the prime reference for all matters concerning performance. As with any method of contracting, the public agency will need to retain a strong capacity to evaluate the service for which it has legal responsibility.

Unit-cost monitoring and evaluation focus the review on the provider agency programming and fiscal management systems and away from budgets and expenditure/cost patterns. Since fixed-rate contracts provide an incentive for contractors to contain costs possible at the expense of service quality, program monitoring is essential. Yet balance is necessary. To the extent that detailed control over the provider agency is built into the contract, the adherence to a pure cost system and product-focused benefits will be diminished.

Contract payments can be based upon documentation that the prescribed units of service were actually delivered. Whenever possible, payments should be coordinated with an evaluation of the contractor's performance to date. Contract close-out would require only the completion of payment for the total units of service delivered. Evaluation of contract performance, further need for service, and availability of funding would determine future contracting with a provider.

DEFINITION OF THE UNIT OF SERVICE

Basic to unit-cost contracting is the designation of a precise unit of service and its method of measure. The greater the specificity with which a unit of service is defined, the more accurately a count of the units of service delivered will measure contract performance (Bowers and Bowers 1976).

Frequently, the precise purpose of social services has not been agreed upon by those purchasing services, those delivering services, or the public at large. The former Title XX requirements for a state comprehensive annual services program plan and for the reporting of subsequent services to state and federal governmental authorities assisted in the effort to define services and their standardized unit. However, many Title XX state plans intermingled definitions of services, problems, and target populations (Whiteneck 1975). The United Way of America has also attempted to provide a uniform and comparable service identification through a goal-structured method of defining and conceptually organizing social services. However, service definitions are still in a developmental state, and consensus as to what constitutes a service unit varies greatly for many services.

In the health industry, the prospective payment system/diagnostic related groups development during the last several years has stimulated much greater specificity in the units of hospital-delivered services.

The service definition determines the manner in which the unit costs will be ascertained. In the past, service definitions were frequently input-oriented. Many national standards for human services focused upon inputs (e.g., child-staff ratios for child day care [Elkin 1980]). This meant that the service effort was measured by quantifying resources such as money, personnel, materials, facilities, and equipment applied to a service. Budgets have usually identified this input information.

The development of unit-cost analysis in the human services has provided the methodology to assess a service at the several stages of delivery (ibid.). The components of a service effort are subdivided. For example, management costs are segregated from program activities, and these components, in turn, are separated by service function.

The emphasis in unit-cost contracting is on performance or output (ibid.). The service definition is measured by quantifying what is produced by service delivery unit (e.g., day of care, hours of counseling). The development of unit-cost analysis has made it possible to define service in such a manner. The most difficult service definition to quantify is that based upon the products of service (e.g., adoption of child or maintenance of an elderly person in his or her own home ([Elkin 1980]). This is due to an inability to collect the necessary information about outcomes and the complexity of the service provision.

In the medicare prospective payment system, the hospitals are paid a predetermined fee subject to the diagnosis, controlled by patient characteristics, sex and age, and sometimes whether there are complicating factors. The measurement unit is the complete hospital stay (Altman 1986).

Interest in the further refinement of service definitions has arisen out of a recognized need for greater accountability of service accomplishments in order to justify social service expenditures. The unit-cost concept permits decision makers to more accurately plan, budget, and match services to citizens' needs.

By altering the unit measurement in Medicare, changes in the acute care general hospital system were substantial. Unit-cost contracting can indeed be very powerful.

The mechanism for setting rates is a crucial element in the unit-cost contracting system, not only because of its obvious implications for cost, but also because it can influence the quantity and quality of service. Most human service unit-cost contracting in the past has been on a cost reimbursement basis. Under unit-cost reimbursement procedures, a cost per unit of service is established for each agency individually by use of budget projections and/or historical cost data. Such a method results in as many different unit costs as there are agencies selected to deliver contracted services. This system results in high administrative costs since it requires a separate contract to be developed with each service provider.

Rate-setting procedures should maximize the funds available for service by minimizing the time and effort spent on individual examination of provider costs. Fixed-rate schedules, which are applied equally to all vendors providing a defined service, remain constant during the contract and are not subject to renegotiation or adjustment either during or after the contract period.

States vary greatly in their methods of rate determination. Rates paid to provider agencies reflect such factors as the number of available service providers (supply), service or client priority (demand), industry average price, provider network historical operating cost data, geographic costs factors, amount of funds available and/or appropriated, service complexity, and other related elements.

When Not to Use Unit-Cost Contracting

Unit-cost contracting is not applicable in all cases. Other contract processes such as cost reimbursement are more suitable when the costs and performance are so uncertain that a reliable price estimate cannot be established. This may occur because a service is needed immediately or it is impossible to determine in advance the precise quantities or location of service delivery. Other contract methods would also best serve unique, hard to define, services.

When to Use Unit-Cost Contracting

Unit-cost contracting is likely to be appropriate for the purchase of the bulk of health and social services. Those services that are the most easily and precisely defined are the most vulnerable to unit-cost contracting. Also enhancing is an environment in which there exists adequate competition among responsible contractors.

As with all accounting tools, the unit-cost concept is only another step in the human services overall contracting process. Yet it meets a number of objectives necessary for government purchase of service programs today. Chief among these objectives are the opportunities to

More appropriately refocus the emphasis in purchase of service arrangements to service delivery (output) and away from rigid

180

    scrutinization and regulation of budget, expenditure, and pro-
gramming activities (input);

Achieve major improvements in realization levels of provider agency
accountability; and

Utilize a system capable of being effectively administered when the capabilities of administrative staff are reduced.

PART FOUR

Implementing Purchase of Service Arrangements: Case Examples

In this section five case examples are offered of purchase of service arrangements "in action." The implementation phase of contracting refers to "real life" experiences, in which alternative delivery methods are put to the test and the public-private sector relationship becomes an actuality.

The implementation phase of purchase of service (or any policy or practice, for that matter) is dynamic in nature, involving the interplay between public and private agencies and their staffs at all levels. The relationship takes on life as the particular program or service that is the subject of the contract becomes a reality. It is the question of what happens in the implementation of the contractual relationship that is the focus of concern in the case studies presented in this section. In fact, it is primarily (if not exclusively) through the study of specific cases of contracting that we are able to gain insight into and draw conclusions from the issues and problems that may arise.

The articles in this section focus on the implementation of purchase of service arrangements from the perspective of both the public and voluntary sectors. In any relationship perceptions about issues, benefits, and problems arising during its course are likely to vary, e.g., what is seen as highly problematic to one party may be seen as a less severe problem to the other. There may also be areas in which there is a convergence of views regarding problems and issues. What we do know from human interactions is that, no matter how good the relationship, it is inevitable that it will evidence both strengths and weaknesses. The case studies presented in this section substantiate the notion that contractual interactions, too, give rise to tensions, even though they may rest on a solid relationship base.

Kettner and Martin maintain that the use of POS requires systematic planning, with consideration to price, quality, and effectiveness.

Reviewing five major studies of decision making in state human service agencies, they detail a series of factors and questions for consideration in the use of contracting. They argue that, on the basis of known priorities, traditions, and conditions, decision-making criteria can be devised and applied to the selection of the optimal mode of service delivery in a given situation.

The authors share in common an interactional view of the purchase of service relationship, e.g., although they may approach their subject from the perspective of one sector, it is the concept of partnership that is used to analyze the nature and cause(s) of implementation issues or problems. Wolock focuses explicitly on these organizational dynamics as the analytic framework for assessing contractual relationships. She sees contracting as an important vehicle for changing the orientation of the public agency from that of "people changing" to "people processing," the latter referring to a primary role of classifying and referring clients to other organizations that will actually provide the service(s). The experiences of one public welfare agency with contracting for child protective services are examined by Wolock to determine whether and to what degree POS is consistent with and encouraging of new sector role orientations. The findings suggest that the extent to which POS can successfully contribute to a changing agency orientation depends, in large part, on the clear articulation and fulfillment of new roles and functions by each of the organizational partners and their degree of collaboration.

Ten Broeck (using a descriptive framework) and Roberts-DeGennaro (using a political-economic framework) both view the contractual relationship from the primary perspective of the public child welfare agency. Roberts-DeGennaro concludes that, in the case of contracting for special needs adoption services in one state, the program implementation was marred by poor or miscommunications, lack of trust and lack of knowledge about the respective roles of the public and private agency partners. Ten Broeck, studying the implementation of a new state law mandating that private child foster care services be used when such compare favorably in quality and cost to those the public agency is providing or could provide, notes a history of similar contractual relationship problems. On the other hand, she highlights the extent to which POS arrangements can be used to stimulate private sector change and ensure that the services delivered under POS are in keeping with the needs and intent of the public contracting agency. These two authors reach the similar con-

184

clusion that clear role delineation, specification of procedures, processes, and expectations, proper maintenance of the case management functions by the public sector, and clear accountability and reporting requirements are essential ingredients of a successful contractual partnership.

The premise that POS can serve to influence or change the mode of operation, performance, or even mission of one or the other sector is important, as it implies that expectations about the contractual relationship may go behind its utility and value as a service delivery mechanism. This premise suggests that POS, through the "power of the purse" and the desire of private agencies to win contract awards to support, expand, or modify their programs, may place the public agency in the position of, or at least condone, exercising a control function. It is clear that the public sector's ever-increasing demands for contract specificity (what will be delivered by whom and to whom and how often), documentation of how the contracted program will help meet public goals, and accountability and reporting requirements are based on the premise that alterations in the operating modes of voluntary agencies is a reasonable exchange for the receipt of public dollars. Either it is assumed that the voluntary providers can easily and willingly make these procedural accommodations or, perhaps, such matters are not even considered. At issue for the not-for-profit sector are the nontangible costs of such intrusions into operations, including the perceived risks to their autonomy, mission, and philosophy.

The case studies offered in this section suggest that there is real concern on the part of the public agency about the process by which private agencies will provide contracted service(s), as well as the products they will deliver and their outcomes. The appropriateness of such process concerns may certainly be open to scrutiny. It is somewhat surprising that the voluntary sector has acquiesced to the degree it has; the power of the purse may, indeed, be a major influence on organizational behavior. The end result, however, may be the creation of a "contracted human services system," or quasi-public sector in place of the voluntary sector as it has traditionally been characterized.

The emergence of this quasi-public type of agency is, in part, addressed by Rathgeb Smith, who explores the implications of accepting public funds on the voluntary sector. Using four types of contracted programs that service victims of crime (child abuse, rape, spouse abuse, and crimes against the elderly) as case examples, this author focuses on the changes that occur in the structure, staffing, client populations served, and mission of not-for-profit agencies and how the availability and use of federal funds affects the overall network of services offered by the voluntary sector. With the exception of child abuse, services to victims of crime were by and large of a self-help nature or nonexistent prior to the availability of federal funding. Here, it was not a question of transferring service delivery responsibility from the public sector, but rather initiating or expanding services through the voluntary sector that were otherwise not provided.

Rathgeb Smith found that the not-for-profit agencies providing services to the four types of victims of crimes all experienced problems associated with lack of secure, long-term funding and that start-up and extensive down time due to delays in payment were pervasive. The lack of long-term commitment to these service programs was, to some extent, countered by the legitimacy bestowed upon them. The author also found that even the more established agencies were subject to considerable impact when they became recipients of public funds, including the types of personnel they hired and the degree of professional orientation they manifested. The impact of public funds on these not-for-profit service providers was anything but neutral.

Money is a powerful influence in many, if not most, transactions, and the nature and dynamics of public-private sector relationships are surely not exempt. Purchasing services has, in fact, often been justified on the widely based (but largely unproven) assumption that such arrangements lead to dollar savings over public sector provision. From the very outset, then, one intent of forming "partnerships" is to ensure cost benefits for both parties. The "costs" of the cost-benefits, however, may not be as easily conceptualized or measured. The need to accumulate a body of experiential and empirical evidence highlighting the conditions under which POS can and does impact positively upon the "partnership" as well as the efficiency, cost, and effectiveness of health and human services is a given, but as yet unachieved, agenda.

Making Decisions about Purchase of Service Contracting

Peter M. Kettner and Lawrence L. Martin

For the past two decades, purchase of service contracting (POSC) has been the preferred method of delivering services to people in need. Each year literally billions of dollars are expended under POSC contracts, providing services from child day care to home-delivered meals for the elderly.

The phenomenon of POSC for human services descended rather suddenly upon the states in the early 1970s. As a result, most POSC policies and procedures were developed under severe time pressures. Knowledge of POSC for human services was somewhat limited as well. To meet the demand for POSC within the allotted time, most states established their POSC policies and procedures with only two goals in mind: to provide services and to devise a simple and routine contracting system. These twin goals tended to promote a partnership arrangement between states and their contractors. By the mid-1980s, this arrangement had become institutionalized in states as the dominant POSC approach.

Today, however, a new school of thought is arising to challenge the dominance of the partnership approach. This trend addresses factors such as the infusion of competition and the power of market forces in determining costs for human services. A recent study by H. P. Hatry and E. Durman describes the kinds of issues being raised:

What human services lend themselves to competition?
What degree of competition is appropriate?
Who should be eligible to compete as contractors: government agencies, nonprofits, for-profits?
Are there sufficient numbers of potential human services contractors to provide for real competition?
Do the benefits of competition outweigh the costs?

As the impact of declining federal financial assistance to states for human services becomes more pervasive, pressures will increase to stretch fewer and fewer dollars to cover more and more services. Clearly, questions about the price, quality, and effectiveness of POSC will become increasingly relevant in the human services.

To improve decision making in this important area of professional practice, we must turn to the emerging body of knowledge on POSC, including all relevant theoretical perspectives and research findings. This article attempts to create a conceptual framework that can be used by government agencies in systematically thinking about the use of POSC for human services. For a foundation, we draw upon five major studies of decision making in state human services agencies.

WHY AGENCIES USE POSC

To understand the rationale behind government agency POSC decisions, we turn to five empirical studies conducted during the 1970s. They are Booz-Allen and Hamilton 1971; Wedel 1974; Urban Institute (Benton, Field, and Millar) 1978; Pacific Consultants 1979; and American Public Welfare Association 1981.

Booz-Allen and Hamilton, a management consulting firm, studied the POSC activities of the state agencies in California, Pennsylvania, and Wisconsin; these three state agencies were among the first to use POSC for human services. This study represents the first empirical research on the subject of why government human services agencies engaged in POSC. Booz-Allen and Hamilton concluded that there were four major reasons these state agencies opted for POSC.

1. *To provide for client choice and to satisfy unmet need.* The dramatic increase in client caseloads and a decision to provide clients with a choice of services (for example, public or private) were cited. At the time, all three state agencies were unable to respond directly to the rising demand for human services. The agencies also believed that many clients preferred receiving services from private, nonprofit agencies.

2. *To provide services not suitable to government delivery.* Some services appeared to lend themselves more readily to POSC than to direct government provision. Examples cited include: monitoring and evaluation of government-operated programs, legal aid services, services provided dur-

ing nonregular work hours, and certain specialized services such as those provided by the big brother/big sister programs.

3. *To increase the type and amount of services provided through the use of private (for example, donated) funds.* In several instances, local, private, nonprofit agencies provided the 25 percent matching funds, enabling the state agencies to earn the 75 percent federal participation. The report concluded that in such instances the state agencies essentially became "conduits to obtain federal matching."

4. *To convert existing programs to new federal funding sources—the human services titles of the Social Security Act.* The greatest impetus for the use of POSC in California, Pennsylvania, and Wisconsin, the study concluded, was the termination of federal support in some program areas. Coupled with that was a state impetus to shift the financial burden for other previously state-supported services to the federal government.

Wedel. By 1973 all fifty states used some POSC for human services. K. R. Wedel looked at all fifty state social service agencies in an attempt to understand motivations for adopting POSC as a service delivery mode. From the limited literature available at the time, Wedel developed a list of the twenty-three most frequently cited factors used either in support of or opposition to the concept of POSC.

The most prominent and commonly recurring theme in the Wedel study focused on federal-state-private agency relationships as the reason for state involvement with POSC. Other frequently mentioned reasons included increased federal and private funding, increased public control and accountability, increased cooperation between public and private agencies, and the strengthening of the nonprofit sector. A second theme dealt with service delivery issues such as increased consumer choice; greater quantity, quality, and flexibility of service delivery; and the opportunity to provide new talent not previously available to clients of public human services. A third theme was the availability, or lack thereof, of potential contractors; and a desire to reduce the size of the public bureaucracy and payroll was the fourth theme.

The Urban Institute focused on the implementation of the Title XX program, including POSC activity, in eight states: Arizona, California, Iowa, Michigan, New York, North Carolina, Oregon, and Texas. State agencies were asked to comment on the formal or informal criteria used in deciding to provide a service directly or to engage in POSC. The Urban

Institute analysis revealed that cost and match availability were no longer as important in POSC decision making as they had been before. The most frequently mentioned decision criterion was tradition, suggesting that the POSC practices of states had become fairly routine by 1978. The second most frequently mentioned criterion was community policies and pressures. Service system considerations such as the availability of staff, state agency capacity to provide service directly, and the availability of potential contractors continued to be important.

Pacific Consultants studied implementation of POSC under Title XX of the Social Security Act in nine states: California, Colorado, Delaware, Georgia, Indiana, Massachusetts, Oklahoma, Utah, and Washington.

The study identified four key variables affecting when and how state agencies utilize POSC for human services. According to the report the POSC behavior of state agencies only can be understood in terms of the interaction among these four key variables.

The first variable was the nature of the service to be provided. Existing capacity within a given state or community, according to Pacific Consultants, may well be the most powerful determinant as to whether a service will be provided directly or through POSC. The example of child day care supports this contention. When most states decided that day care services should be provided, they also were essentially deciding to engage in POSC since few states operated child day care facilities.

The second variable, the organizational structure of the government agency, pointed out that large multiprogram state human services agencies may use POSC less because they have more internal service delivery options.

The third variable was planning and budgetary considerations. POSC can be affected by seemingly unrelated government decisions such as needs-based planning and hiring freezes. For example, needs-based planning can identify a need for a level of service beyond the government's capacity to deliver it directly or for services not provided by the government at all. In the same vein, a governmental agency hiring freeze to reduce a state budget deficit can have a direct effect on POSC activity by making POSC the only available service delivery option.

The fourth variable identified by Pacific Consultants was organizational philosophy. By the time of this study, philosophy was beginning to influence some POSC decisions of state agencies. The study found that in seven of the nine states, there was a basic philosophy that POSC should be used when it was a more efficient and effective mode of service delivery. The study noted, however, that clearly operationalized definitions of the terms "efficient" and "effective" had not been developed.

The American Public Welfare Association (APWA) study covered five states: South Carolina, Arizona, Colorado, New Hampshire, and Wisconsin. The study focused on six services—counseling, employment, family planning, homemaker, legal services, and transportation, selected because they were considered by APWA to be ones for which state agencies truly have a choice between direct delivery and POSC.

Agencies were asked to rate the relative influence of seven variables on their POSC decisions:

Public-private agency relationships;
POSC experience in their own or another state;
Federal encouragement;
Enhancement of client services;
Availability of contractors;
Cost savings; and
Redirection of the state agency away from direct service to more management-type functions.

The APWA study concluded that only one variable—enhancement of client services—was clearly a high priority in all service areas. Two variables—cost savings and availability of contractors—had a mixed effect. All other variables were consistently rated as having a low influence. While not identified as one of the seven study variables, the state agencies mentioned political concerns as a major influence. Some specific examples included making POSC the only services delivery option and pressures exerted by both public and private sector contractors.

COMMON THEMES

Based on the findings of the five studies, a number of common factors emerge as central considerations affecting POSC decisions. These factors and related questions can serve as guideposts in POSC decision making and policy formulation.

Factors and Questions To Be Considered in the Use of POSC

Factors	Questions
Category 1—Productivity, Fiscal, and Cost Considerations	
1. Lowering the cost of services	Are costs for the service higher than is reasonable? Are funding cutbacks for the service anticipated?
2. Increasing fiscal control and accountability	Have questions been raised about the reasonable use of funds? Are fiscal controls considered adequate?
3. Increasing service outputs	Can the volume of service outputs be increased by either direct delivery or POSC?
Category 2—Planning, Designing, and Funding Considerations	
4. Fit of service type to government or private delivery	Are there special service considerations, such as monitoring or evaluation of government programs, advocacy, potential political involvement, etc., that indicate a better service fit with direct delivery or POSC?
5. Flexibility in targeting resources to meet need	Are there seasonal variations in the demand for service? Does the service intervention emphasis change over time (e.g., from treatment to prevention, from therapy to medication)?
6. Availability and capability of contractors	Are there adequate numbers of existing or potential contractors for the service?
7. Utilization of multiple funding sources	Is there reason to believe that the total dollars available for the service could be increased (a multiplier effect) as the result of either direct delivery or POSC?
Category 3—Improving Services to Clients	
8. Improving the quality and outcome of services	Does evidence exist that service quality or outcome is better via direct delivery or POSC?
9. Improving client access to services	Have questions been raised about getting the "right" services to those most in need? Are services located where need is greatest?
Category 4—Government Organizational and Policy Considerations	
10. Government agency philosophy regarding POSC	Is there a formal or informal agency preference for either direct delivery or POSC?
11. Capacity of the government agency to directly deliver services	Is there an adequate direct service delivery capability within the government agency to provide, or would the capability have to be developed?
Category 5—Legal Requirements	
12. Legal requirements	Does law, statute, regulation, or ordinance require either direct delivery or POSC?
Category 6—Politics and Loyalties	
13. History and tradition	Is there a traditional pattern of direct delivery or POSC?
14. Politics and community pressures	Who wins and who loses as the result of direct delivery or POSC?

Toward a Conceptual Framework. We can conceptualize POSC decision making as a series of three sequential decisions. The first involves choosing between total direct delivery, a mix of direct delivery and POSC, or total POSC.

If a mix of direct delivery and POSC or total POSC is called for, the next decision is to select a POSC approach. The final decision is to select the POSC administrative mechanisms to be used.

The First Decision—Determining the Service Delivery Mode. Utilizing the common factors identified as affecting POSC decisions in the five studies, questions can be formulated to serve as a guide in determining which delivery mode is most appropriate. Clearly it is necessary to make an independent decision for each individual service. The factors presented in Table 12.1 can apply to any service.

It is unlikely that clear-cut, definitive responses can be given to many of the questions that affect POSC decisions. A "no" response, however, should not be interpreted as ruling out a particular service delivery option. Rather, a "yes" response indicates that a particular service delivery option is more appropriate than another.

While logic and previous experience may support a particular perspective, a good deal of testing remains to be done. The guidelines set forth in Table 12.1 ideally should be viewed as hypothese, requiring revision in light of subsequent empirical research. For example, research findings have not established that either direct delivery or POSC leads to a lower cost or better service quality. Some research has shown that productivity went up and cost went down when directly provided services were contracted as well as when contracted services were subsequently directly provided by government. Why? A change itself, a Hawthorne effect, can increase productivity apart from any inherent characteristic of either direct delivery or POSC.

Finally, certain factors such as laws or regulations can themselves determine the service delivery mode. In most situations, however, a mix of factors must be weighed to develop a sense of the optimal service delivery mode.

The Second Decision—Selecting a POSC Approach. If examination shows total direct delivery as the most viable option, no further consideration of POSC decision factors is required. If, however, there is to be

Table 12.1. Guidelines for Decision Making in Purchase of Service Contracting

Factors	Total direct	Mix of direct and POSC	Total POSC
Productivity, Fiscal, and Cost Considerations			
1. Lowering the cost of services is a high priority	No clear service delivery pattern indicated		
2. Increasing fiscal control is a high priority	Yes	No	No
3. Increasing service volume is a high priority	No clear service delivery pattern indicated		
Planning, Designing, and Funding Considerations			
4. Nature of service raises problems for:			
—direct delivery	No	No	Yes
—POSC	Yes	No	No
5. Flexibility in targeting resources is a high priority	No	No	Yes
6. Availability and capability of contractors:			
—there are an adequate number of capable contractors	No	Yes	Yes
—there are few capable contractors	No	Yes	No
—there are no capable contractors	Yes	No	No
7. Funding considerations:			
—total direct delivery will increase resources	Yes	No	No
—a mix of public/private funding will increase resources	No	Yes	Yes
—total POSC will increase resources	No	No	Yes
Improving Services to Clients			
8. Improving quality and outcomes of service is a high priority	No clear service delivery pattern indicated		
9. Improving access is a high priority	No	Yes	Yes
Government Organizational and Policy Considerations			
10. Governement agency philosophy promotes:			
—direct delivery	Yes	No	No
—POSC	No	No	Yes
11. Limited agency resources prohibit direct delivery	No	No	Yes
Legal Requirements			
12. Law or regulation requires direct delivery	Yes	No	No
Politics and Loyalties			
13. History and tradition promote collaboration	No	Yes	Yes
14. Politics and political pressures promote POSC	No	No	Yes

Figure 12.1. **The Partnership Model/Market Model Continuum**

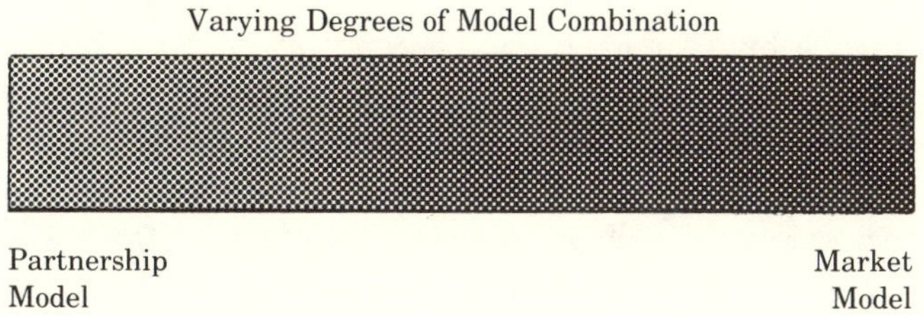

Varying Degrees of Model Combination

Partnership   Market
Model   Model

a mix of direct delivery and POSC, or total POSC, then an approach to POSC must be selected.

We have found that approaches to POSC for human services fall between two extremes—the partnership model and the market model, as illustrated in Figure 12.1.

We define the partnership model of POSC as a set of policies and practices—on the part of the public contracting agency—that view government and the private sector as a part of a comprehensive human services system and where the determining factor in selection of contractors is a concern for the development and maintenance of the human services system. A public contracting agency pursuing the partnership model would emphasize the strengthening of working relationships between government funding sources and contractors and would be flexible and compromising in the development, negotiation, and administration of contracts. Normally the agency would make POSC decisions primarily on the basis of concern for the stability of the human services system and therefore would promote specialization, rather than competition, among contractors in order to capitalize on public/private sector strengths.

In our partnership model, the government and the private sector interact as partners in a joint venture. The POSC process is founded on two equal partners attempting to maximize the human services system's outputs. This approach calls for a high degree of cooperative interaction between the public contracting agency and contractors, particularly in planning, designing services, budgeting, and monitoring and evaluating progress.

We define the market model as a set of policies and practices (on the part of the public contracting agency) that encourages competition

195

among potential contractors; and, where like contractors are competing to provide a like service, price is the determining factor. The market model places a high value on cost efficiency. An agency following the market method would emphasize development of criteria for measuring efficiency and effectiveness and negotiate with a high degree of specificity on issues of performance expectations, program design, budget, and cost. The agency would make POSC decisions primarily on the basis of cost and price and would encourage experimentation with alternative methods of service delivery. Under this model, resources would be marked for the recruitment and development of a pool of potential contractors.

In the market model of POSC, the public contracting agency is seen as a purchaser of human services and the contractor as a supplier. The POSC process becomes a procurement process, with both sides attempting to maximize efficiency and effectiveness through precise definition of contract expectations. The infusion of competition and market forces into POSC is a primary goal of this market model.

The partnership model and the market model are rarely, if ever, put into operation as pure types. In practice, the overall POSC approach of a public contracting agency would tend more toward one approach or the other. For this reason, the partnership model and the market model are conceptualized as extremes on a continuum (see Figure 12.1).

The Pacific Consultants study suggested that the nature of a service might cause a public contracting agency to select the partnership model in one instance and the market model in another. For example, a partnership model might be selected for use in POSC for adoption services, given the intensive nature of this service. A market model, however, might be used for child day care services, given the large supply of potential contractors. Within any public contracting agency, the range of POSC services might fall along a continuum, as depicted in Figure 12.2.

The POSC decision factors and questions derived from the five studies also can used by government contracting agencies to determine whether a partnership model or a market model is most appropriate for a particular program (see Table 12.2). The relationships between the fourteen POSC decision factors and the partnership model/market model are not offered as definite answers but more as logical conclusions in the absence of empirical evidence.

The Third Decision—Selecting POSC Administrative Mechanisms. Ideally, the development of a conceptual framework for POSC for human

Figure 12.2. **Where Services Might Fall on the Partnership Model/Market Model Continuum**

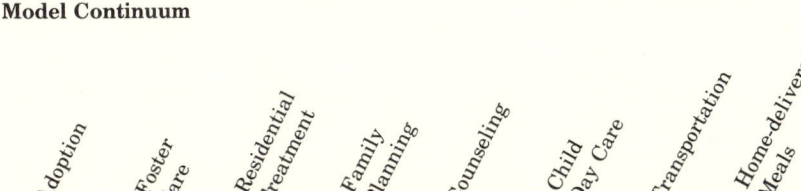

Partnership
Model

Market
Model

services should address both theoretical and technical issues and their interrelationships. We have found that certain administrative mechanisms are more compatible with the partnership model, while others are more compatible with the market model. Consistency between the choice of POSC model (goal) and the use of POSC administrative mechanisms (means) should be maintained.

The administrative mechanism of the request for proposals (RFP) is a characteristic of the partnership model; service considerations usually are given priority over cost and productivity concerns. Conversely, the invitation for a bid (IFB) is more characteristic of the market model because it makes cost the primary decision criterion and usually requires that the contract be awarded to the lowest bidder.

Cost-reimbursement contracts are more characteristic of the partnership model because the financial risk associated with contract performance is removed from the contractor: the contractor's service delivery costs are guaranteed under the terms of the contract. Unit cost, fixed-fee, and incentive contracts force contractors to assume responsibility for cost control and productivity. These types of contracts are considered to be more characteristic of the market model.

We associate multiyear contracts with the partnership model because of the increased stability they bring to the human services system.

197

Table 12.2. **Guidelines for Decision Making in Selecting an Approach to POSC**

Factors	Partnership model indicated	Market model indicated
Productivity, Fiscal, and Cost Considerations		
1. Lowering the cost of services is a high priority	No	Yes
2. Increasing fiscal control is a high priority	No	Yes
3. Increasing service volume is a high priority	Either model depending on availability and capability of contractors	
Planning, Designing, and Funding Considerations		
4. Nature of service raises problems for:		
—direct delivery	Yes	No
—POSC	No	No
5. Flexibility in targeting resources is a high priority	No	Yes
6. Availability and capability of contractors:		
—there is an adequate number of capable contractors	No	Yes
—there are few capable contractors	Yes	No
—delivery capability needs to be promoted	Yes	No
7. Funding considerations		
—a mix of public/private funding will increase resources	Yes	No
Improving Services to Clients		
8. Improving quality and outcomes of service to clients is a high priority	Either model depending on availability and capability of contractors	
9. Improving access is a high priority	Either model depending on availability and capability of contractors	
Government Organizational and Policy Considerations		
10. Government agency philosophy promotes POSC	Yes	Yes
11. Limited agency resources prohibit government delivery	Yes	Yes
Legal Requirements		
12. Law or regulation requires direct delivery	No	No
Politics and Loyalties		
13. History and tradition promote collaboration	Yes	No
14. Politics and political pressures promote POSC	Yes	No

Administrative Mechanisms

Partnership Model	Market Model
Use of request for proposals (RFP)	Use of invitation for bids (IFB)
Use of cost reimbursement contracts	Use of unit cost, fixed bee, and incentive contracts
Use of multiyear contracts	Use of single-year contracts
Use of government and nonprofit contractors	Use of government, nonprofit, and for-profit contractors

Single-year contracts are typical in the market model since they ensure competition on an annual basis.

Partnership relationships are less controversial when the question of profit is not an issue. We view the use of government and nonprofit organizations as typical of the partnership model. Conversely, the inclusion of for-profit contractors is defined as being more characteristic of the market model, because contracts are awarded to the lowest bidder providing the highest volume and best quality of service.

Purchase of service contracting in human services has become big business over the past decade. In its early years, states often were under pressure to develop POSC systems in a very short time and consequently responded in ways that seemed most expedient at the time. After more than a decade, however, experience has begun to reveal that there are better, more rational ways to design and manage POSC systems.

We have attempted here to develop a conceptual framework for analyzing a state's POSC system to determine if it is achieving optimum objectives. With more empirical study, we hope to move toward a theory of contracting for human services. Such a theory would allow resources to be allocated where they can be of the greatest benefit, not simply where they may be directed by political considerations.

13

Contracting as a People-Processing Mechanism in a Public Child-Welfare Agency

Isabel Wolock

A notable trend in public child-welfare agencies, in response to pressures from local, state, and federal agencies to coordinate services and reduce expenditures, has been to shift from a people-changing to a predominantly people-processing orientation. The primary function of people-changing organizations is to change the behavior of people or remedy some condition or problem. The essential function of people-processing organizations is the classification and disposition of people. *Classification* involves conferring some status or category upon an individual, e.g., mentally retarded, delinquent, child abuser; *disposition* entails facilitating or mediating the placement of the classified person in a special external system or unit, e.g., a school for the mentally retarded, correctional institution, or social agency (Hasenfeld 1972).

Consistent with this shift toward people-processing functions, public child-welfare agencies are increasingly assuming investigative, assessment, and service facilitator roles in protective service situations, i.e., classification and disposition. A concurrent phenomenon is the increased reliance on other agencies to provide services to these clients through purchase of service and other interorganizational arrangements. In this chapter the people-processing patterns of one public child welfare agency, the New Jersey Division of Youth and Family Services, are examined. The mechanisms by which the agency mediates the placement of clients in community agency programs and the effect of the use of these mechanisms on the agency's capability to function effectively as a people-

THE SPECIFIC type and levels of contracted service reported here pertain to the period in which the study was carried out.

200

processing organization are explored. Special attention is given to the purchase of service contract as a disposition mechanism.

THE CONTEXT OF PEOPLE PROCESSING

The response of external or market units to the "products" of people-processing organizations is crucial to their functioning (Hasenfeld 1972). The level of performance of such organizations depends, in large measure, upon the effectiveness of the external units as they work with clients. The effectiveness of a public child-welfare agency in alleviating and preventing child abuse and neglect thus depends, in large part, upon the effectiveness of those agencies working with the families of the public child-welfare agency under purchase of service contract.

For the public child-welfare agency to function effectively as a people-processing organization for protective service clients, a number of prerequisite conditions must be met. First, of course, is that protective service clients must be accepted for service by the contracted social agencies. The contracted (provider) agency must also retain the protective service client in service for the period of time necessary to reach service objectives.

The protective service client is often an involuntary client, i.e., he or she may not want the service believed necessary by the public welfare agency. These clients may have more difficult or different problems compared with those traditionally served by the provider agency. In addition, many protective service clients are resentful, apathetic, or fearful of services as a result of recurring failures, disappointments, disillusionments, and frustrations in past encounters with social agencies. These factors may lead to premature discontinuance of services, initiated either by the provider agency or the client. In order to prevent this occurrence, the provider agency must be flexible about the kind of client with whom it is willing to work and emphasize outreach activities to engage and motivate client participation in the service program.

Another condition is that provider agency services must be relevant to the special needs of protective service families. To illustrate, a common child maltreatment situation involves parental failure to provide sufficient and/or nutritious food to the child, gross inattention to the child's cleanliness and personal hygiene, and the neglect of serious medical conditions (Wolock and Horowitz 1978). In such cases it is important that homemaker services be provided to teach the parent how to purchase and

201

prepare nutritious meals within a limited budget, set up schedules for regular bathing and personal hygiene, and provide information and skills to the mother to enable her to better safeguard the health of her child. Day-care services for the same families should involve careful observation of the children to determine whether they are being fed and cared for adequately and whether medical problems improve or persist. Similarly, the material deprivation of many protective service families must be taken into account by the provider agencies. It is important that counseling at mental health centers and family agencies focus not only on the psychological roots of emotional problems, but also on the concrete and tangible bases of these problems such as unemployment, crowded and inadequate housing, and lack of job skills.

Strong lines of communication must be established between the public child-welfare and provider agencies. Public child-welfare agency staff must be kept well informed, for example, of the attendance or participation of the family or family member in the program, the progress being made, new problems that may arise, new incidents of abuse or neglect, and any changes that may have occurred in the family situation. Such information permits more accurate public agency evaluation and monitoring of the services provided to the protective service client based on the changing client situation and allows termination of services when appropriate. Concomitantly, the provider agency needs complete information on the family situation if it is to provide effective interventions.

Finally, it is crucial that the public child-welfare agency carry out systematic and ongoing evaluation to determine which services are delivered to protective service clients and their relevance to and effectiveness in alleviating clients' problems. Evaluation data enable the public child-welfare agency to identify service delivery problems and to take the necessary corrective action.

Protective service clients are typically in the service system involuntarily and come from the lowest socioeconomic strata with the most severe material, physical, and emotional problems. Their special problems and characteristics require intervention styles and strategies that depart in major ways from the more traditional pattern of helping. They represent a "hard to reach" group of clients that many agencies prefer not to service or find difficult to serve. It is argued that the prerequisite conditions of effective people-processing, as outlined above, will be met only to the degree that the public child-welfare agency is able to exercise control over the admission of protective service clients to the programs of other agencies and the kinds of services provided.[1]

Typically, the mechanisms used by the public child-welfare agency to mediate the placement of protective service clients in other agency programs afford the agency little or no leverage over their admission or the types of services provided to them. It is herein contended that the one mechanism that does give the agency control is the purchase of service contract, designed specifically for contracted protective services. These issues are examined utilizing data drawn from one public child-welfare agency, the New Jersey Division of Youth and Family Services (hereafter referred to as the Division). The mechanisms by which the Division mediates the placement of protective service clients (PRS) in other agencies are identified and data presented to assess the degree to which the five prerequisite conditions of effective people processing are met.

SOURCES OF DATA

Top level administrative staff in eleven district offices of the Division were interviewed concerning their own and their staff's experiences in working with other community agencies to provide services to PRS clients. It is recognized that a more complete picture would include the views of provider agency staff and PRS clients. However, independent of the validity of the data, it is clear that the staff believe they are reporting accurately and thus behave accordingly. The interviews were semistructured, two to four hours in length, and tape recorded. They focused on the relationship of each district office with other agencies in the community that were actual or potential providers of service to PRS clients. Questions pertained to the structure and nature of the relationships, problems involved in obtaining services, and the adequacy of services. The emphasis was on three key services recommended for PRS families: homemaker, day-care, and mental health services.

The eleven district offices were located in ten counties in northern New Jersey, a section of the state comprised primarily of highly urbanized central city areas but including suburban and rural communities as well as representing slightly more than half of the state's seven million people.

DESCRIPTION OF THE AGENCY

The Division is the primary child and family social service agency in New Jersey. Its major role stems from its legal mandate to provide protective services to children and families in which abuse or neglect has occurred. The agency is required by law to receive and investigate all reports of child abuse and neglect and to provide appropriate intervention and services in situations in which abuse or neglect was substantiated or in which there is deemed to be a high risk of child maltreatment. Services are provided by casework staff in twenty-five district offices administered through four regional offices and a central office. The majority of families supervised under the PRS program live in impoverished circumstances (Rosenthal 1977; Pelton 1981a).

The Division professes to be a people-changing organization; its primary stated objective is to change the behavior of parents so that they will provide more adequate care to their children and curtail abuse or neglect. The agency is responsible for developing, implementing, and monitoring service plans for endangered children and their families, including the provision of assistance to families with problems associated with child abuse and neglect. Although a number of Division programs provide services directly, federal legislative shifts had influenced the agency to emphasize service facilitator roles. Following the investigation of the reported child abuse and neglect situation and assessment of the family, the agency identifies service needs (e.g., day care, homemaker services, mental health services, or legal services) and arranges for clients to receive these services from another agency, thus functioning as a people-processing organization.

PURCHASING PRS SERVICES

There are several patterns by which the Division mediates the placement of PRS clients in other agency programs.[2] These patterns vary in the extent to which the arrangements with the provider agency are formalized, reimbursement mechanisms and the amount of reimbursement, and the degree of control the Division has over service delivery. The most informal pattern is the referral of a family or family member to an agency program with which the Division has no formal agreement or reimburses. The provider agency has the prerogative of accepting or rejecting the client and determines the types of services to be provided. Any collaboration or coordination that occurs between the two agencies is initiated at the individual practitioner level; it is not standardized or structured.

A second, and more formalized, pattern is the vendor agreement. Under this arrangement the district office is allocated funds from the state aid account to purchase homemaker service, day-care, and diagnostic psychological services, among others, for a small number of clients. In the case of homemaker services and day care, the Division conducts an initial evaluation of the program and develops a simple contract specifying the rate of reimbursement. Because the contract covers only the rate of reimbursement, the provider agency is under no obligation to accept Division referrals, retain Division clients, provide progress reports, or hold case conferences with Division staff. Similar to the first pattern, transactions between the two agencies are not standardized or structured; any joint planning or coordination of services is on an ad hoc basis at the individual practitioner level.

Another pattern for obtaining services is the purchase of service contract. Existing social service agencies are contracted to offer certain types of programs or services consistent with public agency priorities and funded through federal, state, or local sources. Each Division regional office designates a staff member to negotiate contracts with the region's provider agencies, provide technical assistance to contracted agencies, and monitor contract compliance and service delivery. The contract specifies the target population, types, and levels of services, intake procedures, budget and record keeping, personnel functions, and various reporting mechanisms. The provider agency is required to submit a proposal to the Division giving the rationale for the proposed program and detailing its major components. The Division, in consultation with other relevant public agencies, is responsible for selecting proposals, which may be sole source or competitive. State procedures require that contracts be renewed annually. Renewal is based on the performance of the provider agency, service priorities, and the availability of funds. Program modifications may be made at the time of contract renewal.

The Division's purchase of service contracts fall into two categories: those developed for the purpose of serving the general population of eligible residents in the community, and programs designed specifically for the Division's PRS clients. The community-wide programs, which comprise the majority of Division-administered purchase of service programs, seek to provide services to populations other than protective service clients. Although PRS clients are eligible for such programs, they are generally not accorded priority for admission nor are the services designed to meet PRS client needs. Those contracts that target PRS clients tend to restrict referrals to this population, often include mechanisms for public-private sector cooperation, and frequently specify the responsibilities of each of the agencies with respect to shared cases. PRS service contracts have been negotiated with community mental health facilities, day-care centers, a training agency for volunteer workers, and a visiting nurse association.

PROVIDING CONTRACTED PRS SERVICES: EXPERIENCE AND PERSPECTIVE

How do the three basic patterns for placing PRS clients in service programs compare when implemented? District office managers were asked to describe experiences in obtaining homemaker, day-care, and mental health services for PRS clients, utilizing each of the previously identified patterns. Their responses suggest that serious problems arise when either the informal referral or vendor agreement patterns are used.

Although homemaker services are considered essential for many PRS families, it proved exceedingly difficult to arrange for adequate homemaker services utilizing informal referral or vendor agreement. Persuading homemakers even to enter the homes of many PRS clients proved to be a problem; and when they do, they rarely stay long enough to help the family. Most of the families in which abuse and neglect occur live in extremely impoverished housing in rundown and dangerous ghetto neighborhoods. Homemakers are often fearful about visiting these homes. In addition, many clients have emotional problems and tend to be antisocial, hostile, or aggressive. The client family is frequently suspicious of the homemaker, believing her purpose is to report to the Division about the family's activities rather than to help. Furthermore, most homemakers, trained to provide physical care to "patients," are extremely frustrated working with the kinds of situations and problems characteristic of PRS families.

Communication between the Division and the homemaker agencies is reported as virtually nonexistent. Several respondents also noted that they have little choice within the community as to which homemaker program to use. Often only one or two such programs are available; even where there are more, the reluctance of their staff to serve PRS clients is present. To add to the difficulties, most of the programs have a long list of clients awaiting service.

Similar problems are noted with respect to day care, another service considered essential for many PRS families. Managers describe most day-care centers as unresponsive to PRS families and unwilling to accept these children. They suggest that many children who have been abused and neglected also have behavior problems and difficulty getting along with other children, thus posing management problems for day-care center staff. In addition, these children often arrive late, are not picked up on time by their parents, and frequently have poor attendance records. Program operations may be disrupted. Also, because many of the centers are reimbursed on the basis of attendance, the high absentee rate poses financial disincentives. Further, although many parents may need special support services, most day-care centers lack sufficient staff or funding to provide them. Long waiting lists were also noted as typical for day-care centers.

Without exception, the district office managers identified mental health services as essential for a large proportion of PRS clients. Many children and parents require diagnostic services. In addition, the participation of one or both parents in a counseling or therapy program through a mental health center or family service agency is often mandatory if the child or children are to remain at home, or a condition to be met for returning children who have been removed from the home. However, enormous problems are encountered in obtaining these services.

One manager described the difficulties of obtaining psychiatric evaluation services. Either the Division provides reimbursement through vendor agreements or clients are covered under Medicaid, if eligible. According to this administrator, whose district office relies on private-practice professionals to conduct evaluations, psychiatrists are reluctant to become involved in these PRS cases. Reasons include insufficient reimbursement levels and the possibility of court involvement. Strong opposition exists to accepting Medicaid clients, perhaps because of the paper work involved. Mental health facilities are also generally resistant to offering counseling or therapy services to PRS clients.

One set of problems, according to these district office managers, arises from the involuntary status of PRS clients. Most parents supervised for child abuse or neglect do not see themselves as having psychological problems and enter treatment in a mental health facility solely because the Division requires it. More overwhelming for many of these clients are the problems associated with poverty, e.g., poor housing, unemployment, "making ends meet," the burden of child care, and poor health. The services offered by mental health facilities may be irrelevant to many PRS client needs, and their staff tend to overlook economic deprivation and other daily living difficulties as "real" causes of mental health problems. Moreover, as the group of administrators observed, psychological counseling relies heavily upon the active participation of the client in a "talking" and reflective process. This technique is often unsuitable for and ineffective with PRS clients.

District office managers also express concern over the lack of information sharing once the family or family member becomes a client of the other agency. The Division, which is legally mandated to receive reports concerning child abuse and neglect incidents, expects the staff of the mental health program to report any incidents that occur while the PRS family is receiving its services. The practitioners of the mental health program, however, regard such reporting as a serious breach of confidentially. Another divisive issue concerns whether children should be removed from the home. Public agency administrators are generally less likely to recommend removal than are staff of provider agencies.

These different orientations, according to the respondents, are felt in the intake and service delivery processes. Mental health programs are initially reluctant to accept PRS clients or, if they do, find it difficult to work with them, often allowing them to drop out or initiate an early termination of services. District office managers argue that mental health services provided to PRS clients have to be modified to meet the needs of this population; greater attention to concrete and tangible factors underlying mental health problems, increased practitioner outreach, and greater emphasis on "nurturing" and supportive services are essential.

PURCHASING PRS SERVICES

In the early years of PRS contracting, district office managers regarded provider agency staff as more qualified than their own staff to develop service programs for PRS clients. The design and implementation of such programs was thus almost exclusively delegated to the provider agencies. This arrangement, however, was not satisfactory, for reasons discussed earlier, and modifications in contractual procedures were initiated. One change was to define a more active role for division staff in determining the content and structure of contracted programs at the local level as contracts were being negotiated. In addition, most PRS contracts now formalize the nature of Division involvement in program implementation. This often includes Division training of provider agency staff, the assignment of a Division staff member as program liaison, and Division staff participation in regularly scheduled case conferences. The stipulation that the contract be renewed annually enables the district office to address problems experienced in the previous contract year.

Most of the PRS purchase of service mental health programs, in operation at the time of the interviews for two or three years, were described as functioning well. Most were comprehensive programs, which provided services ranging from consultation with the public agency to counseling PRS clients and providing child day care, medical and supportive services, practical help, and child care and transportation to help clients keep clinic appointments. Outreach was viewed as a crucial component of service and was mandated in the contract at the insistence of Division staff. One administrator commented, "Going out to the family's home is one of the thing that we were adamant about. We told the provider agency that if they wouldn't do this we didn't need them."

Managers encountered a common set of problems in working with the provider agencies to develop mental health programs. One identified problem concerned staff attitudes and orientations associated with the traditional clinical approach. Typical are the comments of one manager about the first year's contract implementation with a hospital-based mental health facility:

> Although the professionals who were hired were competent clinicians, none had experience with PRS clients and most held extremely rigid

and traditional attitudes about only wanting to work with the most treatable and motivated clients. Staff were upset because they thought we were referring the most difficult families in our caseload. If they had their way they would have worked only with low risk and preventable situations.

Another problem concerned reporting new child abuse and neglect incidents to the Division. As one district office manager recalls: "Hours and hours of meeting time were spent on the subject of reporting incidents of child abuse and neglect to Division staff. They (the provider agency) finally did agree to report these incidents to us although I know that the Director (of the provider agency) to this day still disapproves of the decision."

An additional problem concerned the allocation of control and responsibility for case planning, monitoring, and disposition between the Division and provider agency. The extent of active involvement by the public agency varied among the individual offices. One administrator insisted that caseworkers attend all case conferences and staff meetings of the provider agency.

District office managers generally feel that the contractual requirements for PRS programs have modified the perceived shortcomings of the more traditional mental health agency when serving this population. General satisfaction with the services provided for PRS clients was voiced, though little or no systematic evaluation has been attempted.

EXCHANGE RELATIONS

Exchange theory, as formulated by Cook (1977), provides a useful framework to understand the relationship between PRS purchase arrangements with nonpublic agencies (i.e., mechanisms of disposition) and the level of control the public agency may exercise with respect to the content and delivery of these services. Cook (1977, 64) defines an exchange relation as consisting of "voluntary transactions involving the transfer of resources . . . between two or more actors . . . for mutual benefit." An "actor" may be either an individual or collective, such as a corporate group or an organization. "Resource" refers to any valued activity, service, or commodity.

The dependence of one organization upon another is determined by (1) the extent to which the first organization has a need for, or values, a resource that the second organization can provide and (2) the degree to which the resource is not available from alternative sources. The power of an organization is defined in terms of resource dependencies. The degree to which the resource is available from alternative sources reduces the dependence of the first organization on the second and increases the first organization's influence over the nature of the exchange. Moreover, "the power of an organization in an exchange relation is increased as the scope of the resources (or the number of different resources) mediated by the organization increases . . . The expansion of an organization's resource base is thus defined as a mechanism for gaining power through increasing the dependency of other organizations which value or need the resources" (ibid., 66–67).

The accounts of district office managers suggest that the use of informal referral patterns (referral to a regular agency or community "purchase of service" program) or vendor agreements decreases the Division's power in the exchange relationship. The Division's ability to influence the nature of the exchange is severely constrained, thus leaving the public child welfare agency with little or no control over the types of services provided to PRS clients by external agencies.

A key factor affecting the limited bargaining power of the Division in PRS arrangements is the negative value accorded the PRS client by the actual or potential provider agency. Many agencies are simply not interested in providing services to this population. Another factor contributing to the power imbalance is the control exercised by the provider agency over the intake process. As Hasenfeld (1972) has observed, the more discretion market units (recipient organizations or systems) have over their own intake, the more dependent is the people-processing organization on these units. Provider agencies also have access to alternate sources of clients with preferred or more desirable characteristics; for example, clients who voluntarily seek service are cooperative, have problems that are more readily amenable to treatment, and have educational and economic backgrounds that make them receptive to services.

The commodity or resource that the Division seeks is service for PRS clients. Although these services may be inadequately provided by non-public agencies, the Division nevertheless depends on those agencies because it lacks the internal capacity to directly provide such services and has limited choice of alternative providers.

The limited influence of the Division is particularly pronounced under informal referral and vendor arrangements, where it lacks the "power of the purse." Referral to a community agency does not involve reimbursement by the Division. Under vendor agreements the level of funding is relatively small and may be insufficient motivation for providing services to PRS clients. In contrast, PRS contract requirements may allow the public agency far greater influence on how and what services are delivered. The Division assumes a prominent role in the design and implementation of a service program responsive to PRS client needs. In an era in which many human services funding sources have been eliminated or cut back, contract funds come to be highly valued by nonpublic agencies. Even though the negative perception of the PRS client is essentially unchanged, the Division's ability to effectively procure, through contracting, services to meet the needs of PRS clients is significantly enhanced. The public agency may insist on contract requirements that insure responsive programming and can withhold funds when agencies are out of compliance. The financial needs of the voluntary sector heighten the influence of the Division and allow greater flexibility in the nature of the contracts negotiated.

DESPITE some shortcomings, PRS contracting has proven to be a viable mechanism that enables the Division to function more effectively as a people-processing organization; contracting affords it some degree of control over provider agencies. Contracting ensures the access of the PRS client to various service programs and facilitates client continuance in service through outreach efforts. District office managers perceive the services to be more relevant and comprehensive than those provided by noncontracted programs. Patterns of communication between the Division and provider agency are stronger as a result of contracting, because the contracts generally include requirements about the frequency and nature of interorganizational linkages. However, it is difficult to determine from the data whether these communication systems are adequate and the extent to which they are actually used. Perhaps the most serious gap in PRS contracting has been the failure to establish an ongoing system for monitoring and evaluating contracted services, resulting in a dearth of information on service effectiveness.

Although PRS contracting appears to be a viable mechanism to provide services to PRS clients, it should be noted that these contracted services are available to only a small proportion of PRS families. For example, mental health services are often recommended for PRS families. With a statewide PRS caseload of 46,851 children, it is obvious that the 1,500 families served by the sixteen contracted mental health programs represent but a small fraction of families for whom such services are recommended or mandated. A related limitation of current PRS contracting practices is the emphasis on contracting for mental health services, to the exclusion of other needed services, such as day-care and homemaking.

A number of questions and issues arise out of an exploration of contracting patterns and their effects. These questions transcend any one service area.

A crucial question concerns the impact that the increased use of governmental contracting for social services has upon the access of clients to services and the responsiveness of the provider agencies to their needs.

There are many client groups who, similar to PRS clients, have a multiplicity of pressing needs and problems but, for a variety of reasons, are "unattractive" to service providers. These include poverty groups, former patients of psychiatric hospitals, discharged residents of institutions for the mentally retarded, and the aged.

The results of this author's exploratory study suggest that public contracting can be a viable method of expanding and strengthening client services, given a number of provisos. Collaboration between professional staff of the public and contracted agencies to develop and implement the service program is extremely important. Here, the public sector's knowledge of client needs can be effectively used. It is essential that provider agencies be monitored aggressively during contract implementation. As recommended by Jansson (1977, 370): "Such monitoring must include analysis of organizational service patterns to ascertain whether members of poverty or minority groups are discouraged from using service whether inadvertently or through obvious patterns of exclusion." Assuring access, however, is only the first step in the process of providing effective service to high-risk client groups. Monitoring must also focus on the specific content of the services and how they are delivered to assess their relevancy to client problems and effective problem solving.

Notes

1. For a discussion of the response of agencies to the lower-income involuntary client, see Brintnall 1981; Cloward and Epstein 1965; Greenley and Kirk 1973; Nagi 1974; Purcell 1964; and Scott 1967.

2. The information in this section was provided by Ann Baran, Assistant Regional Administrator, Metropolitan Region, New Jersey Division of Youth and Family Services at the time the study was done.

14

Federal Funding, Nonprofit Agencies, and Victim Services

Steven Rathgeb Smith

O ngoing changes in the responsibilities of government and nongovernment units in the delivery of social welfare services are at the center of the debate on the future of American social welfare policy (Kamerman 1983; Savas 1981; Gilbert 1983). One of the fastest-growing examples of this shifting public-private boundary is government financing of nonprofit agencies for the delivery of social services. For example, the recent public policy responses to the problems of hunger (Physicians' Task Force 1985) and homelessness (United Community Planning Corporation and Massachusetts Association of Mental Health 1983) have been largely through nonprofit agencies funded by government.

The expansion of government funding of nonprofit agencies in the 1980s is built upon the precedents established in the 1960s and 1970s, when federal funding of nonprofit agencies grew enormously (Derthick 1975; Benton, Feild, and Miller 1978). During the Reagan administration, federal funding of nonprofit agencies has been substantially curtailed, with the responsibility for the funding and administration of social services shifted, in part, to state and local governments. Even with this defederalization, the expansion of public funding of nonprofit agencies continues (General Accounting Office 1984; Kimmich 1985).

In this chapter federal funding of nonprofit service programs is analyzed for victims of four categories of crime: child abuse, rape, spouse abuse, and elderly crime. Four overriding questions guide this analysis. What happens to the organizational structure of nonprofit agencies when

THIS ARTICLE IS ADAPTED from a forthcoming book on victim services by Steven Rathgeb Smith and Susan Freinkel (Greenwood Press).

they accept federal funding? What are the effects of organizational changes on the staff, clients, and mission of these agencies receiving federal funds? How does federal funding affect the overall network of services offered by nonprofit agencies? And, because nonprofits play a key role in the articulation of social problems, how do organizational changes within nonprofit agencies resulting from the receipt of federal funds affect the representation and conception of social needs within the political process and American society?

This analysis of federal funding of victim services is based upon an in-depth investigation of over fifty nonprofit victim service agencies across the country. Information about these agencies was collected primarily through interviews with agency personnel. Additional interviews were conducted with victim advocates and government officials on the overall development and implementation of federal funding policy for victim services. These interviews were complemented by extensive archival research on the funding levels and patterns of fund distribution. The research focuses on federal funding in the 1970s, although policy developments regarding federal funds for victim services during the 1980s were also tracked and analyzed.

BACKGROUND

Prior to the 1960s, social services to address these four victim issues were largely nonexistent. These issues were, for the most part, "private," outside the realm of politics and active intervention by public and major private service programs. The emotional and financial support of victims of rape, spouse abuse, and elderly crime was considered the responsibility of the family and community. Child abuse was regarded as the quiet responsibility of private, nonprofit, and public agencies. Even in this latter case, though, most efforts to address child abuse involved little more than removal of the child from an abusive situation and placement in long-term stay in foster care.

The first victim issue to undergo transformation from private to public warranting governmental attention was child abuse. During the early 1960s, research funding by the federal government helped publicize the discovery of child abuse as a serious social problem. Federal funds also helped spur the rapid proliferation of state laws mandating the reporting of suspected cases of child abuse by medical and social welfare personnel (Nelson 1984, 32–50).

The publicity surrounding child abuse fueled a growing movement in the late 1960s and early 1970s to obtain federal funds for service programs for child abuse victims and their families. Funding for medical and social programs was deemed especially important because the recognition of child abuse was accompanied by a shift in thinking about appropriate interventions in abusive situations. Abusive parents were considered amenable to treatment through counseling and various support programs. Some scholars also contended that it was possible to prevent child abuse through preventive strategies such as education and early detection (Kempe and Helfer 1972; Cicchetti and Aber 1980).

Advocates of federal funding of child abuse programs were able to win passage of the Child Abuse Prevention and Treatment Act (CAPTA) in 1973. This legislation established the National Center for Child Abuse and Neglect (NCCAN) and authorized federal funding of child abuse service programs delivered by public and private agencies. In addition, state child welfare agencies were eligible for funds to professionalize their staff (Nelson 1984; Hoffman 1979). Subsequently, CAPTA was renewed in 1978 and again in 1984.

The passage of federal child abuse legislation created a climate conducive to consideration of other criminal victimization issues. This interest was facilitated by the growing concern about crime and the neglect of the victim by the criminal justice system (Cook et al. 1981).

In the early 1970s, several groups and individuals called attention to the problem of crimes committed on the elderly. Public pressure, especially from the American Association of Retired Persons (AARP), resulted in a modest federal funding effort for service programs at the local level for elderly crime victims. The major manager of these programs was the Law Enforcement Assistance Administration (LEAA); other federal agencies, such as the Department of Health, Education, and Welfare and the Administration on Aging, also provided funds for various service projects (U.S. Congress 1976). This federal effort occurred despite questions raised by scholars that the elderly were not disproportionately victimized and that elderly crime was not a serious social problem (Cook et al. 1981; Hinderlang 1976).

As elderly crime rose in prominence as a public issue, feminist activists around the country were establishing nonprofit service organizations to help rape victims. These agencies were usually volunteer, staffed by non-professional activists who considered rape a tragic and horrendous symptom of widespread patriarchal violence and oppression of women in American society. These programs deliberately stimulated political consciousness-raising to help rape victims transform their conception of rape and the place of women in society. To encourage the opportunity for individual growth by rape victims, the center founders relied upon a collective organizational structure that minimized differences among the staff and between staff and the rape victims receiving service (Klein 1977; O'Sullivan 1978).

Advocates for these feminist service programs, usually called rape crisis centers, looked to the federal government for funding in the mid-1970s. The push for federal funding was warmly received by the Democrat-controlled Congress, and omnibus legislation authorizing the establishment of the National Center for the Prevention and Control of Rape (NCPCR) was passed by a wide margin over the veto of President Ford in 1975. NCPCR was placed within the administrative structure of the National Institute of Mental Health (NIMH) and given authority to fund research and demonstration projects to address the problem of rape. Although it was not the secure, ongoing support of rape services that the rape crisis center advocates had originally envisioned, they hoped that NCPCR would serve as an important first step and precedent for future legislative initiatives (Largen 1981). Other federal funds for rape services during the Carter administration were provided by LEAA (Brodyaga et al. 1975).

The early rape crisis centers and the success of the women's movement in winning passage of federal legislation authorizing federal funds for rape service programs, albeit on a research and demonstration basis, emboldened advocates of battered women to push for federal financial assistance of shelters in the late 1970s. These shelters had been established shortly after the founding of rape crisis centers, along similar philosophical lines, and were also consciously political, nonprofessional alternatives to established human service professional programs. The shelters were primarily volunteer and collectively organized.

Shelter advocates were unsuccessful in gaining congressional passage of legislation authorizing federal appropriations in the 1970s. However, the Carter administration used administrative funds to creative program opportunities. LEAA launched a Family Violence Program (FVP) in 1977, which funded several service projects to address domestic violence during its three-year existence. In addition, the Department of Health and Human Services (HHS) created the Office of Domestic Violence (ODV), which funded technical assistance, research and demonstration projects, and public education campaigns. Other federal programs supporting domestic violence projects at this time were CETA, Title XX, and ACTION (Schecter 1982, 185–202; Center for Women Policy Studies 1980).

The federal government was not the only public source of revenue available. Child abuse, rape, and battered women programs also received state, local, and private funding by means of contracts and grants. However, federal funding set the context and precedents within which state, local, and private efforts evolved. Because of the reliance of federal policymakers on nonprofit agencies to provide victims services, the development of such services is directly linked to federal patterns and initiatives.

PROGRAM IMPLEMENTATION

Despite important differences in constituency groups, funding levels, state and local involvement in service development, and political strategies employed by program advocates, noteworthy similarities exist among the various nonprofit programs receiving federal funds for victim services.

Short-term Federal Support

The lack of secure, long-term federal funding was evident in total federal spending levels in each victim category and in types and amounts of contracts and grants received by individual agencies. Total spending, which was never generous, rose quickly, peaked, and then declined sharply, even before the Reagan administration assumed office. This trend was most noticeable in spending for elderly crime victims. Federal spending, primarily through LEAA, rapidly peaked and then declined precipitously as the attention of federal policymakers shifted to other losses. Federal funding for rape victims and battered women programs suffered a similar fate. For example, during the Carter administration, spending on battered women programs rose swiftly, and then declined by the end of his term. Child abuse spending under the CAPTA legislation jumped in the mid-1970s, then stagnated in the late 1970s.

Federal spending declined further in the early years of the Reagan administration. Then federal spending for nonprofit victim programs rose once again. In 1984 Congress enacted the Victims of Crime Act (VOCA), which authorized federal funding for victims, including generic programs for crime victims such as crime victim counseling and victim compensation (VOCA 1984). Also, in 1984 Congress passed the Family Violence Prevention and Services Act (FVPSA), which authorized federal spending for services to victims of family violence, including battered women and abused senior citizens (FVPSA 1984). Nevertheless budget cutting pressures have continued to date (1989).

This cyclical funding pattern is possible because of the reliance of federal officials on nonprofit agencies to provide services through research and demonstration grants and contracts. Service programs operated by nonprofit agencies are more quickly established than public programs, which face restrictive civil service rules and regulations. Likewise, termination of a federally-funded project operated by nonprofit agencies is easier than termination of a public program, especially because many of these projects have relied on volunteers for many services. The volunteers who frequently have only a weak relationship with the agency permit relatively quick program termination without a major outcry.

Almost all federal program funds devoted to victim services in the 1970s were for research and demonstration (R & D) projects; the only exception was funds earmarked for the professionalization of state child welfare agencies under the CAPTA legislation. Moreover, R & D funding was usually of a one- to three-year duration, and rarely were extensions granted. As a result, tremendous instability was created within the service system for these victim groups. A common lament of staff of coalition organizations for rape victims and battered women was that as soon as a service directory was published, it was out-of-date. This unstable pattern continues into the late 1980s.

Ideally, R & D projects are designed to stimulate and test innovative and novel means of addressing service needs. In fact, R & D funding was often a back-door method of funding direct services, allowing government policymakers' to respond to political demands for service initiatives by victim advocates without making a substantial long-term commitment.

Nonprofit agencies, with their organizational flexibility, provided the convenient and politically attractive vehicle for the rapid distribution of this R & D money. Nonprofit agencies, then, were an essential part of the political response to interest group pressure for victim services.

Containing the Issue

Thus, federal funding of nonprofit agencies for victim services provided a "safe" political response to the potentially adverse social and political implications of criminal victimization: crimes against the elderly, rape, spouse abuse, and child abuse. In each case some scholars and victim advocates argue that these victim issues are the function of underlying problems of class, race, and gender.

Criminal victimization of the elderly is associated with social isolation and poverty, and is therefore an example of broader issues of social and economic injustice (Cook et al. 1981). Rape and spouse abuse raise the serious problems of social and economic discrimination against women (Schecter 1982). Spouse abuse and child abuse can be viewed as the most tragic indicators of the oppression of women and children within the family. And, because child abuse occurs with much higher frequency among lower income groups, this phenomenon can be conceptualized as the inevitable consequence of the lack of adequate income and economic opportunities (Gil 1970).

The effect of federal funding of victim service programs in the 1970s was to exclude or "marginalize" these potentially explosive definitions of victimization. This definitional boundary-setting process was accomplished through the pattern of federal funding distribution and the organizational changes within nonprofit agencies precipitated by federal funding.

The legislative and administrative regulations governing the distribution of federal funds for victim services were actually quite vague, usually expressing admirable, important goals, such as the prevention and treatment of rape or spouse abuse. However, the distribution of funds favored projects within mainstream professional practice. Thus, federal financing for elderly crime programs tended to favor traditional law enforcement projects operated under the aegis of nonprofit agencies or an affiliate of a local law enforcement agency. Support went typically for conventional programs; security improvement in the home, escort

221

services, and courtwatch programs, which tried to identify and give publicity to those judges deemed too lenient toward criminal offenders (Stein 1979; Carter 1980).

Child abuse funds were distributed to a wide array of medical and social welfare agencies. Indeed, federal funding became a mechanism for subsidizing the work of professionals already operating in the child abuse field. These professional projects tended to focus on treating the abused child and his or her family, reinforcing the view that child abuse was the product of aberrant behavior rather than underlying economic inequality.

The dominance of professional treatment meant that prevention programs, such as community education, were neglected. However, under the Reagan administration, priorities changed dramatically, with innovative prevention programs receiving substantial federal financial support, albeit on a research and demonstration basis (Clearinghouse on Child Abuse and Neglect 1986).

In the case of rape services, the nontraditional rape crisis centers operated by feminist volunteers found it extremely difficult to obtain federal funds from the National Center for the Prevention and Control of Rape (NCPCR). Consistent with the professional human service orientation of NIMH, the parent agency of NCPCR, the nonprofessional alternative rape crisis centers were largely excluded from NCPCR funding. Instead, funding for rape services from NCPCR was channeled primarily to such professional organizations as hospitals and social service agencies. The lack of federal funds for rape crisis centers contributed to their organizational instability: without secure funding, the centers experienced staff burnout, service cutbacks, and closure. The prominence of the political feminist critique of rape within the services offered to rape victims suffered accordingly.

Shelter programs for battered women were more successful than rape crisis centers in gaining federal funds, probably because the women's movement had learned from the experience of rape crisis centers. Nonetheless, federal requirements encouraged the professionalization of services for battered women. First, professional human services organizations received federal funding, primarily for nonresidential services, such as counseling. These programs emphasized treatment of the abused woman and her spouse and/or crisis intervention to resolve the immediate abusive situation. Second, many residential shelter programs were

222

forced to reduce the collective structure of their agencies and supplant it with a traditional hierarchical chain of command. In many cases funders preferred the agency to be headed by a trained human service professional. And third, many federal grants and contracts were awarded with the stipulation that the shelters develop cooperative arrangements and linkages with professional service agencies.

In sum, federal practices pushed the delivery of victim services toward the mainstream and helped create an image of the perpetrators of victimization as deviant and the victims as needing professional treatment. Of course, nonprofit staff were not coerced into accepting government money and the accompanying regulations and program requirements. On the contrary, nonprofit staff willingly sought and accepted federal money, even if the effect was to change the agency's character. Two important factors account for this nonprofit-government relationship. First, the professional staff of nonprofit agencies often shared the same professional norms as the federal grant administrators. And second, nonprofit agencies were particularly vulnerable to government influence either directly or indirectly, because they usually lacked secure funding, depended on volunteer help, and were staffed by individuals committed to expanding service to victims and their families. Because the federal government was a major political supporter at the time, agency staff viewed this source as a realistic way to financial health and service expansion for the agency.

Federal Funding as a Liability

Social welfare advocates often portray the federal government as the ally of clients of social programs. Yet, the evolution of victim services in the last fifteen years indicates that those victim program categories with the most dependence on federal support in the 1970s fared the worst in terms of long-term viability.

Elderly crime programs, for example, were almost exclusively financed by the federal government. In contrast to other victim programs, policymakers and national senior citizen lobbying organizations created a network of programs with federal funds; these programs did not exist prior to federal support. When the short attention span of federal policymakers shifted to other issues, as it inevitably does, elderly crime programs were drastically curtailed.

Rape crisis centers began with small private donations and volunteer help in communities across the country. Center advocates directed their fund raising to the federal, rather than state and local government, level. Consequently, these centers were also hit hard when substantial secure federal funding failed to materialize (New York Times, 31 August 1981).

In contrast, battered women programs have weathered the federal cutbacks substantially better than the rape crisis centers, largely because advocates for battered women actively undertook grass-roots political lobbying for state and local funds even as they sought federal funds. Indeed, informal surveys indicate that the number of battered women programs has increased by over two hundred nationwide since 1980 (Moore 1986).

Child abuse programs, long the recipients of state contracts, fared the best. State funding for both public and private child abuse programs rose sharply in the 1980s (GAO 1984; *Boston Globe,* 12 June 1985; DSS 1985).

Service Fragmentation

Federal funding of nonprofit agencies may also stimulate service fragmentation by spurring the proliferation of programs sponsoring varied approaches to victim interventions. For example, federal funding for spouse abuse services went to law enforcement agencies, mental health centers, social service organizations, alternative feminist shelter programs, and hospitals. In each of these settings, the predominant ideology or professional outlook of the staff shaped the type of service offered by the agency. Yet, these diverse approaches to the same problem rarely intersected, although it is certainly arguable that many different types of services are needed by abused women.

This fragmentation led to different service responses to victims, some of whom had similar circumstances. Law enforcement agencies emphasized the criminal act of victimization and offered services that tried to integrate the victim with the criminal justice system: help for the victim in testifying in criminal prosecutions, improved reporting of crime by victims, and educational efforts to avoid victimization. Social service agencies provided counseling and information and referral services toward the goal of helping the victim regain an emotional equilibrium. Hospitals offered medical treatment and crisis intervention. Alternative feminist agencies for rape victims and battered women tried to provide a singular, nonprofessional service for women that focused on peer support and the fostering of emotional and economic independence. Mental health centers focused on long-term therapeutic treatment because many victims needed more than short-term crisis intervention. Mental health centers were less involved in victims' services than other types of service agencies.

Federal Funding and Volunteers

Federal grant administrators in the 1970s looked askance at volunteer programs, preferring instead professional service delivery. This professional tilt is most noticeable in rape and battered women services. As noted, rape crisis centers were rarely awarded funds from the NCPCR in part because of the reliance upon volunteers within the centers. Although battered women shelters fared better in the competition for federal funds, the grant stipulations often required shelters to limit the role of volunteers.

Elderly crime programs, despite the widespread use of volunteers, continued to be recipients of federal funds. However, this funding success appears related to the way in which volunteers were used in elderly programs: the volunteers, who were predominantly elderly, usually deferred to the professionals in charge of the programs. Volunteers implemented a professionally designed service program. Despite this accommodation to federal policies, this program too lost popularity. This volunteer role contrasts with that of volunteers in rape crisis centers and battered women shelters, who were, at least initially, on the front lines of service delivery and making their own independent judgments about client needs. Monitoring occurred under nonprofessional administrators.

In the 1970s child abuse programs supported by NCCAN were overwhelmingly professional. However, the Reagan administration moved instead to a heavy reliance on volunteers. In part, this change is related to the increased emphasis on preventive and educational programs according to NCCAN.

The extensive use of volunteers also created obstacles to access. In general, volunteers are middle-class citizens in stable economic situations, or college students. Thus, most volunteers within victim programs were middle-class and white, tending to discourage poor and minority victims from seeking services. In some cases the paid and volunteer staff of these programs tried to overcome this problem through special outreach efforts or, if funding was available, they paid poor and minority volunteers a wage to "volunteer" in the program. These special initiatives were hampered by a lack of adequate funding and the distance between the agency location and poor and minority communities.

Federal Funding and Victim Advocacy

Despite a cyclical, partially symbolic funding pattern, federal funds permanently transformed the politics of criminal victimization. Each of these victim issues were at one time private; federal financial support gave legitimacy to victimization as a serious social problem requiring governmental attention.

Federal initiatives both responded to and reinforced a network of victim advocates who were eager to establish a more active government role on behalf of victims. For example, the Victims of Crime Act (VOCA) and the Family Violence Prevention and Services Act (FVPSA) of 1984 were enacted, in part, due to the groundbreaking efforts of federal victim initiatives in the 1970s. Also, many advocates worked for more service funding at the state and local levels, not only for specific victim categories but for more generic programs of victim compensation and restitution programs. Moreover, many advocates, especially for rape victims and battered women, lobbied for changes in the legal system to redress long-standing discriminatory practices and statutes toward victims (Bienen 1980; Hamos 1980). Many victim service programs also function as a rally point for local activists who serve as informal watchdogs on legal and political developments that affect victims.

VICTIM service programs underscore the policy dilemmas of using non-profit agencies funded by government contracts and grants to achieve public objectives. Maintaining the "private" character of nonprofit service delivery once these agencies accept government funds is one problem.

Elderly crime victim programs were a prime example of the use of nonprofit agencies as instrumentalities of government policy. These programs existed to fulfill a vague mandate by federal officials to address the crime problem among the elderly; they lacked a preexisting, private, raison d'etre. When the attention of federal policy shifted to other issues, these programs disappeared.

Rape crisis centers and shelters for battered women, on the other hand, were in place prior to federal financing through the efforts of committed volunteers and activists. Moreover, these agencies offered an explicitly private alternative to prevailing public policy; indeed, these agencies openly challenged the established political and professional order. Over time, however, federal funding undermined the distinctively private and ideological character of these programs. The result was greater integration between government and not-for-profit priorities. In the process social services to rape victims and battered women became professionalized. What was gained was a more educated, more experienced staff, more client equity, and greater standardization of services. What was lost was the unique alternative character of these services.

The evolution of victim services also underscores the use of nonprofit agencies, funded by government grants or contracts, as a mechanism for expanding the sphere of professional influence and service delivery responsibility. The rise of professional service delivery eclipsed alternative services and politically controversial conceptions of victimization; professionalization became government policy—an essential element in the federal government's response to victims.

Thus, federal financing was not a neutral, technical means to achieve social welfare objectives. On the contrary, the use of federal funds to support nonprofit agencies for victims' services was highly political, with certain organizations and treatment philosophies favored over others.

The future course of federal policy toward victims is uncertain. At one level, public interest in the problems of crime victims is at an all time high, as symbolized by the VOCA legislation and the continued attention to victim concerns throughout the country. However, current public policy toward victims contains many of the same disturbing, destabilizing features of federal policy in the 1970s: short-term, research and demonstration grants, fragmented system of nonprofit agencies, and a weak federal funding role. Consequently, victim services are likely to continue to experience threats and obstacles to their long-term survival.

15

Contracting for Adoption Services for Special Needs Children

Maria Roberts-DeGennaro

The scope of the problem of foster children waiting for adoption who have special needs, i.e., older, handicapped, or of minority background, is extensive and serious in many communities. The majority of the five hundred thousand children presently in the foster care system are physically, emotionally, or medically handicapped, over ten years of age, and/or nonwhite (National Commission on Children in Need of Parents 1979).

Historically, the public child welfare sector has been regarded as the "appropriate agencies to assume the care for children who are to be permanently separated from their families" (Folks 1902, 245). Since the early 1900s, legal responsibility for foster children has been assigned to the public agencies by the courts. As a consequence the public child welfare sector has been given the predominant fiscal responsibility to provide long-term care for foster children with special needs.

A relatively recent phenomenon in most of the fifty states is the emerging pattern of shared responsibility between the public and private child welfare sectors for finding adoptive homes for children with special needs. This shared responsibility has been operationalized through the contracting of private adoption services for special needs children.

A study conducted by this author focused on the intra- and inter-organizational forces that were affecting a joint adoption program in the state of Texas (Roberts 1981). This chapter presents the issues, major findings, and recommendations concerning contracting for adoption services.

STATEMENT OF THE PROBLEM

At the time this study was conducted, there were about fifteen hundred Texas children legally free for adoption in any one month. Approximately 70 percent of these children had special needs. As part of a permanency planning effort in 1978, the state child welfare agency began to negotiate purchase of adoption services' agreements with Texas-licensed, private, child-placing agencies. Because the supply of infants needing adoptive families was decreasing, this contract arrangement appeared to serve two objectives. It enriched and expanded the private sector's adoption program and reduced the number of children with special needs drifting in the public foster care system.

Difficulties ensued, however, in implementing this joint adoption program. Three major problem areas evolved: first, uncertainty in the private agencies about reimbursement for expenses incurred in recruiting and studying adoptive applicants, because the public agency had the final authority for selecting the adoptive family for a special needs child; second, the public agency adoption staff were suspicious that this contract arrangement would change their role from direct service providers of specialized adoption services to purchasing agents for these services. The third problem had to do with sharing the responsibility for placing the special needs children in adoptive homes.

These problems in developing a working relationship were associated with the ineffectual outcomes of the contract arrangement. It was suspected that this relationship was affected by both political and economic forces operating within each agency and between the agencies (Zald 1970a, 1970b; Wamsley and Zald 1973a, 1973b; Benson et al. 1973; Benson 1975).

THE POLITICAL-ECONOMY PERSPECTIVE

Because the public sector has been given the legal responsibility for special needs children requiring out-of-home care, public funds have traditionally been allocated to maintain these children in the public foster care system. In addition, these funds assist the public sector in employing staff to provide a full range of child welfare services (Geiser 1973).

As a consequence of traditional roles, the public sector maintained an

Table 15.1. **Political-Economy of the Focal Organization and a Member of Its Organization-Set under Purchase of Adoption Services' Agreements**

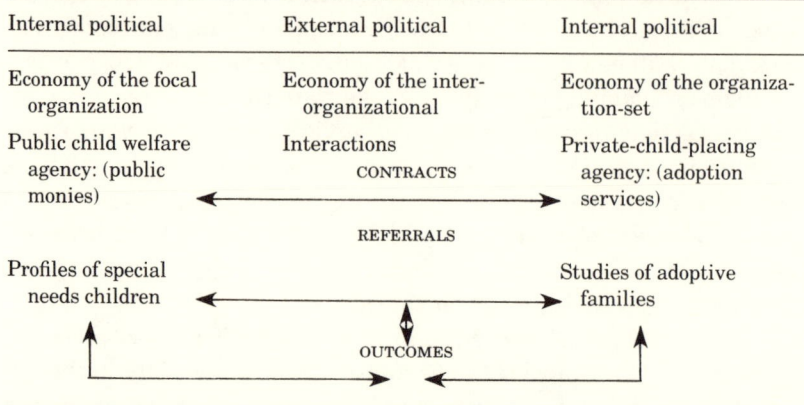

established claim to government-financed child welfare services, including adoption services for special needs children. This claim is actualized in a set of procedures and operating modes on the part of the public agency to find families for special needs children. Those outside the public sector who may provide similar adoption services are often viewed by public staff as inexperienced or incompetent. The institution of a contractual arrangement in this service area was perceived as threatening the public sector's ability to acquire and maintain a reliable flow of resources for its adoption program (Benson et al. 1973). The new policy failed to anticipate the threat to the employees of the public agency.

The decision by public sector administrators to contract for adoption services appeared to enhance the private sector's market and status position in the child welfare field. In light of the decreasing supply of infants for adoption, an increase in the private sector's role in this specialized area of child welfare would diminish the public sector's capacity to practice in the area of specialized adoptions.

To explore the political-economic forces impacting upon this contract arrangement, the unit of analysis employed was the organization-set (see, for example, Evan 1972). The relationship between the focal organization, the public child welfare agency, and members of its organization-set, i.e., the private child-placing agencies providing purchased adoption services, was analyzed from the political-economy perspective, as illustrated in table 15.1.

This conceptual model depicts both the internal and external operations of the focal organization and a member of its organization-set as affected by the purchase of service contract. The perceptions of key informants within these agencies were investigated with regard to the operations of their respective adoption programs, and the operations and performance of the other agency's adoption program under the contract agreement.

CASE STUDY

A key question for investigation centered on the outcomes of the purchase of adoption services' agreements as they were affected by the impact of the political-economic forces involved in interactions within and between public and private agencies. A case study approach was utilized, with four subsets of data from two regional and two subregional sites in the state of Texas. These sites were selected on the basis of their diverse characteristics (i.e., urban, rural, urban-rural). All of the selected regional/subregional public child welfare agencies operated independently of their state agency in terms of administrative structure. All private child-placing agencies that were contracted for two consecutive fiscal years were included in the study, as were eleven private child-placing agencies and four regional/subregional public child welfare agencies.

In two of the sites, only one private child-placing agency was contracted by the regional public child welfare agency. In the third site, four private child-placing agencies contracted with their subregional public child welfare agency. In the fourth site, five private child-placing agencies contracted with their subregional public child welfare agency.

Four independent variables grounded in the political-economy perspective were used: (1) domain consensus or agreement on the role and scope of each agency participating in this joint adoption program, (2) ideological consensus or agreement on the strategies in finding adoptive families for special needs children, (3) the cooperative efforts between the public child welfare agency and the private child-placing agencies, and (4) evaluation or the judgment of the work of each agency participating under the contract agreement (Benson et al. 1973).

Interviews were conducted with four levels of staff: program director, adoption supervisor, caseworker, and contract manager, in both the public and private agencies, for a total of forty-three interviews. Organizational documents were used as a secondary data base.

RESULTS OF AN ORGANIZATIONAL ANALYSIS

The organizational analysis yielded significant data on the "state of the purchased adoption services' arrangement" in Texas during the start-up period in implementing this joint adoption program. A high proportion of similar responses was found among both private and public agency informants across the four sites and were classified for analysis as representing either the private sector or the public sector's perceptions. Several important intra- and interorganizational forces affecting this joint adoption program effort were identified.

First, special needs children were defined categorically in the contract. Reimbursement to the private agencies contracted to place special needs children in adoptive homes was restricted to children fitting specific categories, e.g., age, race, handicapped, and sibling group. On the other hand, the public agency primarily placed special needs children who were Caucasian and under nine years of age. Thus, the public adoption staff referred the harder to place child to the contracted private agencies.

Even though the public and private agencies used basically the same criteria for studying applicants interested in adopting a special needs child, most of the applicants referred by the private agencies were rejected by the public agency adoption staff. The public agency may have been "screening out" rather than "screening in" the adoptive applicants referred by the private agencies, perhaps due to resentment of the contractual arrangement or negative beliefs about the capabilities of private agency staff in this service area. As a result, private agencies were incurring a financial disincentive to renew the contract agreements, especially for those agencies that studied adoptive applicants but made no reimbursable consummated adoptive placements during the contract period. Each private contract agency was placed in a position of competing with other private agencies, as well as with the public agency, for an approved adoptive placement for a particular special needs child under the contract arrangement.

A compounding problem was the ineffective tracking system existing under this contract arrangement. Consistent information was not available on the numbers and types of children who were waiting to be adopted, children who were referred to the private sector, and adoptive applicants who were referred by the private agencies. Without knowledge of the characteristics of the special needs children and the adoptive applicants, effectively developing, monitoring, or evaluating this adoption program was, at best, difficult.

Referral and follow-up procedures were not systematically outlined. The status of the referral of a special needs child to the private agency, or of an adoptive applicant to the public agency, was often not shared between the agencies. Thus, a major burden for both the public and private sectors under this contract agreement was the staff time required to communicate with the "other agency" under a set of nonspecific guidelines.

The contractual arrangement to implement a joint decision-making process was not activated. The prevailing attitude among public agency adoption staff was that the private sector was encroaching upon the public sector's turf. The private sector was perceived by the public agency adoption staff as having expertise only in the area of infant adoptions. As a result, agency adoption staff were reluctant to develop a joint decision-making process to determine the appropriateness of the referred adoptive applicants for a particular special needs child.

In conclusion, this interagency contract relationship seemed to be disorganized, uncoordinated, and disjointed. Impressionistic evidence suggests that the public agency adoption staff was not fully committed to this joint adoption program. The lack of commitment to share responsibility for child placement was perhaps the single most critical problem leading to poor contractual outcomes.

LEARNING FROM MISTAKES

The eleven recommendations that follow in relation to improving the purchase of adoption services emanate from this case study. Many of these recommendations may be useful in developing contracts for other human services.

1. A functional, rather than categorical, definition of a special needs child should be employed. All children who are under public conservatorship waiting to be adopted should be eligible to receive private adoption services. Because the private sector's expertise has been in the area of

younger (under six years of age) and nonseverely handicapped children, its skills should be utilized to place some of the children drifting in the foster care system; usually these cases remain solely within the public agency. The public agency adoption staff could then concentrate on the children who are more difficult to place and who have tenure in the foster care system. A more utilitarian distribution of case loads would be achieved in relation to the respective agency areas of expertise.

2. Information should be collected systematically on the availibility of children for adoption under the public sector's conservatorship. Knowledge of the characteristics of children, particularly those who are older, handicapped, and/or of minority parentage, would assist in planning and evaluating a joint adoption program. A foster child's record should be traced to assess adoptability.

3. Staff training on placing special needs children under public conservatorship should be simultaneously provided for both public and private agency adoption staff. These training events would offer an excellent opportunity for the development of informal networks. The nurturance of these informal networks could become a key bonding tool to promote the commitment and cooperation needed for effectively implementing this joint program.

4. A coalition of private agencies providing contracted adoption services should be formed. Collectively, these agencies could communicate their interests to the public sector in contract negotiations and program planning. A public agency representative could act as a liaison between the public and private agencies. Michigan's Federation of Private Child and Family Agencies is an exemplary model of such coordination.

5. Referral procedures under the contract agreement should be standardized. Specific information relating to the child and adoptive applicant should be identified and documented in each referral. Time limits need to be specified for staff of both sectors to respond to interagency referrals.

6. A contract coordinator in each of the public and private agencies should be designated and should be responsible for processing and following through on each referral. This would serve to reduce the lack of continuity and coordination in interagency communication.

7. A mutually agreed-upon decision-making process is needed to deter-

mine adoptive applicant parenting capacities. Placing special needs children as a shared responsibility needs to be developed.

8. The respective roles and responsibilities of staff of both sectors from the date of placement to the date of adoption consummation should be clearly specified.

9. The private agency staff should participate in a training and orientation session sponsored by the public agency. At this training session, information would be provided on contract terms and referral procedures. Program issues might be explored, including examples of the profiles of children for referral to the private sector and characteristics of adoptive families of special needs children.

10. An analysis of the direct costs incurred by private agencies for adoption services should be conducted. Most services, such as day care and home care, are reimbursed at full cost. The goal of securing permanent homes for foster children would be furthered if the contract payment mechanism provided full cost reimbursement incentives (Young and Brandt 1977; Young 1978).

11. A differential analysis should be conducted to compare the costs of foster care and adoption services. The cost savings associated with adoption placement has been estimated to be equal to two years in foster care. The average stay in foster care is around five years (Children's Defense Fund 1978; Fanshel and Shinn 1978). This type of cost analysis could be used to support requests for increases in states' budget allocation for adoption services.

SIX ISSUES can be identified as impacting upon a system of contracting for adoption services for special needs children. First, contracting requires the development of a working relationship that consists of the following three tasks: reaching a common understanding, clarifying roles, and specifying procedures to reach shared goals. The development of a working contract relationship is a process of building a congruence of expectations (Hartman 1979). A lack of clarity in coordinating efforts between agencies can result in ineffectual performance, especially by the contract agency (Litwak et al. 1970). A high level of outcomes from a purchase of service program depends on the activities contributed by each participating agency under the contract agreement (Pfeffer and Salancik 1978).

Due to its impact on the ability of agencies to achieve their desired outcomes, the second issue is interdependence. Each agency must perceive that its own goals can be achieved most effectively with the assistance of the other agency (Emerson 1962). In Texas, the performance of appropriate, reimbursable action on the part of the private agency, under a contractual agreement, was expected to facilitate the achievement of the public sector's goal to reduce the number of special needs children drifting in foster care. In return, under the contract terms, the private child-placing agencies could fulfill their adoption program objectives, maintain agency domain in adoption practice, and ensure a continuous flow of financial resources (Yuchtman and Seashore 1967).

Sharing responsibility with the private sector to place special needs children could, however, decrease the public sector's leverage for obtaining funds and authority in the area of adoption services for children with special needs, as the private sector also becomes an "expert" (and thus competitor) in placing special needs children. This threat to agency domain is the third issue. The diversion of funds to sponsor direct public sector service provision into funds for contracted private services could enhance the private sector's market position in the child welfare field, thus threatening the public sector's near monopoly. Some degree of dissensus is expected when the public sector seeks to defend its domain while the private sector is interested in domain expansion.

The issue of control must be considered along with the issue of domain consensus to properly understand the problem around contractual arrangements (Hall and Clark 1974; Hall et al. 1977). There is frequently a trade-off in contract negotiations between the need to acquire the resources and the desire to maintain control (Rogers and Molnar 1975). In the case of contracted adoption services, control by the public sector over the selection of adoptive applicants referred by the private sector permits its continued fiscal and authoritative sustenance. As long as the public sector maintains legal responsibility for these children, it can claim public monies for their long-term foster care, thus holding constant fiscal and role security.

The fifth issue is related to the assumption that both public and private sector staff perform their work according to a set of norms. These norms form an interrelated set of domains internalized by staff within both of the participating agencies under the contract agreement. As a consequence, the public sector not only gives up some control to contracted agencies for placing special needs children but also needs to adjust to changing interorganizational boundaries. No longer applicable boundary sets may still operate at the staff level. To some public agency staff, the private sector may be an "illegitimate intruder into an established inter-agency order" (Benson et al. 1973).

Finally, the issue of client ownership overshadowed the intent of this joint adoption program effort. The public agency adoption staff was concerned primarily with the best interests of their client, the child, whereas the private adoption agency staff focused on the best interests of its client, the adoptive applicant. The concept of shared responsibility for placing children in adoptive homes did not appear to work toward the best interests of the adoptive family, which includes the child.

In conclusion, based on evidence from one state, the outcomes of a contracted program may depend on not only a systematically organized set of program procedures but also on the attitudes, skills, and degree of commitment of participating agency staff. Organizational readjustments are needed, as well as interorganizational procedures to develop effective contracting systems.

16

Public-Private Contracting in Child Welfare: The California Family Protection Act Experience

Elsa Ten Broeck

In 1976 the California state legislature passed the California Family Protection Act (FPA) to reform an expensive and ineffective foster care system. A key section in the law required that "each demonstration county shall utilize available private services in the county prior to developing new county operating services when such available private services are at least as favorable in quality and cost as those operated by the county" (SB 30, Section 16526).

FPA was implemented on a pilot basis in two California counties, rural Shasta and urban San Mateo. Due to its small size and limited resources, Shasta County did not provide its services through contracting. On the other hand, San Mateo had many resources available through private, nonprofit community agencies and was able to deliver most of the mandated "Family Reunification Services" through contracts. The FPA project began in the San Mateo County Department of Health and Welfare, Children's Service Section, in October 1977. It took approximately one year to establish all of the mandated services. Due to the need for immediate implementation (the legislation was passed effective 1 July 1977), seven initial contracts were signed without a competitive bid process.

In-home services were required by FPA to prevent removal of a child from the home, and included training of homemakers, housekeepers, and in-home caretakers. After serious consideration of the advantages and disadvantages of contracting out these particular services, Children's Services decided to provide them directly as an extension of its existing shelter care program for children. Shelter care staff, familiar with the needs of children in crisis, were trained to provide care for the children in their own homes rather than in emergency foster homes. Training of

238

shelter care staff also included skill development on how to work with parents to increase their household and parenting skills.

After the first year of implementation, the county and state established a competitive bid system for continuing FPA services. A request for proposals (RFP) was developed and four services were bid competitively: family counseling, parent support groups, therapeutic day care, and respite care and atypical day care. Legal services were continued with the original contractors, but the Parent Aide Program and the Respite Care Program for Adolescents were discontinued.

The following discussion of issues involved in contracting between public and private (nonprofit) child welfare agencies is based upon the author's four years of experience negotiating and monitoring the above contracts as project supervisor of the Family Protection Act Demonstration Project in San Mateo County.

LEGAL REQUIREMENTS OF FPA

All of the contracts were negotiated in accord with county regulations and state law governing Title XX monies; the FPA program was included in the state Title XX Plan and therefore had to conform to Title XX requirements. In addition, the FPA law placed stringent procedural and programmatic limits on the contractors, including the following:

Services could be provided only to families certified by Children's Services for FPA.

Services provided to clients on a voluntary basis were limited to a total of six months. If a family continued to need services beyond six months to keep the child at home, a petition had to be filed in juvenile court by the Children's Services worker and the child placed under court supervision during service continuation.

If a family of a child in out-of-home care could not resolve its problems to the point that the child could return to the home within a legally mandated period of time, FPA required an alternative permanent plan for the child, even if progress in treatment was evident. These strict parameters on contracted service provision under FPA had implications for program operations, roles assignments, and public-private relationships: the private agencies could not develop their own intake.

239

Children's Services' staff assumed the role of case manager and made all decisions regarding placement of the child, provision of services, and service termination.

The private agencies had to develop mechanisms by which to contribute to the public agency's decision-making process and concurrently accept the limitation of not being the final decision maker.

Private agency staff was accountable to the Children's Services' worker regarding services provided or recommended.

Private agency staff was obligated to treat all clients referred and generally worked with families not requesting services.

Private agency staff was required to report on clients' progress in treatment and could be called upon to testify in contested court hearings regarding that treatment.

PUBLIC-PRIVATE RELATIONSHIPS BEFORE AND AFTER FPA

The San Mateo experience highlights some of the impacts of federal policy, specifically P.L. 96–272 (the Adoption Assistance and Child Welfare Act of 1980) on public and private child welfare agencies and their interrelationship. FPA was a prototype of the implementation, on a state and county level, of this federal program. The initiation of preplacement services under P.L. 96–272 was likely to increase the interrelationships between private and public child welfare agencies, in light of the law's specific mandate to use private services when available.

The San Mateo experience provides evidence that the development of formal contracts that delegate responsibility and service financing from the public to private agencies is an effective and efficient way to provide such mandated services. Prior to FPA implementation, San Mateo county had contracted with private agencies to provide treatment whenever possible. However, it was sometimes difficult to obtain the types of services needed by the referred clients. In other instances the community agency would provide services to clients but refuse to release information about the progress or utilization of those services to the public agency. Too often, referrals would result in a conflict of interest between the parents' right to confidentiality and the children's right to protection. With some exceptions San Mateo Children's Services staff found it more efficient to provide services directly or to utilize a select few cooperative agencies and professionals. With the exception of Guadalupe Mental Health Center, the contractors selected under FPA were not used to any large extent by Children's Services prior to the establishment of formal contracts.

The contracting process under FPA changed how the public children's services agency interacted with the private agencies. Rather than referring clients and losing all control over client treatment, Children's Services was able to contract with the private agencies for a specific service and maintain control over decision making and case determination as well as the types of services offered. In turn, private agencies received financial reimbursement for all activities connected with the service, including outreach, preparation time, and failed appointments. Contracting also made it possible for private agencies to obtain formal agreements about the nature of their contributions to decision making and the degree to which they could exercise controls over the services provided.

REDEFINING ROLES THROUGH CONTRACTING

One result of contracting under FPA has been a redefinition of roles for the staffs of the public and private agencies. This redefinition corresponded with the new clinical approach to child protective services developed under FPA. The legal limits placed on the behavior of clients/families by the new juvenile court law made it crucial to assign one professional to work with the family in the role of case manager. This case manager was responsible for informing the parents of the expectations they must meet to keep or be reunified with their children. As the monitor, the case manager assisted the family in obtaining resources, assessed their progress, and reported to the court. This role was delegated to Children's Services staff. The private agency worker, on the other hand, was delegated the responsibility for direct service provision, helping the client deal with the issues identified by the case manager and facilitating change in accord with the client's desires and abilities.

The relationship between the private provider and the client was significantly different from the relationship the private agency had with its traditional clientele. The public agency, as contractor, held the private agency accountable for its services. It was understood and made clear to the client before services began that the private agency had to report to Children's Services and, where appropriate, to the juvenile court about the progress of treatment and the parents' ability or inability to parent their children.

Expectations about client behavior in treatment with the private agency were also communicated. It was made clear that the client was expected to deal with the specific problems resulting in protective service intervention. Even if the parents made use of services and progress in other areas of their lives, clients were informed that the contract agency would have to provide a report on the specific issues related to the care of their children and the extent to which progress had occurred in these areas.

This role delineation between public and private agencies did not occur immediately. Initially, staff at both agencies functioned as they had in the past, with the public agency making a referral and the private agency providing treatment to the client in a manner similar to all other referrals. Through contract monitoring and the results of court proceedings, it became apparent that further guidelines were needed for staff of both public and provider agencies. It was recognized, for example, that Children's Services staff needed to be more specific about the nature of its referrals, including identification of parental issues and problems requiring priority attention in the treatment process. Children's Services workers needed to specify the limits to be set on both counseling and direct services and to elaborate on the intended focus of counseling activities.

Both public and private agency staff had to deal with significant role changes. For the Children's Services worker, this role shift meant assuming a monitoring function and giving up direct treatment responsibilities to the private agency. For the private agency worker, decision making and control over who would be seen and what problems would be addressed were forfeited.

METHODS USED TO REDEFINE ROLES

To deal with the changes in role definition and to facilitate cooperation between the staff of public and private agencies, Children's Services devoted a significant proportion of time to joint staff contacts. Joint training was conducted on how to treat abusive families, and joint staff meetings were held on a monthly basis to discuss cases and administrative problems. Each contract was monitored on a quarterly basis to review the quality and quantity of services. Contracts were renegotiated annually and service descriptions were revised to incorporate changes based on the experiences of the previous year.

Contract monitoring focused on both administration and program. The contract monitor was responsible for authorizing services requested by Children's Services staff and monitoring ongoing services. Frequently, the contract monitor served as the link between public and private staff to resolve issues that could not be addressed on an individual staff basis. These issues included differences in perspective about how services were delivered, whether services were delivered, what disposition was needed in a case, and who should carry responsibility for particular aspects of a case. Generally, these problems stemmed from misunderstandings between professionals of the two agency types or from manipulations by the client. The most common solution to these problems, particularly that of client manipulation, was to clearly state goals and objectives for the service and establish regular meeting times for professional staff to confer about the case plan and progress in implementation.

Impact of Contracting on Clinical Services Confidentiality

The use of contracting most profoundly affected client confidentiality procedures for both the public and private agencies. As discussed earlier, Children's Services staff was used to working with private agencies under conditions in which they had only limited access to information unless the client signed a release. Private agencies considered the confidentiality of the worker-client relationship to be a key ingredient in fostering a relationship of trust. Under FPA, clients were informed that the signing of a release was a precondition for receiving service and that information would be freely exchanged. Clients were further informed that the private agency staff was accountable to the Children's Services agency that was financing the service. This change in approach to confidentiality was disturbing to some private agency practitioners and was initially resisted. Staff from both agencies eventually developed specific ways to deal with confidentiality that did not impede the treatment process. These included the following:

> Parents were informed by Children's Services before a referral was made to the private agency that the information would be

shared. If the client was willing to use the service under these conditions, he or she signed a release to that effect.

During the first contact, staff from the private agency reviewed the agreement about confidentiality with the parents and again committed the parents to that agreement.

Where appropriate or possible, clients were given copies of written reports submitted by the private agency to Children's Services.

If sharing of the reports was deemed inappropriate, the private agency staff discussed with the client the nature of the information being communicated to Children's Services.

Clients were informed when private agency staff attended meetings pertinent to them, such as multidisciplinary team reviews, and were provided information of what occurred at those meetings.

It is interesting that positive case outcomes occurred most frequently when guidelines about the sharing of information were clear and understood by all parties. In these instances clients were generally under court order to participate in treatment. Clients receiving services on a voluntary basis were less successful in treatment, and, in general, guidelines for information sharing between the public and private agencies were more ambigious.

Client Involvement

The degree of involvement was generally a result of the actions and initiatives of the individual workers rather than the outcome of specific agency policy or regulations. Workers were encouraged to involve the client in case planning, but this was often difficult to accomplish due to the types of interventions and the involuntary nature of clients' participation. Children's Services staff was expected to develop, for each family/client, a contract for services that included problem identification, needed areas of change, and the consequences of change or lack of change. Private agency staff frequently developed a secondary contract with parents specific to the treatment issues.

Clients were not involved in program development or selection of contract agencies. Clients also were not given much choice regarding the nature of services available to them under the provisions of FPA. The services available were identified, and the client either chose to accept such services or obtain them on his or her own, thereby also assuming financial responsibility. Most clients who utilized FPA services had input into the nature and process of treatment at the individual provider level.

Client Manipulation

Abusive and neglectful families may evidence manipulative behavior. Contracted agencies, without experience serving such populations, may need to learn that protective services clients may seek to use a system of service to their own advantage. It was not unusual in the FPA program to have contract staff "hook" a client in treatment by identifying with the client against the "system." Clients often tended, with much expertise, to project their problems onto the bureaucracy. To the extent that their projections influenced the course of treatment, private agency staff resources were diverted to battling the court and Children's Services' workers rather than helping the client deal with his or her role in that struggle.

All practitioners of protective services need to be cautious about parents' ability to convince the worker that the struggle lies outside the client. Unfortunately, the real limitations of public systems to effectively address human problems may inadvertently encourage a focus on the service system, as well as on the client. The division within the service system created by a manipulative client was the most destructive client implication stemming from the public-private contractual relationship.

Contract monitoring and training of staff were critical factors in dealing with realized or potential client manipulations. Public and private agency staff needed time to develop relationships that would encourage mutual trust in their judgments and establish communication systems that would facilitate exchanges about the accuracy of client feedback on the other system and its personnel. In addition, staff required training on recognizing and intervening with the manipulative client, such as when the client would present himself one way to one professional and the opposite way to another. Workers needed to know that a mother who appeared overwhelmed and resistant to the Children's Services worker could a few days later appear in control and cooperative in treatment with a private agency practitioner. Training sought to develop workers' understanding of the validity of both aspects of the woman's behavior and that neither could be ignored or totally accepted. Finally, staff had to learn to work together with the client to develop an appropriate case plan that protected the children and helped the parent increase his or her ability to either care for the child(ren) or relinquish them for foster care or adoption.

INGREDIENTS OF A SUCCESSFUL CONTRACT

Based on the FPA experience, the following ingredients can be identified as important for the success of public-private agency contracting:

A carefully negotiated contract that includes definitions, a detailed service statement, clearly defined roles, and reasonable methods of payment

Sufficient rate reimbursement to cover all aspects of the contracted services

Regular contact between staff of the public and private agencies to discuss clinical and administrative issues (generally, once a month)

Designation of a contract monitor who meets regularly with all parties and is available to resolve disputes

Clarification and specificity with the client about the nature and scope of information exchange between the public and private agency

Regular reports from the private agency on progress in meeting the service goals identified in the referral

Administrative commitment from both public and private agencies to contracting and the contract process

The FPA project in San Mateo county met with considerable success over a four-year implementation period. The foster care rate has been decreased by 35 percent, and family reunification or maintenance in the home has been achieved for 94 percent of the children served. A major component of the program has been the use of purchase of service contracts for the provision of services. The development of a contractual process based on the ingredients delineated above contributed toward FPA achievements. In 1981 FPA was extended an additional three years by the California state legislature at a time when few demonstration programs received any funding. The success of FPA can be attributed, in large part, to the contractual service delivery model linking public and private agencies.

PART FIVE

The Impact of Purchase
of Service

In this section the focus is on some of the major policy and practice implications that arise from our collective experiences with purchasing services. Relevant questions include, What are the organizational, structural, and personnel implications of purchasing services? What is the impact of purchasing services on the public-private sector relationship? What are the types of service available to targeted clients/patients, and who receives these services? Does purchase of services promote or hinder equity, equality, and efficacy in the provision of services?

The authors of the four chapters in this section share in common the view that purchase of service (POS) has not, in actuality, proved to be a panacea. Experience with POS implementation suggests that this system of service delivery is flawed. Some of these flaws are structural in nature; others have to do with interorganizational relationships; issues of power and turf; a growing bureaucracy to substitute for earlier, rejected bureaucratic forms; and unrealistic expectations. What is perhaps most telling however, is that all of these authors conclude that, despite the flaws, the purchasing of services should continue.

The subject of expectations is important in explaining the evolving attitudes toward and changes initiated in the procedures and practices associated with POS. The frequent and consistent deviation between intended and actual social policy outcomes is quite pervasive in this country. Time after time, the expectations about new policies and programs intended to change or solve identified problems or social issues are so high that their realization is virtually impossible. Implementation is often marred by insufficient time to test new approaches and, perhaps most important, inadequate funds. We seem often not to learn from our mistakes. Sometimes, there is an inherent lack of clarity about what the new policy is intended to accomplish (e.g., absence of clearly defined goals) or insufficient attention to the degree of consistency between a new policy and existing policies, (e.g., goal conflict). One likely result is that new approaches that are initially perceived to be a means to solve old problems (such as overcoming bureaucratic rigidity, reducing the size of government and decreasing the costs of services) come to be seen as problems themselves. Not only is the original intent not met, but now policymakers and administrators must address the failures or inadequacies of the new policy or practice.

Purchase of service has, in many respects closely followed this cycle of high expectations—implementation problems—disillusionment—reassessment and modification—renewed expectations that several observers of the policymaking process have identified. (See, for example, Pressman and Wildavsky 1973; Edwards and Sharkansky 1978.) As the authors of the following chapters note, there certainly have been modifications in how purchase of service arrangements are planned and carried out, and the call for further reforms is quite consistent. Unlike many of the new programs and service approaches of the 1960s, however, POS has borne the test of time in many significant ways. Foremost, its fit with a major policy agenda of the Carter and, especially, Reagan administrations—privatization—is so evident and strong that, rather than abandoning POS, there is substantial consensus about the desire to resolve the weaknesses of the system.

The conclusions reached by the commonwealth of Massachusetts' Senate Committee on Ways and Means, excerpted here, about the need to improve the administration of contracted services are instructive of the many unanticipated issues that may emerge from the use of POS. The convening of this special committee to examine and make recommendations about the commonwealth's POS system is itself evidence of the perception that problems exist in relation to contracting. The goal of using POS to achieve specified ends (in this case, community-based care) was very much accepted by the committee but, in a series of recommendations, a substantial change agenda to improve the system was detailed. The major problem identified was state government's neglect of the administrative apparatus needed to plan, implement, and oversee this system. The condensed report includes discussion of the reasons accounting for the identified problems, their effect, and how they may be addressed.

Lacking hard data on which to make decisions, the choice about

248

whether, when, and with whom to purchase may, too often, be based more on happenstance than on its potential or proven effectiveness. The internal and external pressures upon the public agencies to contract out services left too little time for planning the necessary procedural systems. The retrospective view, not surprisingly, is that the public sector's lack of preparedness to assume its redefined functions under POS has seriously impacted on both the administration and outcomes of this system.

Addressing the question of the impact of contracting on those receiving services, Gibelman sought to empirically determine what, if any, differences exist in child protective services delivered to clients directly by the public agency or through contracted, voluntary agency providers. Although she, too, found that relationship problems affected the climate and process in which the contracted program was implemented, the findings suggest that POS can positively impact upon the services that clients receive. Compared with the services delivered to clients under public agency auspices, those served under contract with voluntary agency providers received a greater diversity (types) of services, were seen more frequently, had more phone and collateral contacts with their caseworkers, and were seen by personnel with more professional qualifications.

Gurin and Friedman, also drawing on actual experience garnered in the commonwealth of Massachusetts, take a broader systems perspective in their discussion of the efficacy of purchasing services, with primary attention to the question of whether contracting promotes better and more economical human services. Unfortunately, the quest to achieve and measure "better services" is thwart with problems. Subjectivity may be inevitable at this stage in the development of evaluation science. Quality may be "in the eyes of the beholder", e.g., differentially defined depending upon one's perspective. What constitutes "good services" is thus subject to values and interpretation. Only when we can achieve a standard definition of "good services" can we begin to address the nature and measurement of "better services." (Gibelman addressed this issue by looking at factors assumed to be positively associated with quality, according to expert opinion.)

The "soft" nature of human services seems to be responsible for some of the problems that emerge in contracting, ranging from determining the "true" costs of units of services, to monitoring contracts, to the enforcement of and accountability for contracted services. Viewing the larger context of POS, Gurin and Friedman argue that the selection of this service delivery mechanism may have more to do with exigencies than with merit or need, and that the true costs of contracting are not taken into account. With increased use of POS comes increased public agency costs for negotiating, monitoring and case managing. They conclude that the increasing formality and specificity of contracts has not resulted in the delivery of high-quality services, in part because the public agency lacks monitoring capabilities. Given the neutral impact of POS on quality of service and the higher than expected real costs of contracting, they suggest that alternatives, such as voucher systems, be considered.

Based on a sizable number of case experiences with contracting, it is fair to conclude that the public-private relationship manifest in any POS arrangement will be an important determinant of the relative success of both its process and outcome. As Giovannoni concludes, in examining the contextual and relationship factors impacting upon child welfare contracting in a western region of the United States, the continued and ever-expanding use of these arrangements is perceived as a given. However, the articulation of questions about the most desirable scope and mix of public and private services is pronounced. These same relationship issues are repeatedly echoed as a major cause of disillusionment and dissatisfaction with contracting.

These themes, of course, merely reiterate the basic questions about public-private sector relationships that have plagued social welfare experts since the beginning of this country's history. The pendulum-like attitudes about respective roles and responsibilities between the two sectors and the debate about the appropriate degree of intermingling are likely to continue unabated. Although resolution of these basic questions is not likely, it is perhaps the ongoing debate itself that lends a dynamic quality to American social welfare and allows for adaptation and change within the context of the political, moral, and philosophical climate of the times.

17

Protecting the Promise of Community-Based Care

Patricia McGovern

O ver the past twenty years, there has been a gradual change in the mechanisms used to deliver social and rehabilitative services to needy Massachusetts citizens. Formerly, the mentally ill, substance abusers, juvenile offenders, or the mentally retarded received care in large, state-operated institutions. These same populations are now treated in small, community-based facilities or in their homes. The premise on which this change is based is that social and rehabilitative services must allow service users the least restrictive environment and the greatest opportunities for integration into society.

The program that make up the community-based system are as varied as the needs of the populations they are intended to serve. This community movement is national in scope, cutting across state lines, agencies, and populations. The thread uniting the diversity of the movement is the desire to see disabled, disadvantaged, or isolated citizens lead productive lives. A basic tenet of the community approach is that the community must accept and participate in the rehabilitation of the individual, if the individual is to eventually lead a full life within their broader environment.

The growth in the movement from institutional to community-based service has been both dramatic and rapid. In 1975, for example, the Massachusetts Department of Mental Health targeted 84 percent of its direct services budget to hospital and state school programs, whereas only 54 percent of its fiscal year 1986 budget is so allocated. The balance, for FY 1986, of $280 million is targeted for community-based programs and facilities. In 1965 the direct services budget of the Department of Youth Services was allocated, in total, for the maintenance of state-operated regional training schools; in FY 1986, 57 percent of the department's direct

251

services budget is spent on noninstitutional care. The community services budget of the Department of Social Services has increased by $146.8 million, or 180 percent, over the last ten years.

Although the state government has acknowledged community-based care as a successful service model, implementation problems have plagued the movement. Basically, these problems concern the demands to expand and upgrade the community-based system rapidly and to the resulting pressures on the administrative structure. In the past all social and rehabilitative services rendered through institutions were most frequently provided directly by state government. Services in the community, however, are more commonly rendered through contracts with provider organizations. Thus, over a twenty-year period, state government has moved not only from institutional to community-based care but also from direct service provision to a contracted service system. State government no longer directly controls the provision of these services but holds contractors accountable for achieving the public goals of community-based care.

The problem encountered most frequently by the state government is its own neglect of the administrative needs of this new system of contracted service provision. The successes of community-based programs are heralded by state agencies, advocates, families, the press, and service recipients, but the contracted service providers, often the object of suspicion and concern, have not received appropriate attention from state policymakers. The complaints about contracted organizations are frequent and strong. Rarely is it heard that the provider system is operating efficiently, that all parties are content, or that a consensus regarding the future of the system has been achieved.

The contract system seems to breed concern from all sides. Providers are concerned about what they perceive to be burdensome, confusing paper work, believing that the state administration is more interested in paper than in the achievement of program goals. Reimbursements are seen as inadequate and late. State agencies, for their part, are concerned about provider accountability, provider interest in maximizing profits, state government's dependence on outside contractors, and ineffective negotiations. Legislative, audit, and advocacy concerns focus on the expense of the system and its failure to deliver what it should. It is also believed that public funds are spent for services that are badly defined or to meet questionable contract agency charges, Finally, public employee concerns center on the threat posed by the private provider system to public service.

Despite these concerns, annual appropriations for continuing or developing new contracted programs continues to rise. In FY 1986 Massachusetts state government spent in excess of $614 million on contracted social and rehabilitative services, or an amount roughly equal to the state share of the federal medicaid program. Over forty-seven hundred separate contracts were negotiated between state agencies and over twelve hundred provider organizations during FY 1986. For FY 1987 it was expected that these figures would increase, with the total state obligation approaching $700 million.

There are several reasons the community-based system of care developed as a contracted rather than state-provided system. When government made the decision to support local rather than regionally based services, there already existed a strongly entrenched network of charitable, nonprofit, and advocacy organizations interested in providing heretofore government-provided services. Rather than compete, government availed itself of these experienced and willing providers. The decentralized administration of local service delivery, especially by existing organizations, dovetailed with the fundamental goals of community-based services. Decentralization and community-based care shared in common an interest in involving home communities and their citizens in the delivery of social and rehabilitative services.

Perhaps the most important explanatory factor of why community-based care evolved into a contracting system has to do with the incompatibility of the state government's administrative structure and system with the community-based service delivery needs and with the "normalizing" intent of community care. State government's administration of direct services had traditionally addressed institutional needs and were (and are) highly centralized and standardized. For example, state positions carry job titles and descriptions that reference institutionally-based duties. More often than not, use of traditional job titles in community-based care resulted in grievances by state employees called upon to perform tasks not specified in their job descriptions. Furthermore, because the state did not own, and was not capable of maintaining, a network of local facilities to house residential and day programs, early community program developers had to negotiate leases for private residences and facilities from landlords who were expected to wait many months for requisite approvals from central state authorities. The purchase of supplies and equipment also involved central office approval, which often required the use of highly standardized items that were unsuitable for creating a "normalized" environment for clients. The centralized payment policies of the commonwealth, involving batched invoices, a multilayered approval process, and monthly payment of invoices, posed a major obstacle to inducing small, local vendors to provide services to community-based programs. Given all of these factors, the use of a contracted system became the only viable alternative.

The contract provider system has grown dramatically over the past twenty years and now constitutes the primary mechanism used by the commonwealth to deliver community-based services. Even today, state administrative procedures suggest their unsuitability to a local, direct service delivery system. A large network of nonprofit and for-profit service providers has developed to conduct the business of the commonwealth. Unfortunately, this fact is often ignored by central administrative authorities and policymakers. Administration of the contract system has, accordingly, developed in a piecemeal, contradictory, and duplicative manner, with primary decisions left to contracting agencies. The system has not benefited from the kind of consistent and coordinated central oversight that is necessary to ensure effective and long-term viability. At best, the relationship between central administrative authorities and the contracted providers has been one of mutual tolerance.

PROFILE OF THE SYSTEM

The following questions are often asked: What constitutes social and rehabilitative services? How much is the commonwealth spending to contract for such services? How many contracts are there? Who are the providers and how many are there? It is an indication of both the relative newness of the system and administrative neglect of it that such questions frequently arise. Until recently, there was no comprehensive reference document on human services agencies, the largest group of purchasers, and no data on all state purchasing agencies and contractors.

As of FY 1986, fourteen state agencies spent more than $614 million annually to administer more than forty-seven hundred contracts with more than twelve hundred providers of social and rehabilitative services. In excess of two hundred discrete program types have been developed and defined and are routinely purchased by contracting agencies. It is a measure of the rapid growth of the contracting system that in 1971 the commonwealth spent only $25 million annually on social and rehabilitative service contracts.

Types of Service

In terms of both dollars and number of contracts, the largest group of contracted programs are those that provide special populations with the opportunity to achieve the highest level of social functioning. Approximately $300 million annually is spent by the Department of Mental Health, Social Services, Public Health, Youth Services, and Elder Affairs, as well as the Parole Board, the Commission for the Blind, and the Rehabilitation Commission, and the Executive Office of Communities and Development to provide services to various special populations. Such programs include residential centers designed to provide a home-like social, rehabilitative, or therapeutic environment; half-way houses, group homes, community residences, and staffed or cooperative apartments; day programs; and special supporting programs for targeted groups, such as home care for the elderly, personal care assistance, housing services, or radio reading services for the blind. The number and type of such programs are potentially limitless, but they share a common goal: to improve the ability of special populations to function normally within society. Approximately 48 percent of all dollars spent for social and rehabilitative service contracting by state agencies are directed to this purpose.

The second largest group includes contracted programs that strengthen and preserve, or provide a substitute for, family life. Approximately $160 million is spent annually, most of which by the Department of Social Services, to provide these services. Programs serve needy families and children and include day care, substitute care, respite care, case management, homemaker, specialized home care, and parent aid programs, among others. Day care accounts for almost half of the total, and when combined with substitute care (group care, foster care) accounts for roughly 75 percent of the total.

Other significant groups include programs that seek to promote or maintain mental or physical health and programs that seek to improve educational or employment opportunities for special populations. Approximately $70 million is spent annually by the Departments of

Public Health, Mental Health, Youth Services, and Corrections on health improvement; approximately $22 million is spent by the Department of Education on special education programs; and approximately $30 million is spent by the Departments of Mental Health and Public Welfare and the Rehabilitation Commission to assist special populations in securing employment. Programs include a variety of crisis intervention, psychiatric, residential and day treatment, emergency shelter, outpatient counseling, detoxification, nutritional and preventive programs related to health; special education, counseling, and developmental day-care programs in the education arena; and supported work programs, sheltered workshops, transitional employment, and work activity in the area of employment. These three categories account for approximately 20 percent of all social and rehabilitative contracting.

Finally, a number of programs serve specialized purposes such as public safety, provision of basic material needs, or effectiveness of service. A variety of halfway houses, secure detention or treatment programs, counseling programs, and shelter care programs for offenders, ex-offenders, and detainees are funded by the Parole Board and the Departments of Youth Services, Public Health, and Corrections to ensure the safety of the public. The Department of Public Welfare's shelters for the homeless fall within the category of provision of basic material needs, and almost all agencies fund programs designed to improve the effectiveness of services, e.g., case management, information and referral, consultation and education, and transportation services.

State Contracting Agencies

There are currently fourteen state agencies that fund contracts for social and rehabilitative services, eleven of which are with the human services secretariat. These fourteen agencies directly or indirectly administer more than 4,700 contracts totaling $614 million annually. In terms of volume, the Department of Mental Health is the largest state contracting agency, with 2,163 contracts totaling $204.6 million annually. The Departmennt of Social Services, with 1,701 contracts totaling $172 million, is the second largest contractor. The Departments of Mental Health and Social Services, taken together, account for 61 percent of all social and rehabilitative contracting activity statewide. Other large contracting agencies include the Department of Elder Affairs, with 27 contracts totaling $103.7 million annually, and the Department of Public Health, with 597 contracts totaling $53.6 million.

The organizing structure of the contracting agencies varies considerably, ranging from a centralized organization to local administration through a network of area offices. The Department of Mental Health, the largest contracting agency, administers contracts on the local level, through forty-one area offices, whereas the Departments of Youth Services and Public Health administer contracts centrally. Some agencies have developed unique contracting structures. The Department of Elder Affairs, for example, contracts directly with twenty-seven home care corporations, which in turn subcontract for the provision of direct services to elderly persons within their service areas. The organization and structure of contract administration has grown independently and reflects the needs and concerns of individual contracting agencies, rather than a coordinated state policy.

Some agencies purchase relatively few of the more than two hundred existing program types, whereas others purchase a significant number. The Department of Mental Health, for example, can identify eighty-six program types that it routinely purchases, including residential, day care, outpatient, crisis intervention, case management, workshop, and foster care programs, among others. The majority of Department of Mental Health contracts are intended to provide an opportunity for mentally ill or retarded individuals to achieve the highest possible level of social functioning (62 percent of total dollars are so allocated). Programs that promote or maintain the mental health of service recipients account for 20 percent of total contract dollars, whereas employment programs account for 10 percent.

The Department of Public Health also purchases a variety of different program types, ranking second in number of program types purchased. Included, among others, are detoxification, early intervention, halfway houses, maternal and child health, outpatient counseling, prevention, and nutrition programs. Slightly half of the department's contracted programs provide either substance abusers or disabled children with opportunities for the highest possible level of social functioning. Just under half of all contracts provide these same populations, as well as needy families and the general public, with a variety of programs designed to promote and maintain physical health. These programs range from

257

direct treatment services, such as detoxification or primary care, to preventive programs, such as the Women, Infants, and Children Nutritional Program.

Most agencies, however, administer a limited set of program types targeted to specific populations or designed to promote a specific agency mission. The Department of Social Services, for example, purchases only seventeen discrete program types, the majority of which serve the agency's primary mandate to strengthen and perserve, or provide a substitute for family life. Such programs include substitute care, day care, casework, parent aid, and respite care. Similarly, the Department of Elder Affairs, which ranks third in total contract dollars, contracts almost exclusively for homemaker or chore services for the state's elderly population. The Department of Youth Services purchases seventeen program types, with a focus on public safety. The Massachusetts Rehabilitation Commission contracts for seven types of programs, the majority of which provide physically disabled individuals with employment opportunities. The Department of Education contracts exclusively for special education services, and the Department of Welfare and the Executive Office of Communities and Development primarily fund housing services, day care, or employment and training.

The Providers

Over twelve hundred provider organizations, public and private, proprietary and nonprofit, routinely contract with the commonwealth to provide social and rehabilitative services. Although less comprehensive information is available on the providers than on the contracting agencies, it is clear that the majority are private, nonprofit organizations, many of which began with the goal of advocacy for populations with special needs. The wide variety of providers, however, reflects the varied needs of state contracting agencies and service recipients. Providers range from newly organized entities with a single contract and an annual budget of under fifty thousand dollars to well-endowed, diversified hospitals or corporations with annual budgets exceeding $80 million. As might be expected, provider types often reflect the special populations they serve. At the same time, however, a significant number of providers are multiservice agencies serving a variety of needs and contracting with a number of state agencies.

In general, the social and rehabilitative service provider system can be characterized as new, dependent upon state contracts for its existence, undercapitalized, and made up of small organizations. A survey of human service providers conducted for the Executive Office of Human Services in August 1984 yielded interesting data concerning the average provider. Based on the survey sample, 50 percent of all providers are less than fifteen years old, a statistic suggesting that fully half the system came into being as a result of the shift in focus to community-based care and the availability of state contracting dollars. The study also found, however, that 16 percent of provider organizations were over fifty years old, which reflects the involvement of traditional organizations and is suggestive of a mix of new and old contractors.

The average provider was determined to have an annual budget of $528,000, with two-thirds of the providers operating on annual budgets of fewer than one million dollars. The average provider was found to have thirty-four full-time employees and eighteen part-time employees. Fifty-five percent of the providers surveyed also had contracts with more than one state agency. Of particular interest were the findings related to provider income and capital reserves. The average provider was found to receive 56 percent of total income from a combination of all government sources and program fees. Nearly all providers complained of cash flows and/or capitalization problems, with 90 percent reporting less than two months' operating cash on hand. In fact, the average provider was found to have less than one month of cash on hand. Sixty percent of the providers described their cash-flow problems as serious, and 56 percent had ended at least one of the past five years with a deficit. The most common method of addressing cash flow problems was a line of credit or some other form of borrowing. Generally, the provider community is young and still in the process of developing.

With respect to services rendered, the most common types were found to be counseling, education and training, information and referral, advocacy, residential care or treatment, mental health, and day-care services, with most providers offering a range of services.

Although the majority of contractors tend to be nonprofit organizations, the ratio can vary significantly depending on the subsystem under consideration. The residential school, homemaker, and day-care systems, for example, include a large number of for-profit service providers.

259

PROBLEMS WITH THE SYSTEM

The POS system, today, comprises over 1,200 provider organizations offering as many as 200 different types of human service programs and employing approximately 30,000 persons. Recent reports from such diverse sources as the Auditor of the Commonwealth, the Governor's Management Task Force, Massachusetts Taxpayers Foundation, the Blue Ribbon Commission on the Future of Public Inpatient Mental Health Services, and the Massachusetts Council on Human Services Providers, leave little doubt that the community-based movement of the late 1960s and early 1970s has proved to be, in the 1980s, a staggeringly expensive and inefficient system.

The overriding problem of the purchase of service contracting system is the lack of central administrative oversight and planning. Decentralized agency-specific implementation of contracted community-based services, though effective program policy, had given rise to an inefficient administrative machine. Continued neglect of the need for consistent statewide contract management can only result in failure of the system.

The ramifications of this lack of central administrative leadership are many and have produced system-wide problems. These include a lack of clear and consistent standards throughout the procurement process and the inefficiencies and burdensome paperwork requirements of a multilayered, decentralized bureaucracy. System-wide planning problems include failure to develop a long-range financing strategy for the current system, failure to develop a comprehensive training program for agency contract staff, and the failure of the state to address the needs of the provider system. Contracting agency problems center around lack of training, lack of necessary administrative resources, and insufficient central office oversight. Provider problems include the failure to access capital markets and the failure to train, recruit, and retain qualified personnel.

System-Wide Problems

A number of historical factors have contributed to the state's failure to provide centralized contracting oversight. The community system of care developed not as the result of centralized policymaking, but as the consequence of piecemeal decisions that resulted in gradual, unmonitored growth. Second, the nature of the service delivery system itself, with its focus on decentralized, community-based administration, has allowed contracting agencies to neglect central controls and concentrate on field-based operations. Third, service contracting authority has traditionally resided with state agencies responsible for service provision, rather than with a central purchasing office. Although a central office of the purchasing agency has responsibility for state agency purchases of materials, equipment, and supplies, this office has played no role in the purchase of social and rehabilitative services. As a result, contracting agencies have development contract administration systems in a policy vacuum. Each system reflects the definitions and perspectives of an individual agency and is not necessarily compatible with the system developed by any other agency. Fourth, the contracted community-based system of care was developed, in many respects, as an alternative to the state's centralized, institution-oriented administrative system. Contracting agencies were only too happy to avoid an overly restrictive bureaucracy, which was perceived as fundamentally insensitive to the needs and goals of community-based care.

As the volume of state contracts grew and as more and more agencies decided to contract for social and rehabilitative services, central state administration could only react to the growing administrative problem. At first, the comptroller's division, where contract documents are filed and to whom provider requests for payment are submitted, was the only central oversight agency for contracting in existence. In 1975, however, the Rate Setting Commission, within the Executive Office of Human Services, was given authority to set rates for social and rehabilitative service contracts. In the late 1970s, regulations were promulgated by the Executive Office for Administration and Finance to establish a contract authorization system involving not only the contracting agency, the Comptroller's Division, the Executive Office for Administration and Finance, and the Rate Setting Commission, but also the secretariat with jurisdiction over the contracting agency. Since then, the secretariats have gradually expanded contract management and auditing activities. In 1982 the state auditor was given the authority to audit contracts with service providers.

Central oversight of social and rehabilitative service contracting has therefore developed, like the community-based system itself, in a piecemeal and generally uncoordinated fashion. The result is a system that gives a number of independent and organizationally diverse state agencies oversight of a $614 million system.

261

The Contract Authorization System

Oversight of state agency contracting for social and rehabilitative services is inefficient, contradictory, and fragmented. The multilayered bureaucracy, which has been pieced together to bring order to the system, has failed to produce either standards or contracting accountability and has simply increased the level of confusion. Far from reconciling differences between contracting agencies, the central oversight agencies have generally failed to agree among themselves. Instead of simplifying the contracting process, the oversight agencies have magnified the paperwork burden for contracting agencies and providers and have generated policy disputes that debilitate an already unstructured administrative system.

Perhaps the most compelling demonstration of the problem can be seen in viewing the system from the perspective of the contracting agency or provider. Conventional wisdom would assume that once the contracting agency and the provider have negotiated terms and signed an agreement, the terms are set. In the state's social and rehabilitative services contracting system, however, a signed contract marks only the beginning of the process. The state contracting agency is first required to prepare an authorization form providing details about the proposed contract. The form is then submitted to the governing secretariat for approval and eventual filing with the Comptroller's Division of the Executive Office for Administration and Finance. The date of filing with the comptroller establishes the beginning date for services reimbursement under the contract, even if this date disagrees with that on the contract document, itself. Many state contracting agencies have faced unexplained delays in authorization or have neglected to initiate the process in a timely way. So, too, many contractors have provided services in accord with the contract terms, only to find out that services were not reimbursable due to the date they were rendered.

Authorization involves even more steps. The Rate Setting Commission must also file written rate approval with the Comptroller's Division, thereby authorizing payment at the approved Commission rate, even if this rate is inconsistent with the contract specifications. Only when the secretariat authorization form, the contract itself, and written rate approval from the Rate Setting Commission have been filed with the Comptroller's Division, and the content of each judged to be identical, is the comptroller permitted to authorize the first payment. Because the three documents take three completely different bureaucratic routes to the Comptroller's Division, the date of authorization for initiation of services and for first payment are usually unknown to the contracting agency and the provider at the time of contract signing. Often, the first payment under a contract executed in April for July 1 has not been received until September or October because the secretarial authorization form was not filed on time.

Uncertainty and delay with respect to starting date and first payment are serious deficiencies creating cash flow problems for providers, but this problem is only one of many resulting from the state's fragmented oversight system. Contracting agencies and providers are subject to conflicting state oversight agency policies in almost every contracting area and are often uncertain about the validity of significant terms of a fully executed contract. It has not been uncommon for the Comptroller's Division to disallow payment under a fully executed contract after services have been rendered. Such disallowances have occurred when the division took exception to the reimbursement policies of the Rate Setting Commission or the billing terms approved by the secretariat. Similarly, because of rate-setting mechanisms employed by the Rate Setting Commission, the terms of a contract are frequently overturned by the commission in the process of approving a program rate. Contracting agencies and providers also routinely face unforeseen authorization problems for contracts that have received rate approvals and are ready to file with the Comptroller's Division, due to secretarial policies of the Rate Setting Commission or the Comptroller's Division. Such contradictions only demoralize and undercut the effectiveness of contracting for community-based services.

Lack of Standards

Because no single oversight office has an exclusive mandate to administer the social and rehabilitative services contracting system, few clear procurement, contract administration, rate-setting, or auditing standards exist statewide. Depending upon the state agency, or in some cases even the field office of that agency, there can be a variety of interpretations of such contracting fundamentals as to when and if to follow competitive bidding, what costs are reimbursable under the contract, whether the provider can retain surplus funds generated under the contract, what constitutes a billable service unit, or how the contract is to be monitored. There are many, many instances in which providers whose contract program is purchased by multiple state agencies (or by multiple field offices within the same state agency) are subject to conflicting interpretations of "state policy." One extreme example of this problem is a mental health provider operating a residential program with a capacity of eight, funded by eight different Department of Mental Health area offices through eight separate contracts with eight sets of compliance requirements and eight different cost reimbursement budgets, all requiring the submission of expense verification.

Payment standards are particularly unclear and inconsistent. The Rate Setting Commission, which is supposed to price the services purchased under social and rehabilitative service contracts, administers many different regulations governing such contracts, but actually sets rates for only two specific services. The majority of services are reimbursed on the basis of budgets negotiated between contracting agencies and providers. Even budgets, however, are subject to independent rate determination by the commission. In many instances a budget negotiated by agency and provider will be overturned by the Rate Setting Commission, based upon information submitted directly to the commission by the provider; this occurs after a contract has gone into effect. The ultimate absurdity can occur when, two years after a contract has expired, a state audit team is prevented from resolving an audit because of disputes between the contract agency and the Rate Setting Commission over rate jurisdiction. Within the past two years, for example, audits conducted by the Executive Office of the Department of Human Services have found that some providers have billed thousands of dollars in excess of actual, allowable costs or, pursuant to policies sanctioned by the Rate Setting Commission, have purchased properties through state contract funds and profited upon resale of these properties. Such anomalies persist because there has not been any reconciliation of the administration of pricing authority by the Rate Setting Commission with the contracting authority of state agencies.

Another example of the lack of clear and consistent standards for the contracting system is that each of the fourteen separate contracting agencies administers its own program definitions (currently totaling over two hundred program types), even though many programs are clearly similar. The scope of services, monitoring process, billable service unit, and compliance terms for similar service contracts differ from agency to agency, and can differ within the same agency or definitional category depending on field interpretations. At every level of the contracting system, there is opportunity for state agencies and providers to establish nonstandard, even unique, contracting practices.

Inefficiency and Excessive Paperwork

An immediate repercussion of the lack of standardization is inefficiency and excessive paperwork. The contract authorization process can take from one month to a year, and the terms of a completed contract may not be clear upon audit, even two years after the fact. Similar inefficiencies exist in the billing process. It may take several months to be paid, particularly when there are disputes over contract terms, documentation, or proper authorization. In such cases the billing issue may move from area to region to central office to comptroller and back again. Requests for proposals, which are intended to inform prospective providers of the availability of funds for particular program services, are often narrowly circulated or written in a confusing, jargon-ridden manner. (See Chapter 10, this volume, for a discussion of RFPs.) A contracted organization can be audited by a private accounting firm, agency auditors, secretarial auditors, Rate Setting Commission auditors, and the state auditor—all requiring different sets of records and applying different standards. The result is a mass of paperwork at the expense of monitoring or evaluating services.

The paperwork burden for any provider operating more than one program and doing business with more than one state agency can be enormous. Different contract documents must be signed with different sets of attachments and supporting documentation. Different billing practices are employed from office to office and from agency to agency. A twenty-eight page cost report must be filed annually for the Rate Setting Commission, and expenditure and contract monitoring reports must be filed with contracting agencies. The contract authorization process administered by state agencies generates secretarial authorization forms, rate filings, legal checklists, copies of contract documents, and numerous sets of regulations, guidelines, and procedural memoranda. The lack of a consistent approach to contracting state-wide generates a mountain of paper that makes it very difficult for providers to do business with the state and for state agencies to administer the system.

Lack of Long-Term Planning

Perhaps the most damaging effect of the absence of administrative standards and the resulting inefficiencies is the failure of the state to initiate the planning needed to ensure the long-term viability of the contracting system. There is no effective planning because no state office has been given an exclusive mandate to oversee the contracting system. State agencies, therefore, address only immediate problems created by an inefficient bureaucracy. This lack of planning affects every aspect of contract administration from financing to provider assistance to training of contract agency personnel.

The question of how, ultimately, to finance the contracted system of community-based care is one example of the failure to plan systematically. Currently, the state is funded almost exclusively through annual state appropriations. Over the years state funding for community-based care has dramatically increased, but federal support has declined. Yet no comprehensive effort has been made to diversify the sources of revenue for community-based care, even though potential revenue sources exist that could offset the need for continuing increases in state appropriations.

No statewide policy exists relative to charging private individuals or their families for social and rehabilitative services rendered under contracts. Although specific program types, such as home care or day care, are funded under contracts that require the provider to administer a sliding-scale charge system, these are neither uniform nor universally applied. Most contract programs do not administer private charge systems, and in some cases residential programs costing as much as seventy-five thousand dollars per placement per year are underwritten entirely by state appropriation, even though service recipients may have considerable personal or family resources. In many cases donations are not accepted from individuals and families who have expressed a willingness to contribute toward the cost of care.

Efforts to secure third-party revenues by state contracting agencies are also isolated and ineffective. Lack of central coordination and chronic interagency disputes have prevented the state from realizing the potential of the Medicaid program as one source of revenue for community-based services. At present, few program types have qualified for Medicaid reimbursement, even though discussions have continued for many years. Without central policy coordination, the needs of contracting agencies to offset state costs through Medicaid participation are difficult to reconcile with the need of the Department of Welfare to control Medicaid spending. The result, too often, is paralysis.

A special Medicaid waiver program for community-based programming has been in existence since 1981, and although limited use has been made of the program in the Departments of Mental Health and Elder Affairs, no central statewide effort to take full advantage of the opportunity has been mounted. Innovative revenue initiatives, such as a role for the insurance industry in underwriting a portion of the costs of community-based care and treatment, reallocation of under-used state institutional resources to offset expansion of the community system, or coordination and maximization of local government and private foundation monies have not been adequately pursued. Nor is there a clear policy regarding the commonwealth's role in funding community-based services; that is, should the state be the payer of last resort or is it state policy to provide services to special populations as an entitlement, without a test of ability to pay?

Another planning issue neglected by state officials is the question of the overdependence of state agencies on contractors and of contractors on the state. A number of root causes, related to lack of central policymaking, can be identified for this overdependence. For example, the desire of state contracting agencies to avoid the state's central administrative system results in decisions to contract merely because contracts are easier to administer. There are no consistent policies or purchasing criteria outlining the conditions under which contracted services should be authorized instead of direct service provision. The result is often a "knee-jerk" decision to contract and an overdependence by state agencies on contractors. In many cases, such as day care, residential schools for special needs students, group care, or community residential services for the mentally retarded, few state-operated alternatives exist to contracted services.

Another cause of the state's overdependence on contractors is the general lack of standards in the decentralized contracting system itself. Because oversight of agency contracting activities is fragmented, enforcement of contracting standards is weak. Requests for proposals can be poorly drafted and narrowly circulated, thus discouraging competitive proposals. Contract negotiation can be nonexistent, with providers themselves creating their own terms. Monitoring and evaluation procedures can be strict or lenient, predictable or arbitrary, as the contracting

267

agency, or field office of the agency, desires. The result of this unmonitored decentralization of contracting is that too often the awarding of contracts is made to the same providers from year to year, until the existing contractor is believed by the state agency to be the only known provider of services. Of the 585 contracts subject to competitive bidding within the Department of Mental Health for FY 1986, for example, only 34 contracts were awarded to new service providers. Such dependence leaves state agencies in a poor position to effect necessary changes in the service delivery system.

Many providers are overly dependent upon state contracts for their existence, particularly the small, nonprofit provider organizations. Again, the lack of central leadership within the state's contract administration system is the primary cause. Until very recently, for instance, providers were effectively discouraged from fund raising by a state rate-setting policy that required the cost of state contracts to be offset by unrestricted donations and other proceeds of provider fund-raising efforts. This policy was a major disincentive to raising revenue and to diversifying revenue sources for providers, because they received no direct benefit from their fund-raising efforts. Small, nonprofit organizations, already severely undercapitalized, were prevented from establishing new revenue sources by this policy and were therefore made more dependent on state contract funds. Chapter 761 of the Acts of 1985 prohibited this rate-setting policy, thereby creating an incentive for providers to diversify their funding base.

Second, state government had not adequately addressed the chronic undercapitalization of the provider system. The majority of the system comprises new, small, nonprofit agencies that are not well endowed and cannot successfully enter commercial markets for long-term capital financing. The result of the state's failure to creatively address this capitalization problem is that the majority of contract providers seek necessary capital through surpluses accrued under state operating contracts, in turn increasing their financial dependence on state contracts.

Third, the decentralization and fragmented oversight of contracting itself fosters mutual dependence on the part of both providers and state agencies. The failure of contracting agencies to define adequately the services they purchase, which results in the inability of the Rate Setting Commission to set standard rates for similar program types, has led to a parochial, field-controlled system of contract administration, under which providers are subject to the neglect or the overly restrictive interference of agency contract officers. In either case the provider organization cannot be sure of what it is being asked to do under the terms of the contract and is prevented from functioning confidently and independently. With no prevailing standards against which to appeal, the contract provider can be subject to spontaneous policymaking and inappropriate operational control by state contract officers. Conflicting policy statements and uncoordinated activities of the state's oversight agencies may further obscure the contracting environment. Small, undercapitalized providers, who may be subjected to the parochial policies of stage agency field officers, are not helped by contract authorization delays, retroactive rate changes, multiple audits, or policy conflicts that make it impossible for providers to feel confident about the terms of their contracts.

This mutual overdependence is the source of much of the concern and suspicion surrounding social and rehabilitative contracting at the state level. This unhealthy relationship promotes a chronic confusion over the status of contractors and their employees. Questions arise, for example, about whether providers are really "wholly-owned subsidiaries" of state agencies and whether their employees are really quasi-state employees. Charges of conflict of interest in the awarding of contracts, of "sweetheart" contracting arrangements, of agencies taking advantage of providers (and vice versa), are fueled by overly close contracting relationships at the agency level. These relationships are, in fact, based on the overdependence flowing from the state's neglect of contract administration and the lack of long-term planning.

State Contracting Agency Problems

Problems specific to contracting agencies include the lack of necessary administrative resources, lack of trained contracting personnel, and ineffective organizational structures to administer contracts. In general, these problems stem from the ad hoc and unplanned development of contracting at the state level. Although strong, centralized oversight of the contracting system would signify a first step in rectifying these problems, specific attention is needed at the agency level to ensure that contracting agencies have the capacity for effective performance.

The lack of administrative resources for contracting is obvious in the percentage of dollars devoted for such. Direct service dollars have increased by over 2,000 percent since 1971 for state agencies, however, funding increases for administration of contracts have not kept a proportional pace. In part, this deficiency reflects a reaction to, and an attempt to offset, the cost of ever-increasing demands for program dollars. The problem is also one of a fundamental lack of understanding about the resources needed to administer a contract system.

The Department of Public Health, for example, which contracts for fifty different program types at a cost of $53.6 million annually, has a staff of ten devoted, full-time, to contract administration. The approximately $200,000 spent annually by the department to administer contracts is inadequate by any standard. Within the context of an administrative and oversight system that is primarily manual and generates needlessly complex requirements, contract administration in the Department of Public Health can scarcely achieve more than compliance with paperwork requirements. The Department of Social Services, which contracts for $172 million in services per year, has a central office contracting staff of fifteen who are responsible for overseeing field activities. The Department of Mental Health, with annual contracts of $204.5 million, has a central office staff of twelve with full-time responsibility for contract administration. Although both departments contract through field offices, it still remains that staff time in the field offices is devoted to program development and service problems rather than contract administration.

The lack of central contracting standards has resulted in differing organizational patterns in the field. Some regional or area offices attempt to focus on contract administration, but others do not. It is common that contract administration is afforded no special status and is treated as a subcomponent of the budget office. In most agencies contract administration means little more than achieving authorization for contracts and exercising budgetary control. Formal needs assessment, procurement, contract monitoring, program evaluation, and audit activities are often secondary functions.

Those staff members assigned to contract administration usually have not received formal training for their job. Prior experience and education are difficult to obtain in an area that is as new and lacking in explicit standards as social and rehabilitative services contracting. Most state agency contract personnel have learned on the job and have previous tenure in the budget offices or program divisions. The State Auditor's Institute, a recent creation of the Auditor's Office, is the only state sponsored in-service training available to both state agency and contracted providers' personnel.

Oversight agencies do offer technical assistance to contract agency personnel, but this is generally limited to an explanation of current policies and procedures of the individual offices, such as the Comptroller's Division or the Rate Setting Commission, and can result in uncoordinated policymaking, as previously discussed. Although clarification of annual regulations, policy guidelines, and so forth are helpful, this does not constitute training. Contract officers need to be proficient in the procurement, negotiation, administration, monitoring, evaluation, and audit of contracted services. The same officer must understand the program of services being purchased, the fiscal basis for the purchase, and the laws and regulations governing contracting. In other words, the skills required of a contract officer are broader than those of other administrative staff. Without proper staff training, the contract administration system can be nothing more than a paper processing exercise, casting doubt about the accountability for the $614 million spent annually through contracts.

The absence of organizational standards for agency-level administration of contracts poses yet another weakness in the system. Contracting agencies have had to adapt contracting activities to existing central administrative requirements and, in some cases, to unique structures that do not promote good contracting practices. An example of this structural problem is found within the Department of Mental Health, which currently contracts for social and rehabilitative services through forty separate federal and state appropriation accounts and a network of forty-one area offices. The many appropriation accounts, which are established annually by statute, are subject to separate appropriation ceilings, which can be changed only by legislative action. Surplus funds in one account cannot be administratively transferred to another account to offset deficits. Most providers contracting with the department have more than one contract at a given time, and many of these are funded through separate appropriation accounts. A provider may therefore generate a surplus in one contract and a deficit in another, but the contracting agency is unable to authorize a transfer of funds. The administrative structure is in need of an overhaul to simplify and fine tune the system.

PROVIDER ORGANIZATIONAL PROBLEMS

Undercapitalization

As noted earlier, the existing provider system includes many small, newly created nonprofit organizations with few capital reserves. Many of these providers must borrow to obtain working capital or funding for expansion. Because of the decrease in federal funds and the constraints upon local government stemming from Proposition 2½, most of these providers are dependent for their existence on income from state contracts. The ability of providers to compete in the commercial capital-borrowing marketplace is often severely limited by lack of collateral.

Providers' fiscal dependency on state government has made them victims of the overall fragmentation and short-sightedness of the contract administration system. Until recently, for example, Rate Setting Commission policies have effectively prevented providers from undertaking independent fund-raising efforts. The failure of contracting agencies to define services and of the Rate Setting Commission to set rates by service has led to reliance on contract funds, which do not offer providers the incentive to render services efficiently in the hope of retaining surplus income. Perhaps the most compelling obstacles to reasonable treatment of provider capital expenses are the multiplicity of appropriation accounts and the general pressure on contracted providers created by statutory appropriation ceilings, which prevent agencies from reimbursing capital costs even when circumstances would suggest that this be done. Although government-backed financing authorities exist, social and rehabilitative service providers are generally ineligible for assistance, favoring the for-profit businesses or the more well-established nonprofits.

Without significant assistance in the form of government-backed capital, and without reform of a contract administration system that fosters provider dependence, the contracted system of community-based services will deteriorate as providers gradually exhaust meager capital reserves.

Compounding all of the problems cited above is the inability of the providers to recruit and retain qualified direct service employees. In part, this problem is aggravated by low salaries, reflecting chronic underfunding of contracted programs by state agencies. In recent years, concerted governmental efforts have been made to upgrade the funding for direct service workers' salaries. In FY 1986, for example, over $10 million was appropriated to address this problem.

The turnover rate among provider staff is remarkably high. A Department of Mental Health study conducted in the early 1980s, for instance, found that it was common for direct service positions to experience turnover every six months. Such turnover is not solely related to low pay. Lack of career ladders, fringe benefits, training, and other features of a sound human resources policy are to blame for the failure of provider organizations to build a qualified workforce. Given the integral relationship between provider organizations and the state agencies, it is reasonable to assume that such policies should be jointly developed.

Because the system, as a whole, has developed in a piecemeal fashion, employees of provider and state agencies have had to rely on on-the-job training as their primary source of preparedness for their jobs. No organized education or training system, public or private, exists to supply provider organizations with qualified community workers, and few personnel systems offer young employees the opportunity for career advancement. Unless the community-based system offers a tangible career future, its long-term viability will be threatened as surely by a lack of personnel as by a lack of capital resources.

RECOMMENDATIONS

A reasonable reaction to the above litany of problems would be to question the effectiveness of contracting as a mechanism for administering community-based services. The failures of the contracting system can certainly lead to the argument for a new administrative approach. Abandoning contracting for another approach, however, may prove counterproductive. The contract system has developed in tandem with the community-based system of care and has become inevitably linked to state-funded social and rehabilitative services. The central administrative systems of state government are not suited for community service delivery, whereas the flexibility of contracting allows state agencies and community-based providers to achieve, cooperatively, the goals of community care. In addition, the provider system has developed an expertise in administering community services that the state agencies, were they to provide services directly, would need to develop. Moreover, it has generally been the case that small provider organizations render more effective community care at lower cost than state government, which is burdened with high overhead costs.

The cost of ignoring the contracting system's problems are likely to be much higher than the costs of resolving them. It is not just a matter of organizational ineffectiveness; ultimately, it is the recipients of services who suffer from the system's bad performance.

The following recommendations are proposed by the Massachusetts Senate Committee on Ways and Means to improve the capacity of oversight agencies, contracting agencies, and providers to perform their roles effectively.

Strengthen the Role of the Executive Office of Administration and Finance

The failure of state government to effectively administer the contracted system of community-based social and rehabilitative services has been primarily a failure of the Executive Office for Administration and Finance (EOAF). Only EOAF has the jurisdiction and mandate to coordinate the activities of the various contracting agencies, secretariats, and oversight agencies involved in the contracting process. EOAF must begin to recognize the problems of contracting for social and rehabilitative services and address issues of administrative coordination and the system's long-term viability. Although an active EOAF role is essential, the committee believes that this role should involve policy-setting and administrative oversight rather than direct purchasing responsibility. Although decentralization and fragmentation in the contract system pose significant administrative problems, the committee also believes that purchasing authority rightfully belongs with state agencies charged to serve special populations. With proper coordination of policy development and implementation, the community-based contract system of care can be made more effective and accountable.

The creation of a central purchasing agency within the Executive Office for Administration and Finance is not considered necessary. Rather, it is recommended that resources be provided to that office to allow it to begin to address the needs of the social and rehabilitative services contracting system. The creation of a new office of purchased services to conduct long-range planning, set standards, and coordinate the activities of contracting and oversight agencies, is recommended.

274

Create Office of Purchased Services

The committee recommends that two hundred thousand dollars be included in the FY 1987 budget for the initial cost of an office of purchased services within the Office of the Secretary for Administration and Finance. The office, as a division of EOAF, will perform a coordinating and standards-setting function, similar to that performed by the Office of Management Information Systems, as well as undertake research, planning, and evaluation efforts on progress with, and future development of, the social and rehabilitative services contracting system.

The office will have administrative oversight responsibility for the purchase of service activities of state agencies, including the activities of secretariats, the Rate Setting Commission, and the Comptroller's Division. Although the office will not be authorized to directly contract for the purchase of social and rehabilitative services, it is recommended that its oversight responsibilities include coordination of the procurement, selection, contract negotiation, rate-setting, contract administration, contract monitoring, contract compliance, and postaudit activities of state agencies. In addition, the office should be authorized to develop administrative procedures consistent with laws and regulations governing purchase of service; to design and implement standardized contracting forms and issue a procedural manual for use by all state agency employees; to audit state contracting agencies and oversight agencies to ensure compliance with purchase of service laws, regulations, and procedures; to conduct training programs for state agency employees; and to authorize interim administrative processes, including interim payment mechanisms, in the event of conflict between the activities or policies of state agencies.

The purpose of the new office of purchased services is to ensure the implementation of a consistent, efficient, and accountable system of social and rehabilitative services contracting, with the goal of simplifying and streamlining the contracting process for state and provider agencies. It is anticipated that the office will function both as a central administrative oversight agency, with responsibility for ensuring the consistent implementation of standard procedures and as a troubleshooting office capable of solving the many administrative problems that occur in a decentralized system.The planning and evaluation responsibilities of the Office of Purchased Services will include

1. The elimination of the overdependence of state contracting agencies on contractors through the following two mechanisms:
   a. The development of so-called "make or buy" policies that clearly define those functions and activities of state agencies that may be contracted out and those that must be provided directly
   b. The development of state administrative procedures that facilitate the direct provision of community-based social and rehabilitative services by state agencies
2. The creation of a long-range plan to finance the contracted community-based system of care through the development of revenue sources other than state appropriations, including but not limited to the following:
   a. Developing a universal system of charges for community-based services
   b. Maximizing potential third-party revenue sources such as Medicaid and other federal programs, Blue Cross/Blue Shield and other insurance programs, and other public or private funding sources
   c. Reallocating underutilized resources to offset the cost of providing community-based care
   d. Coordinating existing generic resources to provide necessary support services in the community, such as medical or transportation services
3. The creation of a human resource plan for both state agency and provider employees, including, but not limited to the following:
   a. An assessment of the need for staff technical assistance and training programs and a plan for developing training
   b. A plan for the provision of educational opportunities for staff through the development of programs, through institutions of higher education, focused on purchase of service administration and direct social and rehabilitative service provision. The potential role of the community college system in providing such educational programs should be examined.
   c. Extension of technical assistance to provider organizations to develop recruitment strategies; career ladders; personnel policies; and group insurance or retirement programs and, as appropriate, tuition remission programs.
4. The development of policies and procedures for the creation of public

276

instrumentalities designed to assist provider organizations to obtain necessary capital funding to ensure the financial stability of the contracted system, including, but not limited to the following:

a. The use of multiyear contracts and other administrative means for strengthening providers' ability to borrow collateral

b. Developing, in conjunction with the Rate Setting Commission, accelerated depreciation, return on investment, and other legitimate capital reimbursement policies that provide an incentive for provider organizations to make service-related, long-term capital investments

c. Developing standard contracting and reimbursement policies and technical assistance programs designed to encourage and assist provider organizations in their fundraising efforts, with the goal of diversifying provider revenues and preventing overdependence on state contract revenues

d. Rendering, if necessary, direct capital financing assistance to providers through existing state financing vehicles, such as the Health and Educational Facilities Authority, the Massachusetts Industrial Finance Agency, or the Community Development Finance Corporation, or through other new or existing capital financing mechanisms designed to strengthen the ability of social and rehabilitative services providers to access necessary capital financing

e. Developing payment procedures that ensure continuity of payment for providers and minimize the need for working capital borrowing to finance state contracts

f. The exploration of innovative alternatives to existing service contract mechanisms, such as "performance" contracting, under which provider organizations would be reimbursed and held accountable for achieving performance goals set by contracting agencies, or grant mechanisms, under which providers would receive lump-sum payment for specified programs or projects, subject to routine program and financial audit.

In addition to coordination and planning, it is expected that the Office of Purchased Services will act as liaison with other offices of state government, such as the Department of Personnel Administration, the Group

Insurance Commission, the Retirement Commission, and others, to establish a technical and direct assistance capacity within state government to address the human resource problems of provider organizations.

In support of this initiative, funding is recommended for:

1. The Department of Personnel Administration to study problems with provider personnel systems, including classification, career, ladder, salary, and fringe benefit structures; and
2. The Board of Regents to study the development of curricula and the establishment of programs within the public higher education system to train students for careers in the community-based service system.

Strengthen State Contracting Agencies

As centralization and additional resources are needed to improve state oversight of social and rehabilitative services contracting, similar measures are needed to address administrative fragmentation within the contracting agencies themselves. Contracting agencies need to increase their central control of the contracting function through the creation, where appropriate, of consolidated appropriation accounts and through the availability of sufficient administrative resources.

Contract Management Offices. It is recommended that central contract management offices in the departments of Mental Health, Social Services, and Public Health be funded through line items in the state budget. These three departments account for 70 percent of the state's social and rehabilitative service contracting activity and are among the most administratively fragmented of contracting agencies. Although each agency maintains contract management personnel, there has been insufficient attention paid to the need for an ongoing contract management function capable of centralizing and simplifying purchasing activities. Targeting of resources to contract management offices in these agencies will ensure that such administrative resources are used for contract management purposes.

Added Contract Management Resources. It is recommended that $585,000 in new funding for central contract management personnel be provided to three state contracting agencies. Increased administrative funding, in conjunction with centralized control of contract management, will enable state contracting agencies to address the inefficiencies of the current decentralized system.

Consolidation of Contracting Accounts. It is recommended that, in agencies negatively affected by multiple contracting accounts, that there be a consolidation of budgetary line items to facilitate the centralizing of contract administration. Specifically, it is recommended that

1. The existing budgetary structure, within the Department of Mental Health, of forty separate line items funding community-based contracts be consolidated into three central office line items funding mental retardation, mental health, and children's services.
2. The Department of Public Health's contracting activities be overseen by a central contract management division. The department currently funds alcoholism, drug rehabilitation, family health, early intervention, maternal and child health, and dental health services through separate line items and separate agency divisions. It is recommended that the contracting activities of the Department of Family Health Services and the divisions of Drug Rehabilitation and Alcoholism be consolidated into two appropriation accounts.

Strengthen the Provider System

The provider system is directly affected by the fragmented structure and inconsistent policies of state government's contract management system. For this reason, it is believed that provider organizations will benefit greatly from improvements to the contracting system, due to simplification of the process and the reduction in duplicative paperwork that will result. The most important step that state government can take to benefit provider organizations is to administer a fair, accountable, and efficient contracting system.

The two overriding problems specific to the provider organizations that should be addressed by state government are undercapitalization and recruitment and retention of qualified employees. In both cases strategies involving the cooperative efforts of numerous state agencies will be

279

needed to resolve the problems. Attention must focus on capitalization initiatives such as improved payment systems, improved depreciation and other capital-related reimbursement policies, multiyear contracts and other contracting improvements, and, if necessary, the availability of government-backed capital financing for service-related provider investments. In relation to personnel recruitment and retention, areas to be addressed include the extension of training, education, fringe benefit and other human resources technical assistance, and appropriate funding for staff salaries and career ladders.

18

Private Market Strategy for Social Service Provision: An Empirical Investigation

Margaret Gibelman

With positive public backing, the Reagan administration and Congress have implemented sweeping changes in the methods of financing and delivering social services. The ability of the public system to effectively deliver services has been challenged on the basis of the belief that government is more likely to be the cause than the cure of social and economic problems *(Washington Post,* 25 August 1981). To circumvent the weaknesses of government in its service provider role, the Reagan Administration elected to expand the functions of the private sector. A directive issued by the Office of Management and Budget, "Policies and Procedures for Acquiring Commercial Products and Services Needed by the Government," strongly encourages public agencies to contract out much work now being performed in-house by government *Washington Post,* 16 April 1982). Although not explicit, contracting with private sources most likely refers to arrangements with private-for-profit sources rather than not-for-profit, when available.

The use of a private sector strategy within the social services, however, rests on many untested assumptions about the ability of nonpublic agencies to perform to the level expected of them. Are private agencies really the stronger and/or the more efficient and effective providers of service? Can services be provided equitably when the private sector is responsible for screening and selecting those who are to receive services? Cost considerations aside, are clients adversely affected by the shift in service responsibility to the nonpublic sector? This chapter addresses some of the issues that emerge in relation to changing service delivery auspices. Findings are derived from an empirically-based study in a large urban state, conducted by the author to assess the impact of purchase of service

(POS) contracting on patterns of social service delivery. The results of this study suggest reason for optimism about the use of the private market to provide services often considered within the domain of the public sector. The often-heard complaint that voluntary agencies "cream" the "better" clients is refuted, and the benefits that can be derived from an active public-private partnership are highlighted.

In this discussion *purchase of service* refers to formal agreements, usually in the form of contracts, between a governmental agency (the contracting agency) and another organization (the provider). The purpose of this agreement is to purchase care or services for individuals or groups meeting established eligibility criteria as determined by law or administrative regulation. Although public agencies may and do contract with other public, voluntary or proprietary agencies or individuals, discussion here focuses only on purchase agreements with voluntary, not-for-profit agency providers. Voluntary agencies, sometimes referred to as private or nonprofit, provide social services as a primary function under the direction of a board of directors. Such agencies employ professional staff to deliver services, typically including social workers. Financial support comes primarily from direct or United Way contributions, endowments, client fees (often on a sliding-scale basis), and government contracts. Contracts to support specific service activities, however, provide only one source of revenue, and the identification of the agency and its staff is as independent entity removed from external domination or control.

Public agencies are tax-supported organizations whose powers and duties are delineated by statute and administrative regulations. The scope of services provided and the means of provision are decided by a person or group elected by the voters or appointed by public officials. The parameters of activity are circumscribed by enabling legislation or other state and federal regulations.

BACKGROUND

Purchase of service (POS) represents an option about how services will be delivered in the conduct of government's social welfare responsibilities. With current national attention focused on cost effectiveness issues, decreasing the size of the government bureaucracy, and promoting private sector initiatives, contracting with nonpublic agencies has become an increasingly more attractive option for delivering services. For example, one long-standing argument in favor of POS is that such arrangements are apt to be profit motivated and competitive. As a result, greater economy and efficiency can be achieved than in a monopolistic or bureaucratic system (Wedemeyer 1970). Likewise, the management and administrative practices and expertise commonly attributed to the private enterprise system can be brought to bear on quality products. The belief has also been expressed that contracting provides a superior product and specialized skills, permits greater flexibility, and limits the growth of government (Fisk, Kiesling, and Muller 1978).

Both theoretical and practical arguments have been advanced in favor of purchase of service. From a pragmatic point of view, the use of POS addresses the perceived lack of desirability of expanding the manpower and associated costs of direct public provision and the rigidity of civil service regulations and union agreements. From a fiscal perspective, the use of POS may result in cost savings for states, because provider agencies may be required to match state funds in cash or kind. (Prior to enactment of the Omnibus Reconciliation Act of 1981, Title XX regulations provided a 75–25 percent matching formula between the federal and state governments. States could augment their own contributions through the use of donated funds from private sources. With the elimination of state matching requirements, states may institute their own criteria for a match with contracted agencies.)

Are there certain governmental functions that can, indeed, be more efficiently and effectively met through the development of a nonpublic capability, thus producing another kind of cost savings? Certainly, it is no longer believed that public funds should be expended only by government agencies, perhaps, in part, because it has never been so practiced in this country. However, this shift in service delivery responsibility can significantly alter the roles of both sectors, decreasing public agency functions related to direct service delivery while enlarging the scope of responsibilities delegated to the private sector. The growing disillusionment on the part of taxpayers, social welfare professionals, and clients with public agency operations and services encourages the trend toward privatization. A public-private partnership is widely viewed as feasible and the desired direction for service delivery, to the ultimate benefit of both systems and the clientele (Kamerman and Kahn 1976). A core issue, however, is whether the reliance on private agencies will positively or negatively affect the types, quality, and quantity of services clients will receive.

SERVICE CAPABILITY

Can voluntary agencies provide better services to clients heretofore serviced by the public sector? Historically, public and voluntary agencies have been perceived as differentiated by a number of dichotomous dimensions. Voluntary agencies, for example, have been seen as serving a more affluent client population, predominantly with psychosocial services. These agencies have largely been staffed by social work professionals with M.S.W. degrees. Public agencies, on the other hand, have traditionally been staffed by less well-educated practitioners, the majority of whom lack any formal social work education. So, too, because of federal and state mandates, priority for public service provision has tended to reside with the most needy, who have received services largely of a concrete nature in response to immediate, crisis-oriented situations. In the conventional wisdom of the profession, these distinctions in the nature of clients served, types of services offered, methods of financing services, and staffing patterns suggest a two-tier service system, with the higher-status clients receiving the more valued psychotherapeutic services by higher-qualified personnel through voluntary agencies.

Despite the growth in government's responsibility for social welfare services, the private service system has traditionally been the favored provider. This historical preference for the nonpublic sector is in large part due to the residual nature of government services and the pervasive uncertainty regarding the proper role of government in regard to social welfare functions. Public social services were established to serve the residual client, those unacceptable to, or ineligible for, voluntary services. The repeated denigration of the public sector by the media, politicians, professionals, and even the clientele, has reinforced the preference for the voluntary sector as the "better" service delivery system. Contracting with voluntary agencies, the providers of choice for the nonpoor, might eventually assist in blurring the reputation of public services as poor services for the poor (Buttrick 1970). The introduction of the War on Poverty legislation and the 1962 and 1967 amendments to the Social Security Act formally encouraged the practice of public-private contracting (Smith

1971). Incentives to purchase services have been incorporated into successive federal social service initiatives.

The very attributes of voluntary agencies, however, that make them desirable providers may encourage exclusionary practices in regard to those most in need (Hoshino 1979). Specifically, voluntary agencies have a purported track record of "creaming" clientele to fit their mode of services. The term *creaming* has come to be associated with the selection of those clients most closely approximating "desirable" social characteristics, e.g., the less poor, the more verbal, and the less disturbed (Miller, Roby, and de Vos van Steenwijk 1970). When contracting is used to obtain services not otherwise available, there may be increased opportunity for voluntary agencies to exercise discretion in selecting their clients. Particularly when voluntary agencies are delegated the responsibility for client intake, the possibility of favoring a traditional clientele is enhanced. Acceptance of public money by voluntary agencies does not insure the equitable provision of services to those most in need; this is all the more true when contracted agencies have a virtual monopoly on the services they are authorized to deliver (Kramer 1964). In such instances provider agencies may serve as "gatekeepers" into the service system, deciding who is to be served and with what types of services.

The possibility that purchase of service will result in an inequitable service system is perhaps heightened by the pervasive lack of resources for services and the need to limit the population receiving services. Client competition for services may result in more services for those most politically able to make their needs known. This is especially likely when the voluntary agencies have their own constituency that they cultivate and favor. This constituency, if traditional stereotypes hold constant, is likely to differ substantially from those served by public agencies in regard to socioeconomic status, nature and severity of presenting problem, and attitude toward service. The provision of public services through purchase agreement with nonpublic agencies, then, may encourage the exclusion of those most in need.

In the face of a dramatic reduction in the level of service, combined with a preference for the use of the private sector, questions arise about the extent to which voluntary agencies are equipped to offer a wide spectrum of services to client populations with multiple needs. Have voluntary agencies departed from their reputation as the service providers of the less needy, expanding their scope of services to respond to the needs of all socioeconomic groups and types of client problems? What differences can be discerned in public-private service provision, and with what consequences for the clientele? The findings of one case study shed light on these issues.

STUDY DESIGN

To determine the emerging patterns of service delivery resulting from the use of purchase of service contracting, a descriptive, single-state study was undertaken. This study involved the testing of a series of hypotheses related to the socioeconomic characteristics of the clients, the presenting problems and the number of problems, and the types and intensity of services provided across public and voluntary agencies. Interviews with the direct service workers of two contracted voluntary agencies and a district office of the state youth and family service agency in a large, northeastern state served as the primary source of data. Each of thirty-nine workers servicing the 120 sample cases were asked a series of questions by means of a closed-ended data collection schedule.

Child protective services was selected as the focus of study, because it is a service area traditionally provided by both public and voluntary agencies. As well, child protective services represents a "clustering" of services, in that several discrete services may fall within this category, such as family counseling, day care, emergency shelter, and group therapy. Thus, within this service category, agencies and workers have flexibility in deciding how best to meet the needs of their clients. Finally, child protective services are available without regard to income; i.e., there is universal eligibility regardless of socioeconomic status.

The state selected for study met the dual criteria of high urbanization and both direct public agency and contracted provision of child protective services. All cases selected for the sample were opened during a specified nine-month period and had been, or were, receiving service for three consecutive months. In addition, each case was serviced exclusively by either the public or voluntary agency, though the public agency may maintain case management responsibilities in relation to the contracted cases.

CLIENT CHARACTERISTICS

Disclaiming the creaming theory, the client population making up the study sample was found to be relatively homogeneous. The families consist predominantly of households headed by females, with an average of one to two children in the home and, frequently, members of the extended family, particularly grandparents. Mothers are often divorced, separated, or never married. A majority of the families are black, live in a rented apartment or house in an urban area, with neighborhood and structural housing conditions of fair to poor quality. Most families live within close proximity of the agency from which they receive service and have accessibility to public transportation.

Aid to Families with Dependent Children (AFDC) is the primary source of income for the largest proportion of clients. Adult females are most often unemployed, and for those cases in which an adult male is present in the home, there is an almost even division between the number employed and unemployed. For both employed males and females, the majority occupy skilled, semiskilled, and unskilled positions, particularly of a clerical or technical nature.

Since the individual characteristics of clients served by public and voluntary agencies were very similar, a scale of normative social functioning, comprising twelve variables associated with adequate social functioning, was developed to test whether a combination of characteristics would better distinguish the clientele served by both sectors. More statistically discriminating measures were employed, including discriminant analysis, and revealed a slight but nonsignificant suggestion of creaming in relation to those serviced by the voluntary agencies. It was also found that the aggregated normative social characteristics proved to be a stronger predictor of those maintained within the public sector, i.e., those with the less positive social attributes. However, differences in relation to who is served by the voluntary agencies are more reflective of the pattern of client referral from the public to the voluntary agencies than to any gatekeeping activities on the part of the voluntary sector. Though the voluntary agencies did have the right to refuse a case, there is evidence to suggest that once the referral was made from the public agency, the clients were maintained in service. Thus, any difference in who is referred out may reflect the judgment of workers about which clients may better profit from, or be more appropriate to, the services provided by either agency type.

CLIENT PRESENTING PROBLEMS

The presenting problem(s) of clients refers to the condition, symptom, or occurrence related to a family that brings it to the attention of, or comes on its own to the public agency for child protective services. It was expected that significant differences would be found in the types of client presenting problems for those clients served by the public agency and voluntary agencies under purchase of service contract. Presenting problems may range in type and severity from the physical abuse of one or more children, in which actual bodily harm has occurred or is likely to occur, to emotional neglect of a child(ren), which may consist of isolating, ignoring, or otherwise damaging a child through lack of affection, attention, proper nurturing, and so forth.

As indicated in table 18.1, families served by the public and voluntary agencies are similar in relation to the types and number of presenting problems. This similarity in the nature of the presenting problem extends to the rank ordering of the frequency with which problems are identified, e.g., physical neglect is rated second in frequency for both agency types. No significant differences, using chi square, were found between public and voluntary agencies regarding either the presenting problem or the source of client referral. On the other hand, some differences were found to be significant on dimensions related to the severity of the realized or potential abuse and/or neglect. In the view of respondents, the voluntary agencies tend to service the more severe cases in regard to the extent of actual harm and potential emotional harm to the child(ren). This latter finding runs contrary to traditional stereotypes, which hold that voluntary agencies service the "nicer" cases.

SERVICE PROVISION

In relation to the provision of services to clients, a number of dimensions were studied, including the types and numbers of services actually provided, the major focus of service delivery, and the intensity of the services rendered (i.e., how frequently clients have contact with their workers either in person or by telephone). Together, these variables re-

288

Table 18.1. **Nature of the Presenting Problem, Rank Ordering by Number**

	Public		Voluntary		Totals	
Presenting problem	%	(*N*)	%	(*N*)	%	(*N*)
Physical abuse—one child	25	(14)	29	(18)	27	(32)
Physical neglect—one child	21	(12)	19	(12)	20	(24)
Physical neglect—more than one child	27	(15)	14	(9)	20	(24)
Emotional neglect—one child	12	(7)	22	(14)	18	(21)
Mother-related problems	23	(13)	13	(8)	18	(21)
Emotional neglect—more than one child	14	(8)	14	(9)	14	(17)
Marital/family problems	5	(3)	10	(6)	8	(9)
Other	7	(4)	8	(5)	8	(9)
Physical abuse—more than one child	2	(1)	10	(6)	6	(7)
Truancy/runaway	9	(5)	3	(2)	6	(7)
Failure to thrive	5	(3)	5	(3)	5	(6)
Sexual abuse—one child	2	(1)	3	(2)	3	(3)
Total number of presenting problems		(86)		(94)		(180)

The unit of analysis is the family/case.
NOTE: Total number exceeds 120 (number of cases) since families may have more than one presenting problem.

lated to service provision were expected to yield data supporting differences between the public and voluntary agencies under POS contract. It was expected, for example, that clients serviced by the voluntary agencies would be seen more frequently, be provided a wider range of services, and that such services would tend to be more psychologically oriented than concrete or environmental. It should be recalled that voluntary agencies have been faulted for their alleged tendency to focus on verbal, psychologically oriented treatment to the sacrifice of the more concrete needs of clients (Miller, Roby, and de Vos van Steenwijk 1970).

Substantial differences were indeed found in the types of discrete services provided by the public agency and voluntary agencies under contract. Respondents were asked to indicate which of twenty-two discrete services had been or were now being offered to the families. A significant difference in the types of discrete services provided was found for eight of the twenty-two service areas. As indicated in table 18.2, the more intrapsychic services were, as expected, provided to a larger proportion of clients in the voluntary agencies.

Table 18.2. **Services Provided Differentially by Public and Voluntary Agencies**

Service	Public		Voluntary		Totals	
	%	(*N*)	%	(*N*)	%	(*N*)
Information and referral	84	(48)	67	(42)	12	(90)
Individual therapy/counseling	60	(34)	83	(52)	12	(86)
Transportation services	40	(23)	64	(40)	9	(63)
Diagnosis and assessment	21	(12)	76	(48)	8	(60)
Family therapy	11	(6)	52	(32)	5	(38)
Day care	33	(19)	14	(9)	4	(28)
Financial management counseling	4	(2)	22	(16)	2	(18)
Marital counseling	5	(3)	21	(13)	2	(16)

The eight services listed are those found to be significant at or better than the .05 level.

NOTE: Other services provided to families in both public and private agencies, but with no significant differences, include: parent education, medical/health services, crisis intervention, intervention to mobilize extended family and friends, advocacy, placement in foster care, employment and vocational services, recreational services, emergency financial assistance, group therapy, emergency shelter, homemaking services, and placement in residential care.

The unit of analysis is the family/case. The sample was composed of 57 public agency and 63 voluntary agency cases.

Although the public agency tends to provide less psychologically oriented services to its clients than do the voluntary agencies, this situation is reversed in relation to some of the more concrete services such as day-care and health/medical services. In this latter category, the public agency often acts as referral agent rather than direct service provider. Likewise, the emphasis on public agency provision of information and referral services is not surprising; public agencies are often mandated to serve a clearinghouse, resource function. In addition, the public agency's use of POS necessitates that staff have knowledge of community resources in order to appropriately refer clientele.

To further test these differences between the two agency types in the provision of discrete services, the twenty-two service areas were categorized and collapsed. The purpose of this categorization was to ascertain whether there are differences between the public and voluntary agencies in relation to clusters of services provided. A panel of experts was convened in order to determine the extent of agreement on which of the discrete interventions fall into four predetermined categories of advocacy, counseling and therapy, education, and monitoring/case management. Each of the twenty-two discrete services were assigned to one of the four categories on the basis of the classification of the panel of experts.

In three of the four categories of service (counseling and therapy, education, and monitoring/case management), significant differences, using chi square, were found between the public and voluntary agencies. For example, in the voluntary agencies a much greater range of counseling and therapy services are provided to clients. Also, clients serviced by the voluntary agencies receive more educational services than do those serviced by the public agency, including employment/vocational counseling, financial management, and parent education. These findings suggest that, overall, voluntary agencies provide more diversified types of services than is true of the public agency. Apparently, greater efforts are expended by the voluntary agencies to resocialize and reeducate their clients than in the case in the public agency.

In the largest category, advocacy, fourteen discrete services were combined for purposes of analysis, but no significant difference were found between the two agency types. It had been expected that the public agency would provide more advocacy services because this category includes a range of concrete, environmental services such as emergency shelter, homemaking, and placement services. The similarity across agency types in the provision of advocacy services disputes the notion that voluntary agencies are unable or unwilling to address the concrete needs of their clients.

Finally, significant differences were also found in the provision of monitoring/case management services by agency type, including case management and diagnosis/assessment. The findings again show a more concerted efforted in this area by the voluntary sector. In some respects this finding is not surprising since a larger proportion of voluntary agency clients receive diagnosis/assessment services. On the other hand, it would have been expected that case management service would be frequently offered by public agency staff, particularly in light of the contract monitoring role held by this sector. It is, however, possible that workers do not construe case management to be a service on the same order as counseling and advocacy and thus do not report it as such.

In summary, the voluntary agencies provide a much broader range of services to their clients than do public agencies. Although voluntary agencies do provide a heavy concentration of psychologically oriented services, particularly in comparison with the public agency, the provision of more concrete services is not precluded. Thus, clients served by voluntary agencies have a significantly greater opportunity to receive a diverse spectrum of services to meet their needs than is the case in the public agency.

Major Focus of Service Provision

The differences in service provision by agency auspices is further highlighted in relation to the major focus of service. As indicated in table 18.3, voluntary agencies tend to identify counseling as their major focus of service delivery. In contrast, there was a wide range of foci identified by the public agency, with case management/supervision ranking highest. This finding is somewhat inconsistent with data on discrete services provided; case management was not identified by the public agency respondents as a service delivered to many families. It is possible that, in the aggregate, public agency workers view the overall provision of services differently than they do the provision of disrete services. For volun-

Table 18.3. **Major Focus of Service Provision by Public and Voluntary Agencies**

Service focus	Public		Voluntary		Totals	
	%	(N)	%	(N)	%	(N)
Counseling	11	(6)	81	(50)	47	(56)
Case management/supervision	26	(15)	3	(2)	14	(17)
Environmental intervention	16	(9)	3	(2)	9	(11)
Parent education	9	(5)	8	(5)	8	(10)
Placement	11	(6)	2	(1)	6	(7)
Day care	12	(7)	0	(0)	6	(7)
Other	5	(3)	3	(2)	4	(5)
Health	7	(4)	0	(0)	3	(4)
Housing	4	(2)	0	(0)	2	(2)
Totals	48	(57)	52	(62)	100	(119)

$x^2 = 65.64$ $df = 8$ $p = 0.0000$

NOTE: The unit of analysis is the family/case. The sample was composed of 57 public agency and 63 voluntary agency cases. Lower totals signify missing data.

292

tary agency workers, the identified service focus is consistent with the nature of the discrete services offered.

Intensity of Service Provision

It is generally believed that the amount of contact workers have with their clients will affect the process and outcome of service and that greater frequency of contact increases the likelihood of successful outcomes. To determine differences, if any, between the public and voluntary agencies in relation to the frequency of contact with families, respondents were asked about the total number of in-person and telephone contacts held with, or on behalf of, each family since the case was opened. It should be recalled that the sample cases included only those open during a nine-month period of time and for whom at least three consecutive months of service had been provided.

As illustrated in table 18.4, a significant difference was found between public and voluntary agencies in the number of in-person contacts. However, the length of each contact was similar across the agency types, with the greatest proportion of in-person contacts lasting between forty-five minutes and one hour. In relation to phone contacts, significant differences were again found, with voluntary agency workers surpassing their public agency counterparts at a level less than .0001.

Auspice appears to have a dramatic impact on the type and intensity of services provided. In summary, clients serviced by the voluntary agencies, representing a range of client problems and intensity of problems,

Table 18.4. **Worker In-Person Contacts with Families since Case Opening**

Number of in-person contacts	Public		Voluntary		Totals	
	%	(*N*)	%	(*N*)	%	(*N*)
0–10	56	(32)	21	(13)	38	(45)
11–30	33	(19)	41	(26)	38	(45)
31–50	9	(5)	27	(17)	18	(22)
51–100	2	(1)	11	(7)	7	(8)
Totals	48	(57)	53	(63)	101	(120)

$x^2 = 19.91$ $df = 3$ $p = 0.0002$
NOTE: Percentage totals over 100 due to rounding.

received service with greater frequency than their public agency colleagues. One possible explanation related to the intensity of the services provided may have to do with differential caseload size. Indeed, using chi square, a significant difference in the workers' caseload size was found, at a level less than .0001. The majority of workers in the voluntary agencies carried a caseload of ten or less, whereas for public agency workers, the average caseload size ranged from ten to thirty-one or over. Thus, there appear to be some realistic limitations on the frequency with which clients may be seen in the public agency owing to the volume of cases carried. It should be noted, however, that a proportion of public agency cases include those carried for case management purposes only, and that as a result of contracting, caseload size has decreased dramatically.

REFUTING traditional stereotypes, the voluntary agencies studied were found to be extending their services to a client group composed largely of lower socioeconomic families and making available to them a range and intensity of services substantially greater than those available to clients of the public agency. Although some suggestion (albeit, not significant) of a creaming phenomenon was noted, the pattern of referral from the public agency to the contracted agencies seems to account for this nominal tendency. These referral patterns may be based on the perceptions of public agency workers about voluntary agency preferences and practices rather than on concrete experience. Yet, despite public agency attitudes, the voluntary agencies were not found to be "filtering out" the least desirable clients after the referral was made. Additional research may be needed to determine whether, in those instances when the voluntary agency performs the intake function, the exercise of gatekeeping decisions by the voluntary sector is more in evidence.

It is also possible that the similarity in the client population served across types of agencies can be explained in relation to a relatively homogeneous child protective services population. This client group may be drawn more from the lower socioeconomic strata than has previously been claimed by some (Gil 1976). Pelton (1981a), for example, concludes that "both evidence and reason leaves the unmistakable conclusion that contrary to the myth of classlessness, child abuse and neglect are strongly related to poverty, in terms of prevalence and severity of the consequences" (p. 36). If Pelton's view is substantiated by others, voluntary agencies servicing child protective services cases under contract would simply have less opportunity to exercise discretion than might be the case with other client groups. Even if child abuse and neglect is a problem affecting all socioeconomic groups equally, it is still likely that those of lower socioeconomic status would be identified and treated. It is this population that most frequently comes to the attention of, and is visible to, public hospitals and human service agencies, which refer a sizable proportion of protective service cases.

If public and voluntary agencies under contract are servicing a similar population with similar problems, the key question then becomes whether one sector can do a better job than the other in providing services. Although this study did not tap qualitative dimensions of service delivery, it is assumed that staff training and type, range, and intensity of services provided are positively associated with quality service outcomes. The findings suggest that voluntary agencies have adapted their treatment approaches to meet the diverse needs of a child protective services client population. Although the voluntary agencies did emphasize intrapsychic services, this was not to the exclusion of the more concrete services generally associated with public agency provision. On the other hand, the public agency, which was found to focus more on concrete services, did not do so in any greater proportion than did the voluntary agencies.

Inequity, however, may still be an outstanding issue. For those clients retained for service in the public agency, certain services, particularly those of a psychotherapeutic nature, may be increasingly unavailable. It does not necessarily hold that clients served by the public agency need fewer of these services. Such possibilities may provide justification for expanding the scope of purchase of service contracting so that voluntary agencies would assume increasing responsibility for serving the whole of the child protective service population with needed services. If further research indicates that voluntary agencies are, indeed, able to provide the full range of services required, they should be contracted to do so when such agencies are available and accessible and when their track record indicates consistently positive service outcomes. Concurrent with this movement toward additional delegation of service delivery responsibility to the voluntary sector, the role of the public agency would need to be modified to insure agency competence in contract monitoring, negotiation, and evaluation (Capaccio 1978). This may also entail a change in the classification of worker positions and different hiring requirements.

With even scarcer service dollars available, states are likely to opt to provide services to only those with the most pronounced need. In Texas, for example, a priority system has been instituted for child protective services, in which only cases where there is imminent danger of death or serious risk of injury receive follow-up. All other cases simply receive no services (Austin 1982). In many states similar priority-setting activities are being initiated to insure that service dollars are targeted to those most in need. Despite the elimination of the "Fifty Percent Rule" regulation, which mandated that 50 percent of all Title XX dollars received by a state be allocated for SSI, AFDC, and Medicaid recipients, the need to streamline the client population eligible for services may help to ensure that the interests of the poorest and neediest receive some protection. This targeting of services is likely to become a requirement of all contracted programs, as well, thus limiting the discretionary powers of the nonpublic sector in selecting their clientele.

19

Contextual Factors Affecting the Purchase of Services

Jeanne M. Giovannoni

Although the purchasing of services is far from a new practice, both the process and outcome of these arrangements are significantly affected by environmental influences. Contracting between the public and private sectors has certainly not been without conflict, and there is evidence to suggest that participants do not always enjoy satisfactory relationships. In this chapter some of the contextual issues surrounding the use of purchase of service contracting are explored, and a framework for analyzing specific contracting issues in greater depth and within limited resources is suggested. The material for this discussion is drawn from the experiences associated with child welfare services contracting in Federal Region IX, from the vantage point of that region's Child Welfare Training Center.

The expansion in the use of purchase of service arrangements occurred at the same time that management principles derived from the field of economics and productivity models of private industry were permeating all government activity, including the administration of human services. Efficiency, cost-benefit, and accountability goals and principles became the major criteria for defining effective performance and were similarly applied to the management of contracts. Included within this management thrust was the specification of expected results and the measurement of progress toward meeting goals and objectives. The application of these models, developed for use in other fields, to the human services has been fraught with as yet unresolved problems in both the management of directly provided government services and contracted services. The search for clear outcomes in the human services is a far more complex task than is the case with the physical sciences.

A related contextual issue is the demands on and expectations of the voluntary not-for-profit sector. As noted in chapter 2, qualities of innovativeness, flexibility, and creativity have been attributed to the voluntary sector. There has been an inevitable stress placed upon this sector; living up to the "superior image" in the service delivery function has also involved the expectation that public services, through purchase of service contracting, could be similarly innovative, flexible, and creative. Some voluntary agencies, in reaction, have opposed public funding, others have expressed reservations, and still others have seen the public-private partnership as beneficial to all concerned.

There are many arguments for and against public-private partnerships. Unfortunately, more energy has been devoted to arguing controversial issues surrounding purchase of service than gathering hard data by which to substantiate or refute them.

The goal of the project undertaken by the Child Welfare Training Center in Region IX was to identify sources of dissatisfaction among the public-private contractual partners and illuminate ways in which these might be addressed and resolved. The project's scope was limited to key informants in the public and private sectors in Region IX. Eight agency representatives were interviewed in the public sector, including state and county personnel, but excluding federal officials. In the private sector, six voluntary representatives were interviewed and, in addition, self-administered questionnaires were completed. The interview included questions asked in a United Way of California and United Way of Los Angeles 1981 survey, which examined the contracting problems of nonprofit California agencies.

The selection of respondents was based on the recommendations of the center's Steering Committee and other persons knowledgeable about agencies engaged in the delivery of contracted services. Agency directors were sent an introductory letter outlining the project and asking that a respondent be designated for a telephone interview. The interview guide was developed to tap information about respondents' experiences with the contracting process in relation to (1) time constraints, (2) contract structure and content, (3) monitoring, (4) auditing, and (5) client services. The interview guide also allowed for more open-ended responses about respondents' views on the future of contracted services.

TIME CONSTRAINTS

Inquiry about time elements involved in the contracting process focused on the following key points: (1) time allocated for issuance of request for proposals by the public agency, (2) the corresponding time for a response by potential contracted agencies, (3) the time between submission of a proposal and award notification, (4) the time between notification of award and first payment for services, and (5) the time between contract expiration and renewal. Lengthy or prolonged time lapses at any of these points in the contracting process can have a negative effect on the quality of work for both parties to the arrangements. Time delays can also adversely impact upon the interorganizational relationship, e.g., ill will may be created when there are delays in payment to the contracted agency.

In general, respondents indicated that, for both parties, time constraints presented problems. Rather wide variations among public agencies in the time allocated were noted, but even given problem areas, those with serious deleterious effects were the more isolated cases.

Among public agency personnel, two types of pressures were noted. The first concerned the time pressures experienced in issuing proposals, with some respondents reporting that they were often under extreme pressures. A relevant factor, of course, is the volume of contracting in which the public agency may engage, as well as funding cycles and the distribution of work among personnel. In one instance one person carried exclusive responsibility for securing approval on thirty-four contracts within a thirty-day period, each year! An additional source of time pressure occurred in those agencies seeking to take advantage of federal funds; here, federal timetables were added to state and local timetables.

A second source of pressure experienced by public agency personnel results from political pressure exerted by bidders whose proposals have been rejected. This situation, identified as a major source of delay in making contract awards, was experienced at both the state and county levels, with the seriousness of the problem varying on the basis of power differentials between the public and private sectors.

Although respondents from the voluntary sector stated that time contraints were not an acute problem, dissatisfactions were noted. Voluntary agency respondents in the sample population had considerable experience with contracting and had developed, over time, the capacity to

299

respond quickly to requests and weather financial crunches created by time delays in payment. These respondents, however, conceded that these time pressures tended to screen out small agencies from the competitive contracting process. The seriousness of time constraints thus seems to depend on the agency resources that can be brought to bear and the availability of staff experienced in the writing and negotiating of contracts.

Even the more experienced agencies, however, feel the effects of time pressures; respondents indicated that there was a loss in the quality of proposed programs and a sacrifice of innovativeness. One recommendation called for a pattern established by the U.S. Department of Health and Human Services, Office of Human Development Services. Here, an initial screening is undertaken of brief concept papers, and only those considered to be highly competitive are asked to submit full proposals in a second stage process. It was felt that this practice, adopted at the state or county level, would enhance innovativeness.

In sum, the degree to which time constraints are problematic for either the public or private sectors is in part dependent on the adequacy of staff resources. Any increase in the volume of contracting without a corresponding increase in personnel resources could only exacerbate the situation. For the voluntary sector, the competitive disadvantage of smaller, less experienced agencies serves as a screening device but may also perpetuate a lack of innovativeness and preclude potential effective service providers.

STRUCTURE OF CONTRACTS

Respondents were questioned about their experiences with several aspects of the structure and content of contracts, including the degree to which changes could be negotiated, and matters of interpretation, including legal and budgetary. Here, too, dissatisfaction was expressed by both sides and suggestions made for improvement. On the whole, the problems were not considered to be too severe.

Because of variations among the procedures and processes of the public agencies, public agency respondents' experiences with contracting reflected the idiosyncratic patterns of different levels of government and political jurisdictions. Within the public sector, problem were noted about the different kinds of expertise needed and the lack of availability of qualified personnel to efficiently process contracts. Program staff, it was found, usually do not feel secure in handling either the fiscal or legal aspects of contracting; this discomfort also pervades relationships with colleagues in other departments who are experts in these areas. The bureaucratic structure results in a dysfunctional division of labor between departments and agencies. One respondent noted that some of her contracts required sign-offs from three different state agencies.

Public agency program personnel are often placed in the uncomfortable position of mediating between service providers and a system even they find difficult to negotiate. In the words of one staff person: "The most important thing is to learn how 'to grease the system'." Those respondents who seemed to have the least difficulty blending the programmatic and technical aspects had specialized staff to work exclusively on contracts. A partial solution for some is the use of a standard boilerplate, focused on legal aspects. However, one voluntary agency administrator said that although he has not as yet experienced problems, the stipulations in the boilerplates produce uneasiness, especially the numerous "hold harmless" clauses that could place the agency in a precarious position.

An expected result of the complexities of the bureaucratic system is a tendency toward rigidity, often manifest in reluctance to institute contract changes. Most respondents thought that there was some latitude in regard to postaward contract changes, but not a great deal. For example, budget line items could be adjusted and, with respect to program, the methods to achieve goals might be changed. Changes of this order were not found to be problematic by personnel of either sector. All experienced them and found that negotiations could result in agreement, particularly if that process was completed before the final contract signing.

Among provider agencies, there were two prominent sources of dissatisfaction with structural matters, both of a fiscal nature. A majority of respondents reported that their rate of reimbursement seldom equalled their actual costs. Particularly in regard to contracts with counties, it was reported that administrative overhead costs were frequently disallowed or not considered, resulting in the need for providers to absorb some of these costs. Several respondents pointed the desirability of adopting the principle of an assigned administrative cost, such as the indirect cost formula used by the federal government.

A second source of dissatisfaction concerned the unit of service as a basis for cost reimbursement. In some contractual arrangements, the public agency is the sole source of client referrals, and although the rate of referral flow may vary, provider costs remain constant. Hence, providers are at risk of incurring financial losses should the referral flow not be adequate. With the reduction in the number of public agency personnel providing referral services, the rate of referrals to the private sector has become an acute problem in some areas. However, one agency has successfully negotiated at least a partial solution to this problem. Three contracts contain stipulations that the agency will receive payment corresponding to the units of service delivered or the equivalent of one month's allowable costs, thus ensuring that there is some guaranteed level of support for the provider. In residential services, one solution has been to provide for maintenance fees even when beds are empty. One public administrator cited this practice as potentially eliminating the needless maintenance of children in placement, simply in order to ensure bed capacity reimbursements.

MONITORING CONTRACTS

Respondents' experiences with contract monitoring showed greater differences of opinion than expressions of dissatisfaction. Opinion differences were expressed in relation to the functions of monitoring and, consequently, clarity about who should perform this function and how it should be done. The diversity of opinion was as great within the public sector as between the two sectors. One point of view, particularly among public agency employees, is that the primary, if not sole, purpose of monitoring is to achieve contract compliance. Those holding this view believe that the monitoring function should be performed by designated, specialized personnel; the preference is for nonprogram, nonsocial work staff, unless appropriate training is made available. The objection to the use of program staff is based on the perception that these staff represent the users of services and are therefore likely to overlook compliance problems.

A second point of view is that monitoring is composed of multiple functions and is a mechanism for establishing collaborative relationships to enhance program development and quality improvement. The appropriateness of this model of monitoring is debatable, but if it is to be at all viable, there must be a sufficient number of trained personnel within the public sector to carry out these functions. Some public agency respondents voiced awareness of their inability to give providers the type of assistance they wanted; this was attributed to staff shortages and high work loads. It would also appear that monitoring to enhance program development must occur in an interorganizational climate of cooperation, or, as one provider put it, "in an atmosphere of mutual trust." This is not always the case.

Providers criticized public agencies for inconsistent and lax actions. Both sides agreed that the most severe problem in monitoring was the failure to address evaluation of the quality and effectiveness of services. (This problem, however, is not unique to contracting, but pervades all of the human services.) Although many agencies were able to demonstrate quantitative results in reducing costs and the number of children in foster care as a result of purchased services, questions remain as to whether clients are actually better off. Respondents saw the need to produce evaluative data above and beyond compliance and cost-effectiveness measures as a result of the monitoring process.

It is possible that the expectation that monitoring will produce program development and evaluate data may be unrealistic given an already overburdened system. Qualitative evaluation would demand the collection of more complex data than is true for monitoring.

FISCAL AUDITING

Little dissatisfaction was expressed about fiscal auditing of service contracts, most likely because none of the respondents carried accounting responsibilities. It was noted, however, that the lack of uniformity in auditing procedures among different government agencies placed an additional burden on agencies with multiple contracts. This problem did not cause undue hardship, perhaps because no financial losses had occurred as a result of audits. One agency executive cited an example of "unreasonable" auditing. Child care staff had maintained dietary records, but trouble arose because they recorded which children received cereal, but did not note whether there was milk on it!

CLIENT SERVICES ISSUES

The scope of services under discussion is limited to the child welfare area, particularly those services to involuntary clients toward the goal of restoring family functioning (when children and their families are the service recipients) and/or family reunification and permanency planning. Not all respondents were involved in the service delivery area.

There was unanimity among respondents that, in respect to confidentiality of records, the purchasing agency had, at least in principle, the right of access to information, particularly in cases involving legal action. Some public agency officials took the stance that, because the government was paying for the service, everything, including the records, were public agency property. Others spoke of potential problems about information access, especially in regard to client data peripheral to the agreed-upon treatment goals. An example here is information about parents that does not bear upon the protection or safety of their children. In nonlitigious cases confidentiality issues are less clear. One provider, for example, stated that all information is considered confidential when services are provided to youth in crises accused of no crime.

Although there was general agreement on confidentiality parameters, there was some variation in responses about when and how clients were to be informed. One public administrator simply stated, "Tell the client there is none" (confidentiality). Some thought that the clients should be told about confidentiality limitations from the outset, or, alternatively, only when information was to be divulged. A key issue in confidentiality appeared to center on mutual trust by public and private sector representatives. As stated by one provider: "There doesn't have to be a problem. Setting it up with the client that we are the guys in the white hats and the public, the guys in the black hats is something we create; it doesn't have to be there."

Questions about the autonomy of providers in selecting clients elicited considerable, but not total agreement. In general, public and private agency respondents agreed that the provider should accept for service all clients referred. Exceptions to this principle, it was felt, should be spelled out in the contract. Once a population of service recipients was identified in the contractual agreement, the provider should be held accountable for delivering services to them. Some sentiment was expressed that, in the case of "good professional reasons," a client might be denied service, particularly if the referral is considered to be inappropriate.

Private agency providers expressed some strong reactions to the screening out of clients they were contracted to serve. This reaction was based on the belief that the private sector could serve the public agency clientele only by changing their practice modes and adapting to client needs. One agency director said, "The family agency cannot continue as a form of subsidized private practice. They have to take everybody and learn to work with everybody—and we believe we have demonstrated that they not only can, but also can become enthused and excited about their work." It appears that strict adherence to contract stipulations restricting the selectivity of providers can avoid creaming the "good" clients and the consequent rejection of the less attractive ones. To obtain true compliance in some instances, however, may involve fundamental changes in provider agency practices.

There were some dissenting opinions from providers. Some thought that an agency should be able to state limitations about whom they would serve. One voluntary sector representative, noting that the agency had been accused of being "choosy," offered another reason. Community-based agencies have a commitment to serve a particular community or population group. If this commitment is to be honored, the agency should be able to concentrate its efforts on that population.

Mixed emotions were expressed by respondents about contractual limitations on the frequency of client contact and the length of time they should be served. Public and private agency personnel that had been working within a family reunification/permanency planning service model saw some validity and benefits to these limitations. The problem arose in specifying just what the time limit should be. Some advocated a case-by-case determination or specification of only a portion of that total service population to whom service limitations might be applied. Others thought that when there are specified client outcome goals, time limitations are superfluous. One concern expressed was that the use of service time limits could be manipulated so that in child dependency cases, the public agency could demonstrate in court that parents had failed to respond to services that had been offered, therefore they should lose their custody rights. One public agency representative expressed deep concern that court-imposed treatment time limits, combined with severe fiscal cutbacks, had all but eliminated services to the noncourt or voluntary client, in turn essentially eliminating early intervention in child protective services situations.

ADVANTAGES TO PURCHASING

Respondents were asked about their view of the overall advantages and disadvantages of purchasing services and what further practices in this area should or could be. There was consensus that an advantage of purchasing is that it is cheaper than public agency service provision, largely because private agency staff are paid less and have fewer fringe benefits than their public agency counterparts. Purchasing also decreases public agency overhead and administrative costs. In this respect the private agencies might prefer less cost savings, since it has been claimed that the administrative costs to providers are insufficient. None of the respondents cited greater efficiency on the part of the profit-motivated private sector as an advantage of purchasing, a surprising finding in light of the frequent references in the literature posing efficiency as a justification for purchase of service.

Another universally cited advantage of purchasing is that this practice is responsive to the need to establish a diversified service system capable of addressing the full range of problems brought to the public agency. Specifically, all respondents saw a continuing public sector role that could not be delegated: that of social control. Such functions include licensing and eligibility determination, which are seen as clear public mandates and within the exclusive jurisdiction of the public agency.

Although there is agreement on the regulatory/social function role of the public sector, there are outstanding questions regarding the desirable allocation of treatment and service roles. Nor surprisingly, respondents were far from unanimous in their views. Public administrators' responses are typical of the range of opinions. One administrator thought that all case management and crisis intervention services should be handled by the public agency, with all other services purchased. Another administrator in the same agency cited resistance among public sector staff to extending contracted services.

Private agencies were, of course, much stronger in their views of the advantages of purchasing. The ability to raise program money from a variety of sources was cited, as was the private sector's capacity to tailor services to the diverse needs of different communities, particularly ethnic minority communities. Voluntary agencies also saw themselves as more flexible in the use of self-help groups, volunteers, and citizen participation in administration. Greater potential for professional performance was also cited or implied as an advantage of the voluntary sector, as opposed to the perceived bureaucratic orientation of public agency employees. It is not clear, however, to what extent public agency personnel share these views about the advantages of purchasing services from the private sector.

From the perspective of the private agencies, the advantages of purchasing are increasingly recognized, but acceptance of this practice has been hard won. Several respondents noted that legislative action, rather than public agency prerogatives, have led to the expansion of purchase of service. Even with legislation encouraging purchase, some agencies have yet to adopt this practice. Indeed, the major criticism of contracting in the view of private agency respondents is the failure of public agencies to apply purchasing to more services, rather than experiences with contracts already let. Numerous instances were cited of the application of pressure on public agencies to expand their contracted services, particularly in the areas of treatment and counseling.

Given that all of the respondents had extensive experience with purchase of services, they have witnessed, and been a part of, the improvement of public-private relationships. Indeed, the development of a creative partnership between these sectors was cited by many respondents as a chief benefit derived from contracting. One public agency administrator observed that both morale and performance of her overburdened child welfare staff had greatly improved since contracting for treatment services had begun. This person also remarked that objectivity in case planning had been enhanced since workers were relieved of the burden of implementing every aspect of the case plan.

From the perspective of private sector respondents, a continuing benefit of contracting is the influence that can be brought to bear by providers on the service delivery system beyond that involved in specific areas. One administrator, for example, cited the impact of his agency on law enforcement in two counties through a contracted program that demonstrated that youth in crises could be maintained in an unlocked facility. Among those who have successfully developed good working relationships through contracting experience, there has been a diminution of the stereotyping of each other. In the words of one respondent: "There is a validity to different worlds. There are different roles to be performed. If conflicts develop, they must and can be resolved so that the clients don't get caught in between."

Building a relationship between the public and private agencies took time and effort. The achievement of a coordinated child welfare service delivery system involves consideration of coordination as a cost item to be factored into the equation. The argument that service contracting is best because it is cheaper may be limited by the failure to consider all costs and to hold cost efficiency as the highest value. If the public agency is to be more than a conduit for tax dollars channeled to the private sector, adequate resources and personnel must be budgeted. Any inadequacy in the funding or programming of the public sector will impact on the entire purchasing system.

THE FUTURE OF PURCHASING

When asked about the future of service purchasing, respondents differentiated between what should happen and what actually might occur. Not surprisingly, all private agency respondents thought that contracting should be significantly expanded. Public agency personnel were not as unanimous, and responses ran the spectrum of urging more purchasing to reservations about the most desirable mix of public and private service delivery.

Political orientation appeared to be a key factor in what respondents thought would happen with contracting. Some private sector representatives were heartened by the Reagan administration's emphasis on voluntarism, seeing in it the potential for revitalizing the voluntary agency. They saw the political climate as an opportunity to bring pressure to bear at all levels of government to increase the private share of public dollars. One public agency representative took issue with the administration's definition of voluntarism: "They don't mean professionals working under voluntary auspices—they mean volunteer, free for nothing—and that's not going to work with our clients."

Pessimistic views about the future were also expressed, particularly in light of severe budget cuts instituted by the federal government affecting state and local governments. Some respondents see the entire service area shrinking, with the private sector carrying a disproportionate share of the burden. Most thought that the public sector would respond to budget cuts by curtailing purchase of services rather than diminishing staffing or directly delivered public services. The power of public employees' unions was cited as a strong force in protecting their members from displacement.

In an era of retrenchment, arguments that purchasing services saves money can become a double-edged sword. When such information is presented to local county boards of supervisors, a likely result will be to reduce budgets to acknowledge potential and real cost savings. Such reductions are likely to spur greater union activity. Some feared that all services, public and private, might come close to extinction, with only the social control functions/programs continuing. In general, most respondents thought that if contracted services were to continue, even at their present level, it would not be without some severe battles.

309

20

The Efficacy of
Contracting for Service

Arnold Gurin and Barry Friedman

The great expansion of publicly financed human services that began during the 1960s and continued well into the 1970s was accomplished in large part through the use of voluntary or proprietary agencies as the instruments of service delivery. The rapid growth of public-private contracting or purchase of service (terms that are generally used interchangeably) has been documented in a number of studies (Edwards, Benton, Millar & Feild 1978; Fisk, Kiesling, and Mueller 1978). Analysts, researchers, and commentators, in a growing body of literature on this subject, have been exploring both the reasons for the increased use of contracting and the strengths and weaknesses of existing practices (Benton, Feild, Millar 1978; Nelson 1978; Wedel, Katz, and Weick 1979; Savas 1977a). Although some of the literature is based on systematic studies, much of it is more polemical than empirical.

Issues of public-private contracting have a substantial ideological component. They involve and reflect general value differences regarding the role of government vis-à-vis private enterprise. Even before the renewed emphasis on the primacy of the private sector, introduced by the Reagan administration as a major feature of federal policy, arguments in favor of contracting tended to stress the alleged superiority of voluntary or private administration over that of government. On the other hand, those committed ideologically to a dominant role for government in meeting

THIS CHAPTER is based on a study conducted by the authors, with the assistance of Natalie Ammarel and Carole Sureau, Grant No. 18–P-00170/1-01 from the Office of Human Development Services, U.S. Department of Health, Education, and Welfare. The title of the final report is *Contracting for Service as a Mechanism for the Delivery of Human Services: A Study of Contracting Practices in Three Human Services Agencies in Massachusetts*, June 1980.

the needs of people through human services continue to express concern about the abdication of those responsibilities to allegedly noncontrollable and nonresponsible providers, whether profit or nonprofit (Hanrahan 1977).

Although these arguments proceed on a philosophical basis, they rest on explicit or tacit assumptions that are empirical in nature and therefore subject to examination and study. Although proponents of the private sector may sometimes seem to be arguing that there is intrinsic good in private enterprise itself, in some ultimate sense, the major thrust of their position is that the greater use of the nongovernmental sector makes for better and more economical human services. Similar arguments on the other side are implicit in the position taken by those who favor more direct government responsibility. In other words both are making points about efficacy. This chapter deals with issues of efficacy in contracting for human services and how they have been or can be studied.

Efficacy has two aspects that may be characterized, broadly, as *quality* and *cost*. Quality has many dimensions that include not only the character of the service being rendered but also access to those services by clients with varying characteristics. Costs are also multidimensional, since they cannot be considered in isolation but only in relation to varying quantities of service.

In regard to both quality and costs, such questions of efficacy have been posed as: "What is superior: direct service by government or government purchase of service through the private (profit or nonprofit) sector?" In these formulations the emphasis is on a comparison between direct and contracted services. It has proven difficult to subject questions framed in this manner to empirical testing because there are few examples where totally comparable services are administered, in the same time and place, both by governmental and nongovernmental agencies. In addition such general questions may not be very useful to administrators who frequently have no freedom of choice, for a variety of reasons, in whether to engage in contracting. For them, the operating issue is most frequently not whether contracting is more effective than direct service, but rather how to make contracting most effective.

Government agencies responsible, under the law, for providing human services to specified target populations have used the mechanism of purchasing services for a variety of reasons. Some of these may be intrinsic to the nature of the service or the market conditions in which it has to be provided. For example, state rehabilitation agencies purchase many services for individual clients, from training programs in established educational institutions to medical supplies. In these instances there are adequate suppliers in the market, start-up costs for production are considerable, and demand on the part of the public agency is sporadic and relatively small. There is clearly no reason, under those conditions, for government to establish its own direct service capacity and every intrinsic reason not to do so. For most of the services, however, the issue is not that clear cut. Rehabilitation services also purchase medical and psychological diagnostic services from a variety of private practitioners. Here, the volume of purchase is substantial and there are no institutional start-up costs. There is therefore no intrinsic reason why either direct or purchased service would be preferable.

The major reasons for using indirect rather than direct means for delivering services are not intrinsic but are based on the exigencies of particular situations, including tradition and the availability of nonpublic providers. Two major incentives to purchase services are the budgetary and personnel constraints on public agencies. By purchasing services, states have been able, in some instances, to pay only for the services used rather than for a year-round fully employed staff and have been able to avoid start-up costs. They have thus converted their financial obligation from one including both fixed and variable costs to one that is limited to variable costs. At least, that has been the intention and expection. In reality, there is some question as to whether such savings have actually been realized, because the public agencies continue to incur fixed costs for monitoring, accounting, and, frequently, case management. As the volume of purchased services increases, the direct work of the public agency does not necessarily decrease proportionately, since there is a parallel, although not necessarily proportionate, increase in case management and monitoring requirements. Indeed, one of the generalizations that can be made about purchasing is that it requires, if it is to be used effectively, a considerable management capacity on the part of the agency doing the purchasing.

PROGRAM EFFECTIVENESS: ISSUES OF QUALITY, ACCESS, AND ACCOUNTABILITY

Most human service programs aim to treat numerous individual clients, each with somewhat different problems and needs. The real test of quality in the delivery of a social service is what happens to the individual client. For any individual client there is presumably some treatment that is most suitable. Differences among individuals create a major problem in establishing quality control, because outcome criteria cannot be formulated in consistent, uniform terms. In rehabilitation services, for example, an outcome is defined in terms of employment but the specific nature and extent of employment being sought will vary with the individual. In the case of children's protective services, the overall goal is a living situation that will most likely provide physical and emotional security for the child. Individual judgments have to be made, however, as to whether any given living situation meets those criteria.

Because of the the difficulty of standarizing outcomes, social service agencies attempt to exercise quality control by standardizing inputs and processes, relying on these inputs to produce satisfactory outcomes. Major agency inputs involve decisions about the range of services to be provided, the personnel who will render such services, and policies governing priorities in the selection of clients for service. Evaluation (judgment as to quality) is frequently based on determining whether the standards for personnel qualifications are being met, whether agency services are being rendered in the manner prescribed by agency policies and regulations, and whether the priority groups are being reached. Quality control refers to means established by an agency for determining that standards of priorities, processes, and inputs are being met.

FORMS OF CONTRACTING

Contracting arrangements can take a variety of forms, from straightforward purchase of services on a unit basis in the open market to formal contracts between the public agency and the provider in which blocks of services are purchased. Variations occur in the degree of informality or formality of these arrangements. The simplest arrangement, found in rehabilitation services, is the use of purchase orders by counselors or case managers to obtain products or services from providers in the

313

open market. The use of more formal mechanisms of one type or another is designed to achieve certain specific purposes.

One purpose of contracting is legitimation, i.e., to establish which providers may be used. Where licensing or certification provisions exist in law, no such legitimation may be required, because the contracting agency can simply require that the providers must have such credentials. In many areas of service, as in day-care or homemaker services, no such legal requirements exist. A contract therefore becomes the means of establishing that a provider meets the standards that are required as a condition for obtaining government payments.

Moving a step beyond mere legitimation, contracts can and do specify the kinds of services to be delivered and the standards for conducting those services. Such standards can vary considerably in the degree of their detail and specificity. Some public agencies try to make the formal contract very specific as a basis for monitoring and quality control. Others are much more general in their specifications, listing the services to be supplied in quite global terms, such as "counseling" or "clinical services," or concrete services such as "homemaker" or "transportation."

Another function that contracting can perform is to make sure that the provider will, in fact, meet the demand for services. That is the case when the contract specifies that the provider will make available a certain number of service units to the contracting agency. There are many instances, however, in which contracts leave open-ended the amount of service to be rendered, but simply specify the nature of the service, in general or specific terms, and the rate to be paid for a unit of service. They involve no obligation on the part of the provider to furnish a specific volume of service nor an obligation on the part of the contracting agency to purchase a specific volume of service.

It is apparent that there is a wide repertoire of contractual arrangements to be drawn upon selectively, depending upon the purposes to be achieved. Informal, general types of contractual agreements have the advantage of providing the contracting agency with maximum flexibility as to how and how much to use the private providers. That can be an effective approach to contracting when mechanisms are in place to make the necessary discretionary judgments as to both quantity and quality of services needed. On the other hand, if market conditions are such that the agency requires firmer commitments from providers that services will be available, more specific contractual obligations will presumably be sought. It is not equally obvious that more formality and specificity in the content of contracts lead necessarily to more effective quality control. The contract, after all, is signed before the service begins. Whether the contents of the contract matter subsequently depends on the nature of the monitoring. The limited study conducted in Massachusetts (Gurin and Friedman 1980) indicated that decentralized and discretionary methods of monitoring seemed to have a better chance of being implemented than centralized mechanisms based on centrally negotiated contracts. However, there has not been enough systematic study on this point to permit broad generalizations.

ACCESS TO SERVICES: PRIORITIES

Given the universality of limited resources, human services face the need to ration those resources by determining which part of the total potential demand they will try to meet. Some programs have income eligibility requirements. Title XX, for example (now subsumed under the Social Services Block Grant) established specific eligibility income ceilings for some of its programs while making other services universal (open to all). Under the new law (97–35) each state may determine the level of income eligibility required. Other services relate eligibility to condition, as in the case of rehabilitation, which in recent years, has given priority to clients who are the most severely disabled. Another mode of rationing is to service people on a first come, first served basis, but to close intake when the limits of resources have been reached.

One of the problems involved in the contracting between public agencies and nongovernment providers is how to establish and implement such rationing. Two types of arrangements exist. Under one, known as "closed intake," the contracting agency receives the original applications and does the screening, referring individual clients to the provider agency on the basis of its own selection. Under an alternative procedure of "open intake," applications for service are received and acted upon directly by the provider agency, which then reports to the contracting agency and requests reimbursement. Both methods have their advantages and difficulties. Closed intake gives the governmental agency a greater degree of assurance that its priorities will be followed, but requires the maintenance of a substantial direct service operation and may involve some duplication of effort. Open intake may have the advantage of increasing the accessibility of services for clients, but can make it more difficult for services to focus sharply on priority target populations.

The issue of whether contracting increases the accessibility of services merits further investigation. It can be argued, in theory, that the existence of large numbers of providers should increase the possibility that clients will learn about services and be ready to use them if they are under auspices that are an integral part of their natural environment. Such claims have been made in the past, particularly in regard to underserved groups such as ethnic minorities. During periods of program expansion, new providers did appear in such services as day care, small group treatment homes, mental health, and drug clinics. Some of these smaller services were self-help groups that made special efforts to reach out to underserved groups. Because many of these services were fully supported by government funds, they have faced growing difficulty as the period of expansion changed into one of contraction of public service budgets.

In the Massachusetts study (Gurin and Friedman 1980), there was no evidence to confirm that contracting made for any discernible increase in accessibility. In homemaker services the number of providers available in any locality was generally small. In children's protective services, most of the contracting was done with a few large, well-established agencies. It was found that certain groups did have a problem in gaining access to service, e.g., people living in isolated rural areas, or groups in certain sections of the inner city where providers were reluctant to render service. Such limitations were not overcome by the contracting practices used.

CASE MANAGEMENT

The use of a case manager is a frequent contracting practice. An early and influential model for this approach was the rehabilitation counselor, who carried responsibility for working out service plans with individual clients, deciding upon the providers to use and monitoring the results. The rehabilitation counselor has the authority, within budget limits, to issue purchase orders for services, and thus the ability to implement the service plans that he or she had worked out. The counseling and service planning functions, in this mode of service delivery, are not contracted out, although clinical diagnostic or treatment services are purchased. Attempts have been made to use the rehabilitation case management model in other services, such as services to the elderly, children's services, and health and mental health services. It is a way in which a multiplicity of services can be brought together and integrated at the client service level.

The function of case management is not always easy to differentiate from counseling or casework. When a contracting agency purchases counseling or casework services (e.g., in children's protective services) and tries to maintain a case management function as a direct service, there are problems of duplication, as well as conflict over whose case judgments are to prevail. There is thus a dilemma between the obligation of the contracting agency to be accountable for services for which it is paying and the desirability of decentralization, individualization, and lack of unnecessary duplication in the rendering of the services.

These and other issues of regulation and monitoring are difficult to resolve, but they lie at the heart of efforts to construct effective and efficient systems of contracting.

REGULATION AND MONITORING

One approach to regulation and monitoring is to try to build controls into formal contracts, through precise and detailed specifications of the services to be provided, and to hold providers to those specifications through program and fiscal monitoring. That approach presents several difficulties. It calls for a substantial investment of staff resources in contract management by the contracting agency and thus adds a significant factor to the total cost, to the point where whatever economies to be expected from the use of contracting may be compromised. Two Massachusetts studies (Gurin and Friedman 1980, and Massachusetts Taxpayers Foundation 1980) concluded that the governmental agencies did not have the capacity to monitor effectively. Gurin and Friedman (1980) pointed to the paradox that the agency with the most formal contract arrangements, the Department of Public Welfare, was least able to exercise any control over the performance of its contracted providers and even had difficulty in maintaining adequate information about the disposition of cases. This does not imply that they did or did not perform more effectively when they directly delivered services.

Another difficulty with relying on formal contracts relates to the earlier discussion about defining and measuring quality. Given the complexities of the quality issues in the human services, formal contracting, at

317

best, can specify a set of inputs. Centralized monitoring based on formal contracts, given adequate resources, should be able to determine whether providers are in compliance with input standards. Additional kinds of monitoring would be required to form judgments about the quality of outputs.

An alternative to monitoring and regulation is to rely less on formal contracting and more on marketlike mechanisms of consumer choice and decentralized decision making. In a case management system, where the decisions as to which providers to use and how to use them is decentralized to the level of the case manager working with the client, monitoring is based on informal rather than formal methods. Such a system provides quick feedback to the manager about client perceptions and evaluations of the services rendered to them by the providers. It also maximizes opportunities for the client to participate in the choice of the provider. On a day-by-day basis, case managers learn the capacities of providers to respond to client needs and are able to evaluate their availability and reliability.

Monitoring in the human services is a difficult enterprise under any circumstances. Governmental agencies that provide services directly experience substantial error rates, as in the case of public assistance, and have persistent problems in tracking clients, as in the case of children's services. They are beset by quantitative and qualitative limitations in staff, budget constraints, and inadequate information processing, to say nothing of the intrinsic complexities of the human problems with which they try to cope. Contracting does not solve these problems and may in some instances even complicate them. But they can modify contracts annually. They can change vendors. These are tools not available to public agencies when they hire their own staff under civil service regulations. Human services vary considerably, and contracting mechanisms need to be adapted to the specific requirements of each field. In general, however, it appears that some combination of centralized and decentralized procedures is needed for effective operation. Centralization is required for general policy guidance, economies of scale, negotiations with larger providers, identification of resources that exist beyond the boundaries of local units, and for fiscal auditing and control. For monitoring of quality, decentralized mechanisms that maximize client participation and are close to the level of service delivery would seem to have decided advantages. This type of decentralized monitoring was found to take place in rehabilitation services through the use of purchase orders for particular services and in the purchase of homemaker services for particular clients (Gurin and Friedman 1980).

ISSUES OF COST AND PRICING

In the polemical discussions of contracting, the question of cost has played a central role. It is argued, and widely assumed, that the private sector can operate more efficiently than government and that equivalent services should therefore cost less if they are purchased rather than delivered directly by the public agency. In the human services, there is no definitive data to support or reject this argument. For reasons indicated earlier, it has proven difficult to make rigorous comparisons. One study that was able to establish the proper conditions for comparison (Pacific Consultants 1979) found mixed results. Although the direct cost for a unit of service (chore services) was found to be lower for the private provider, the total costs, taking into account administrative expenses of both the provider and the monitoring cost on the part of the contracting agency, were higher than the total cost of providing the service directly.

Friedman, in the study of three Massachusetts agencies (Gurin and Friedman 1980), undertook a theoretical analysis of how contracting would compare with direct service provision, under the assumption that both sectors were performing efficiently. Under such conditions, an agency providing services directly should be able to allocate clients among offices or staff so as to equalize marginal costs, thus minimizing total costs. In using providers, however, an agency pays a uniform rate for all units of service purchased. The marginal cost of getting an extra unit of service from a provider thus depends not only on the marginal cost of that extra unit per se but also on the possible need to adjust the rate on all units of service as an inducement to the provider. The best the agency can do, given limitations in its knowledge of the detailed cost curves of all providers, is to equate these more complicated marginal costs; if these are equated, the simple management costs of an extra unit of service will not be equated, meaning that total cost will not be minimized. In the case of profit-making providers, there is also the factor of profit, which is an additional cost above what the service would cost

319

if provided directly. The amount of this extra cost will depend on the amount of competition among providers: the more providers compete with each other, the smaller this extra cost (profit).

In reality, it cannot be assumed that there is perfect efficiency either in the public or nongovernmental sectors, and there are compelling reasons that make it advantageous for the public agency to seek the services of voluntary or proprietary providers. If it is to obtain the expected benefits from contracting out, the public agency needs to optimize its ability to obtain a given quantity of services at the lowest possible cost. The rate-setting process is therefore a crucial element in the management of contracts.

RATE-SETTING PROCESS

There are several different ways in which rates can be set. The following list, although not exhaustive, includes the following major variations:

1. *Purchases at the market price.* The agency simply purchases services in the open market at the stated price. Sometimes comparison shopping is done if there are price variations, e.g., the use of taxis for transporting clients, with the payment being the meter rate, or the purchase of a medical appliance.
2. *Uniform rates.* The agency establishes a price for a given unit of service and pays that price uniformly to providers who are ready to provide the service at that price and whom the agency is willing to use.
3. *Rate schedules.* Rate schedules are a variation of uniform rates. Instead of establishing one rate for all providers, the agency may have a range of rates, varying with size or other factors. Rate schedules are indicated in services where there may be economies of scale, such as homemakers or sheltered workshops, with the average costs falling as the operation grows larger, at least up to a point.
4. *Individually negotiated rates.* The contractor does not have a uniform rate, but pays each provider on the basis of its own costs. Such rates are based on examination of the provider's costs, with nego-

       tiations to determine what items of expense will or will not be in-
       cluded in the reimbursement formula.
5. *Competitive bidding.* The use of competitive bidding is more compli-
       cated in the human services than in private industry because
       of the difficulties of formulating definitive qualitative speci-
       fications.

Where the government agency is an occasional buyer of a service and
therefore does not have much market power, it will have little flexibility
in departing from the market price. There are many instances, however,
in which the contracting agency does have market power. Gurin and
Friedman (1980) found examples of situations in which the public agency
was in fact paying less than market rates. For example, the agency was
able to obtain diagnostic services from providers who would charge the
state less than their private patients. This is due to the fact that some
markets are segmented. In this example there were some providers willing to accept the state's rates, either because of an ideological conviction
that they should provide services to these clients and/or because they
were just beginning professional practice and did not as yet have private
patients to occupy all of their time. It is thus not necessarily desirable to
rely on competitive bidding for the lowest rate; costs can be reduced
through the self-selection that will come about among providers, in some
instances, in response to a fixed rate. On the other hand, such savings
may be at the expense of both the desired quantity and quality of services, if not enough providers respond, or if those who respond are of less
capability than desired.

If rates are to be set unilaterally by the contracting agency or a rate-
setting commission, it may be necessary to use approximations, through
a trial and error approach, to determine what rates are necessary to obtain the desired quantity of service. In that process a number of considerations must be taken into account that differ, depending on whether the
provider is a profit or nonprofit organization.

In Massachusetts proprietary providers entered the homemaker field
some years ago, when public funding for that service was expanding.
Some of these agencies conducted a relatively large volume of service
that resulted in economies of scale. Given a uniform rate, their profits
would increase the greater the volume of service. The Rate Setting Commission of the state did not use uniform rates but had a rate schedule as a

guideline, where the rate allowed would decline the greater the volume of service. In addition, it negotiated individual rates with each agency, depending on its costs, in an attempt to push rates below the schedule. Beginning in 1981, it gave up the practice of negotiating, relying on the rate schedule alone. The consequence was that the large proprietaries and large nonprofits received low rates while the small nonprofits received high rates. Such a system could be justified if the small nonprofits served special needs or underserved areas.

There are indeed some special and complex issues that arise in relation to voluntary providers. There has been a tendency for some voluntary providers to resist substantial expansion of services, so that they have not met the demand by the public agency for their services. The reasons for this vary in different service fields and among agencies, but usually involve some qualitative considerations. For example, some voluntary agencies have preferred to limit their services so that they may give more professional, intensive services to those clients whom they do accept. A pricing mechanism that is based on meeting the actual costs of the service offers no incentive to such agencies to expand and therefore loses the benefits of the economies of scale that might be derived from expansion. It is possible that, in paying a higher rate, the contracting agency is paying for a higher quality of services, but that is not always clear. Nor is it clear that the quantitative limits have been reached even within the definition of quality service to which the provider is committed.

To the defects of individually negotiated rates that have been described, one must add the administrative costs of the negotiating process. Because there is no uniformity among providers, each rate negotiation involves examination of different accounting practices in regard to the allocation of overhead and other technical problems. These negotiating costs are never calculated into the equation of the costs of contracting, but they are real.

One way to increase the efficacy of contracting as a mechanism for the delivery of service is thus to simplify the rate-setting process through the use of uniform rates or a scale of rates. (For a more lengthy discussion of rate-setting in the human services, see Richardson, this volume.) Just what the rates should be can be determined only through trial and error, which calls, in itself, for a competent administrative capacity on the part of the contracting agency. If both effectiveness and cost efficiency are to be optimized, contracting agencies must be able to specify more clearly than they now seem able to do both the quantity of services being sought and the major qualitative elements that may be related to differences in cost. Contractors would then be able to make targeted departures from uniform average rates in order to achieve a specific objective, such as providing greater service to underserved areas or populations.

THE PRACTICE of contracting by public agencies with nongovernmental providers engenders problems of dependency and risk for both. Many providers came into the field because of the expansion of public programs, are completely dependent on public funds, and face severe problems during the current period of reductions in public expenditures. On the other hand, the Massachusetts Taxpayers study (1980), Hanrahan (1977), representing public employee unions, and others argue that government has become too dependent on providers, having lost its capacity to provide services directly and therefore not in control of its own policies and programs. Whatever the merits of those contentions, it is clear that the contracting relationship, by definition, is a condition of interdependence between the contractor and provider. These concluding comments deal with some of the conditions that need to be met if that interdependence is to function effectively in providing human services to clients.

In most instances where the public agency contracts with nongovernmental providers, it does not delegate responsibility fully to the providers, but retains legal responsibility in varying degrees for both individual cases and the program at large. Frequently, it retains the functions of screening, eligibility determination, and case management. At a minimum the contracting agency is accountable to governmental authorities and the public for effective auditing of the providers' work. In order to carry out these responsibilities, the contracting agency needs a substantial capacity for policymaking, implementation, and management. One of the risks in the proliferation of contracting is that this requirement is not fully recognized and the budgets of the public agencies are not adequate to maintain the necessary capacity at an effective level.

The providers have parallel needs if they are to perform effectively the responsibilities that are placed upon them. Some providers have very substantial resources of their own and are only minimally dependent on the public agencies. This is, however, not the usual case. Most providers, in order to function effectively, rely upon some degree of stability and predictability in program, policies, and funding. Small providers are particularly dependent, for example, on timely payments from the contractors, lacking the resources to handle extensive delays in cash flow. Some may need help in meeting the initial capital costs of entering the field. Both contractors and providers face risks due to uncertainties in regard to utilization. If payments are related to units of service and the capacity is underutilized, the provider may not be able to continue to operate. For the contractor, this involves the risk that the service may not be available when needed. Some way of sharing these risks by reflecting them in the rates paid for service would seem indicated.

Contracting has been motivated in large part by the immediate exigencies of situations facing public agencies, but with a lack of systematic and long-range planning. The pressure has been to take advantage of immediate gains by escaping from government rigidities and by limiting payments to variable costs, avoiding the obligations involved in fixed costs. Policy direction and monitoring tend to be minimal. Given the continuing pervasiveness of contracting as a way of delivering human services, there is a strong case for an intensification of effort to make these practices more effective.

PART SIX

Monitoring, Evaluation, and Accountability in Purchase of Service

In the early period of implementing purchase of human services arrangements, relatively little emphasis was placed on contract monitoring and evaluation. In part, this inattention reflected naiveté about potential problems in the delivery of contracted services. With little experience upon which to draw, public agencies no doubt operated under the assumption that what was written into contracts would, in fact, be implemented. This logic was not inconsistent. Public agencies had no history of systematic evaluation of their own programs. A corresponding issue mitigating against monitoring and evaluation was the lack of specificity of earlier contracts; relatively brief, descriptive, and process oriented (e.g., how services would be delivered versus what the outcomes would be) were the norm. In such instances, considerable discretion about contract implementation was left in the hands of provider agencies. Decisions about contract renewals were often based on relationship and reputation factors rather than hard data.

A combination of factors led to increased attention to the role of the public agency in contract monitoring and evaluation. First, it soon became apparent that public agency expectations about the delivery of contracted services were not always met. In part, the discrepancy between expectations and experience stemmed from differing conceptions of "high quality, efficient, and effective" service delivery held by the public agency and contract nonpublic providers. The different and often disparate ways of doing business was also recognized, with growing concern about both process and outcomes. Often, expectations were not clearly communicated from the contractor to the contractee.

At both the federal and state levels, instances of contract abuse were played up in the press, with allegations ranging from the mismanagement or misappropriation of funds to provision of poor-quality services to the wrong target group. Public agencies were put in the position of responsibility to curtail the misuse of government funds.

As noted in chapter 2, the growing use of purchase of service in the 1960s and 1970s led to the unanticipated spiraling of social service costs; monitoring came to be viewed as one cost control mechanism. The growing emphasis on "accountability" for dollars spent and outcomes achieved also highlighted the real and potential uses of monitoring and evaluation data. To ensure that the dollars spent were in keeping with contract intent and the public interest, the focus shifted from "partnership" to public control of the operations and outcomes of contracted programs.

Although the terms *monitoring* and *evaluation* are often used interchangeably or in combination, they apply to distinct processes and have different objectives. Each of these terms may be used narrowly or more broadly. For example, monitoring is sometimes described as a process to ensure conformity and compliance with contract terms and requirements. In a more global sense, Jansson, in this section, describes monitoring as a management function that spans the entire contracting process and includes preventive, troubleshooting, and ameliorative components. In his conception, contract monitoring is a means to increase the likelihood of high performance on the part of contracted agencies or individuals.

The literature on purchase of service reflects a greater emphasis on monitoring than evaluation. There are several explanations for this phenomenon. First, earlier regulations (foremost, under Title XX) required state agencies to develop and implement monitoring procedures for contracted programs. Tatara and Pettiford describe monitoring practices among select state and local public agencies within the context of federal laws and regulations; such monitoring requirements allowed for the accumulation of experience with various monitoring models. On the other hand, program evaluation, a process to assess the ultimate impact of services and the extent to which program objectives are achieved, has not generally been mandated; thus, the body of knowledge regarding evaluation procedures, their validity and utility, is not well developed. There are exceptions, Head Start, some job training programs, and some early community mental health grants and contracts required program evaluation. In the late 1980s these efforts have been abandoned.

Evaluation of the quality, effectiveness, and goal attainment of con-

326

tracted services involves the development of evaluation designs and strategies, often of a quantitative nature. For example, in evaluating the effectiveness of a program to provide birth control information to teenagers, one design might involve assessing whether participants in a control group show differential rates of knowledge and attitude change. The ultimate test would be behavioral.

Evaluation, in almost all instances, must be geared to the objectives of a specific contracted program and usually involves substantial time, effort, and resources to appropriately accomplish. Although evaluation designs need not require the ultimate in research technology, they do require staff with expertise in design, assessment, and quantitative analysis. Evaluation may also involve longitudinal analyses at predetermined time intervals following the completion of service delivery. However, such evaluations yield results only after considerable time and involve ongoing relationships with contractees, perhaps beyond the point of the contract itself or after renewal has already taken place, e.g., after the fact. From a cost-benefit perspective, public agencies may well conclude that monitoring is a more realistic, immediate, and useful means of assessing contracting than formal evaluation processes.

Monitoring, unlike evaluation, offers more concrete, current, and practical data for assessing contracting. The concern in monitoring is not with the outcomes, but rather the extent to which the provider fulfills the terms and requirements of the contract. As Tatara and Pettiford note, monitoring may pertain to fiscal compliance, as determined through audits, or compliance with the required steps and procedures, e.g., number of clients being served, the types of services being provided, frequency of client contacts, methods of involving the community, and so forth. Such monitoring data can, and often are, used to represent performance rather than outcome measures. An advantage of monitoring is that its procedures can, in general, be applied to all contracts, without the need for program-specific modifications. So, too, once a monitoring system is in place, less skilled, but technically proficient staff can perform the monitoring function; this is not the case with evaluation strategies.

The chapters in this section reflect the general state of the art of contract monitoring and evaluation. Three of the four chapters focus on monitoring, although there is an inevitable overlap in defining the boundaries of monitoring and evaluation. The large supply of theory, data, and experience in contract monitoring stems from its longer history and emphasis when compared with the status of evaluation technology, implementation, and experience.

The authors of the three articles on monitoring purchase of service contracts approach this subject from different vantage points. They share in common, however, an essential agreement that the monitoring function resides with the public agency and is an integral component of the contracting process. In defining monitoring from the broadest perspective, Jansson provides a theoretical base on which to view the public agency's functional role within the context of interorganizational relationships. Addressing the monitoring role from a pragmatic point of view, Tatara and Pettiford detail some actual experiences of, and models employed by, public agencies based on their interpretation of legal and regulatory mandates. Using data derived from a sample survey of state and local practices, these authors highlight the most commonly used monitoring methods without attempting to evaluate their merits or shortcomings.

Wedel and Chess also assume a pragmatic posture to explore the rationale and objectives of a monitoring system. Issues addressed include who should do the monitoring, when it is to be done, and what methods may be employed. Practical monitoring strategies are offered and corrective action alternatives are identified by the authors when problem areas are recognized through the monitoring activity.

Addressing some of the evaluation strategies available for use by public agencies, Schlesinger and Dorwart focus primarily on benefit-cost analysis and client outcome monitoring. Noting the many weaknesses associated with the use of these methods, they also propose the use of alternative contracting procedures, including competitive models and selective contracting, to augment formal evaluation. The need for formal evaluation, they contend, has much to do with the political context in which contracting takes place and the degree of control the public agency exercises in relation to contracted providers.

Unlike monitoring, it is not altogether clear that the public agency must perform the evaluating function. In fact, many contracts stipulate that the provider agency outline and implement the steps and procedures to evaluate both the process and outcome of the services it is contracted to deliver. Although the validity of such procedures and their results might be challenged on the basis of bias and self-interest, it is also true that a significant amount of information is available from service providers that

328

may allow for comparative and longitudinal analyses. However, no systematic effort has been made by states or the federal government to collect, analyze, and compare these data, with the exception of the dollar value of contracts, types of providers, and other gross characteristics of the purchase of service system.

The dearth of information related to establishing and implementing evaluation systems and their relative merits, as compared to well developed theory, suggests that this area is ripe for exploration and development by researchers, managers, and agency administrators. The feasibility of using third parties—those with evaluation expertise who are neither the public agency nor the service provider—might also be reconsidered. (It was fairly popular at one time.) A mitigating factor is the cost disincentives associated with formal evaluation and the priorities and pressures emanating from Congress and state legislatures to establish accountability for dollars spent rather than outcomes achieved. This emphasis, in an era of scarce dollars, may have the effect of deterring both the public agency and contracted provider from the true goal of the public-private partnership: to provide the highest quality services in the most efficient and effective manner.

21

Purchase of Service Monitoring and Evaluation Policies and Practices

Toshio Tatara and Evelyn Kays Pettiford

As the rate of purchase of service has increased, the issue of accountability in the use of tax dollars has correspondingly become a matter of greater public concern. The Massachusetts Taxpayers Foundation, Inc., in its publication, "Purchase of Service: Can State Government Gain Control?" (1980), charged that the purchase of social services in Massachusetts has become big business over which the state has not established adequate control. Further, the report alleged that the state's purchase system is dominated by providers to an extent that mitigates against the state gaining fiscal and program control. Similarly, a national study by the Urban Institute found that, in general, states have not reorganized their overall management structures and personnel systems in a manner that would allow them to properly monitor and evaluate the contract performance of purchase of service agencies (hereafter referred to as POS agencies) (Benton, Feild, and Millar 1978, 136–137).

Without judging the validity of the above observations, it is important to note that in the late 1960s and early 1970s, a number of factors coalesced to thrust the states into purchase of service agreements with private and voluntary providers prior to the states' development of rational approaches in deciding what to purchase and why. Foremost among these factors was the federal government's encouragement to purchase social services. The 1967 amendments to the Social Security Act authorized public welfare agencies to receive 75 percent federal reimbursement for expenditures on services that were purchased from private, nonprofit, or proprietary organizations. Second, as the demand for social services grew at an ever-expanding rate and the cost of services escalated in an inflation-ridden economy, some states began turning to purchase of service as a means of limiting or reducing the public payroll. Finally, changes in the philosophy and methods of addressing social problems also contributed to increasing rates of purchase of social services. As the concepts of deinstitutionalization, normalization, mainstreaming, and "least restrictive environment" gained increasing credibility as treatment methods for the aged, delinquent youths, and the mentally ill and retarded, many states turned to private and voluntary providers as the most expeditious source of instituting new approaches to service delivery (Massachusetts Taxpayers Foundation 1980).

Thus, the stage was set for a climate in which public social service agencies found themselves playing "catch-up" in an effort to develop, after the fact, appropriate mechanisms and procedures for managing purchase of service systems. Public agencies, which for years had been geared to the direct management and delivery of services to clients, were now forced to refocus a portion of their energy and resources on contract management and oversight.

In an effort to assess the state of the art in developing systems for monitoring and evaluating purchased social services in the state and local public social service agencies, the authors conducted a telephone survey of fourteen state social service agencies and two local (county) agencies. Agencies from the following states and counties were included in the survey: Arizona, Arkansas, Florida, Idaho, Indiana, Iowa, Maine, Michigan, New Hampshire, New York, Vermont, Virginia, West Virginia, Wyoming, Milwaukee County, Wisconsin, and San Joaquin County, California. The authors also reviewed written materials made available by these agencies that detailed their monitoring and evaluation plans and activities. The agencies, selected through random sampling from the categories of high-, medium-, and low-purchase states, represent the diversity exhibited by all fifty states with regard to size, geographic location, and type of system used for administering social services (i.e., either state-administered or county-administered, state supervised). Generally, the survey revealed that all sixteen agencies have implemented systems for monitoring the performance of POS agencies, but that program evaluation efforts designed to determine the effectiveness or impact of purchased services is still a developing art.

GENERAL APPROACHES TO PURCHASE OF
SERVICE MONITORING AND EVALUATION

State and local social service agencies monitor and evaluate the performance of POS agencies in several ways. Although the specific terminologies and definitions of these monitoring and evaluation activities vary from one agency to another, there are three types of activities that are intended to assure the quality, effectiveness, and efficiency of purchased services: (1) fiscal monitoring or auditing, (2) contract compliance monitoring, and (3) program evaluation. These activities are not totally independent of each other but differ mainly in terms of purpose, focus, and personnel involved in the effort.

Fiscal monitoring is directed almost exclusively to the review of accounting and billing practices, whereas contract compliance monitoring is generally concerned with whether service providers are in compliance with the terms and requirements of a specific contract. Program evaluation, on the other hand, focuses upon the processes and outcomes of services delivered to clients from the standpoint of their effectiveness and efficiency. Although the effectiveness or efficiency of a service cannot be determined without fiscal data and contract compliance information, in the strict sense, program evaluation of purchased services is generally considered a distinct activity in many jurisdictions.

This chapter focuses on two of the above-described activities: contract compliance monitoring and program evaluation. The discussion is limited to the monitoring and evaluation of purchased social services from the perspective of the public agencies. Because state and local agencies purchase a wide range of services and the policies and practices related to monitoring and evaluation vary from one type of service to another (even within the same jurisdiction), it was important to limit the study so that valid cross-state comparisons could be made. Thus, the study examined primarily the purchase of social services under Title IV-B and Title XX of the Social Security Act.

FEDERAL REQUIREMENTS FOR PURCHASE OF
SERVICE MONITORING AND EVALUATION

Under Title XX of the Social Security Act, the federal government required both fiscal and contract compliance monitoring of purchased social services, but did not require the evaluation of the outcomes of such services. Under the *Code of Federal Regulations* (CFR), states were required to execute written contracts with POS agencies in order to obtain federal funding on a matching basis. The (purchase of service) contract was to "specify requirements for fiscal and program responsibility, billing, records, controls, reports and *monitoring procedures* (emphasis added) . . . 45 CFR 228.70 (a) (12), until September 1980 and 45 CFR 1396.70 (a) (12) until September 1981."

Based upon this requirement, most state social service agencies have established routine procedures for monitoring the purchase of service process from the standpoint of financial accountability and compliance with contract provisions. Although the specific practice in terms of scope, method, and frequency of monitoring varies rather significantly from one agency to another, all agencies surveyed under the present study have developed written policies for fiscal and contract compliance monitoring, and these policies are, in fact, implemented.

On the other hand, because program evaluation per se has not been required by federal regulation, the decision to include it as a requirement of POS contracts has been left to the discretion of each state. To date, only a few social service agencies have established a formal policy requiring the programmatic evaluation of purchased services. Even those agencies that regularly conduct program evaluations of purchased services rarely specify in the POS contract that program evaluation is required or will be undertaken. Nevertheless, despite the absence of a federal requirement, program evaluation of purchased services is being conducted at state and local levels, as will be reviewed later in this chapter. The extent of program evaluation, however, varies widely from one jurisdiction to another, largely depending upon the capabilities and resources of the evaluation units of the various agencies.

The Omnibus Budget Reconciliation Act of 1981 amended Title XX of the Social Security Act to establish a social services block grant. The new regulations implementing the block grants, in keeping with the basic purpose of the legislation, greatly simplify the process of state grant administration and minimize the federal government's oversight functions. Many of the federal regulations previously governing the Title XX program were eliminated, and instead the new regulations indicate that each state's own laws and procedures for expending state revenues should govern the state's use of block grant funds.

334

Under the Social Services Block Grant, states are now required to meet only three federal reporting requirements: (1) to submit an annual report to the secretary of the Department of Health and Human Services on the intended use of block grant funds prior to receiving the funds, (2) to submit to the secretary at least once every two years the state's report describing how funds were actually used, and (3) to submit a copy of the audit report of state expenditures to the secretary at least once every two years. Further, the block grant legislation means that decisions regarding whether and how to monitor and evaluate social services, including purchased services, are now state matters, devoid of any federal requirements.

STATE AND LOCAL APPROACHES TO
CONTRACT COMPLIANCE MONITORING

Without exception, the surveyed state and local agencies use contract compliance monitoring as a major tool for assessing the performance of POS agencies. In addition to the basic requirement for contract monitoring, the majority of agencies also have written policies and procedures that govern the monitoring process itself. Written guidelines range from formal administrative manuals devoted solely to monitoring POS agencies to social services manuals that contain sections relevant to contract compliance monitoring.

The majority of public social service agencies monitor POS agencies on a sampling basis, with particular emphasis placed upon services receiving high purchase dollars and agencies serving comparatively large numbers of clients. Reviews are generally conducted once a year, though some states monitor particular aspects of compliance on a more frequent basis. Areas most frequently examined by the public agencies during contract compliance monitoring include client eligibility determination, service provision, case record-keeping system, facility review, staffing ratios, administrative practices, compliance with licensing and certification standards, and compliance with federal and state regulations.

A number of public agencies include a provision in their POS contracts that stipulates that the public agency will monitor the contract and specifies the frequency, method, and process for monitoring. A few agencies indicated that they utilize the results of monitoring to modify and/or terminate contracts; however, a greater number of the agencies use the

335

results to provide technical assistance aimed at assisting the POS agencies to comply with contract provisions and improve their services.

By and large, the agencies surveyed assign their own staff to develop contracts and to monitor contract compliance. In state-administered systems, central or regional/district office staff generally develop and monitor contracts. In county-administered, state-supervised systems, local agency staff develop contracts (frequently based upon a model contract developed by the state office) and then monitor contract performance.

Finally, three of the agencies interviewed use a "manager" concept in relation to contract compliance monitoring. In the state of Iowa, a project manager is assigned to oversee each purchase of service contract. As the chief liaison between the state agency and the service provider, he or she monitors contract performance and provides technical assistance to the provider as needed. Similarly, in the state of Michigan, contract owners are designated to develop and monitor contracts. (An example of monitoring by project managers can be found in chapter 16).

Among the three states using the manager concept, Florida has initiated perhaps the most elaborate system for contract development and management. Based on the belief that the state must protect and gain maximum benefit from the funds it distributes, the state agency (the Department of Health and Rehabilitative Services) has established a Contract Management System (CMS), which governs the procurement and management of all purchase of service contracts. A contract manager is assigned to monitor the performance of each contractor, using the monitoring plan as specified in the contract. Each contract manager reports to one of twelve contract administrators (located in the central office and each of the eleven district offices) who have general oversight responsibility for all contracts executed by the state agency. The specific responsibilities of the contract manager are (1) to review and analyze program reports submitted by the contractor; (2) to review and process invoices/requests for payment; (3) to conduct site visits and meet with administrators, service providers, and clients; (4) to develop a written plan for corrective action as indicated; and (5) to document the results of corrective actions taken for submission to the contract administrator.

STATE AND LOCAL APPROACHES TO PROGRAM EVALUATION

Although all of the public social service agencies surveyed use monitoring to ensure that POS agencies comply with the provisions of their contracts, fewer than half of the agencies indicated that they evaluate the effectiveness of purchased services. This finding was not unexpected. Wedel (1979) noted that impact evaluation, which is concerned with the accomplishment of service goals and objectives, is generally an underdeveloped area in social services. Similarly, a national study by the Urban Institute found that "more than half of the jurisdictions administering Title XX across the country have neither completed nor undertaken a single study of the effectiveness of the programs they administer" (Benton, Feild, and Millar 1978, p. 32).

Of the sixteen public agencies surveyed, only six reported that they evaluate the effectiveness of purchased services, and one agency reported that it is developing criteria and standards to evaluate both services provided directly and those purchased. The agencies that evaluate service effectiveness generally do so on a selective basis, with particular emphasis placed on service areas receiving high purchase dollars. Generally, services are evaluated by the evaluation unit of the public agency at the request of public agency program personnel.

Another approach often used by public agencies to evaluate the effectiveness of purchased services is to require that POS agencies develop and implement an evaluation plan as a provision of their contract with the public agency. This approach, though not widely used among the states surveyed, can be used in lieu of an evaluation by the public agency or in conjunction with such an evaluation.

All of the agencies surveyed indicated that evaluation of the effectiveness of purchased services was very limited when compared with the volume of services purchased. This limitation is partly a function of the lack of public agency staff and resources, particularly in the evaluation area, and partly a result of relatively underdeveloped evaluation capacities, technology, and tradition in the public social service sector. Over the past few years, the increased use of contracting has generally provided impetus for program evaluation at the state level. However, as the volume of purchased services has expanded at ever-increasing rates and the resources of states have simultaneously dwindled, many states have found it exceedingly difficult, if not impossible, to assume new initiatives in the evaluation area. At the same time, the limited resources of many POS agencies have not permitted them to take the lead in evaluation efforts either.

Despite the resource problems currently facing public social service agencies, many of the states surveyed expressed a desire to expand their evaluation activities, when possible, to include both services provided directly and those purchased. At the time of the survey, at least one state (Florida) was planning to conduct a comparative study of the effectiveness of services provided directly versus those purchased. Areas under consideration for study were adoption services and the case management of developmental disabilities.

Although not among the states surveyed, Minnesota's Community Social Services Act of 1979 is worthy of mention. This law is basically a "state Title XX Act," which assigns responsibility to the counties for administration of most of the state's personal social service programs. Of particular note is the fact that the act mandates the evaluation and monitoring of both services provided directly and those purchased. Counties must specify in their county plans the methods by which they will monitor and evaluate community social service programs. In addition, the state plan must include a description of how each program's effectiveness will be evaluated in relation to measurable objectives and performance criteria.

One trend among those public agencies that evaluate the effectiveness of purchased services is to periodically interview or survey the recipients of services (i.e., the clients) to determine the level of improvement in their presenting problems and to measure their degree of satisfaction with the services provided. This approach, now commonly referred to as client outcome monitoring, has gained increasing recognition in recent years as an effective and useful evaluation measure. Of particular note is the fact that it is now required by law in Milwaukee County, Wisconsin.

MILWAUKEE COUNTY PURCHASE ORDINANCE

Adopted by the County Board of Supervisors in 1972 and partially revised in 1976, the Milwaukee County Purchase Ordinance (Section 46.09 of the Milwaukee County Ordinances) sets forth the basic policy of the Department of Social Services on the purchase of "care and treatment services" from nongovernmental vendors within the county.

338

Although many other local jurisdictions have ordinances designed to regulate the purchase of goods and services, this ordinance is unique because it mandates the monitoring of purchased social services through the use of client outcome monitoring.

Implementing the purchase ordinance is the responsibility of the Quality Control Unit of the Department of Social Services, which was established by the ordinance in 1972. This unit enforces the provisions of the purchase ordinance by conducting four major "quality assurance monitoring activities": (1) consumer (client) satisfaction survey; (2) agency site visitation, (3) Title XX compliance review, and (4) service verification/documentation survey.

The consumer (client) satisfaction survey requires that the department conduct a survey of persons receiving care or services from a vendor agency (or their guardians) to obtain their impressions regarding the adequacy and quality of the services provided to them. The survey must be conducted at least once a year.

Initially, staff of the Quality Control Unit mailed survey forms to all clients receiving purchased services in a selected month. Currently, questionnaires are sent monthly to a 2 percent randomly selected sample of clients of each vendor agency. Originally, the questionnaire was standardized for use with all clients, regardless of the service received. Several versions of the questionnaire were later developed to allow for variations in client characteristics and types of service received.

During 1980 the department's quality control staff sent questionnaires to a total of 1,235 clients by using the 2 percent sampling method mentioned above. This sample of clients represented a total of twenty-four different service categories and sixty-eight nongovernmental service vendors. The rate of return on the questionnaires was 45.2 percent (N = 558), a very high return rate for a mail survey and apparently indicative of strong consumer interest in participating in assessing service adequacy and quality (James, Jr. 1981). Continued observation and assessment of the results of Milwaukee County's consumer satisfaction survey should prove instructive for other jurisdictions interested in evaluating service effectiveness through client outcome monitoring.

TRENDS IN CLIENT OUTCOME MONITORING SYSTEMS

Client outcome monitoring is increasingly seen by public agencies as an important management tool for evaluating both services provided directly and those purchased. It has taken root in a climate in which major emphasis has been placed on consumer satisfaction and the protection of consumer rights. Client outcome monitoring is also consistent with the increasing attention to management improvement in both the public and private sectors.

Eager both to improve client services and demonstrate service effectiveness to state and federal legislative bodies, public social service agencies have begun to place more emphasis on ongoing data collection efforts, including client satisfaction surveys. The analyzed data, it is believed, will assist administrators and legislators to make informed decisions about program funding and operations. For example, the states of Colorado, Florida, Michigan, and Texas, as well as some local human service agencies are using client outcome monitoring approaches to evaluate the effectiveness of certain social services. Colorado has established the nation's first office of client outcome monitoring within the Department of Social Services and has conducted several studies.

In 1980 and 1981, the American Public Welfare Association (APWA), under contract to the Urban Institute, sponsored several training workshops on client outcome monitoring procedures for public social service agencies. Although the primary purpose of these workshops was to train public agency representatives to design and implement client outcome monitoring systems, APWA also found a strong interest among public agencies in developing and using client outcome monitoring as a major management tool.

Participants, the majority of whom were state and local public social service agency representatives, were asked if a client outcome monitoring system existed within their agencies. Of the 104 respondents to the question, 83 persons (79.8 percent) indicated that either a client outcome monitoring system was already in place in their agencies or the development and implementation of such a system was being considered. Although it is not possible to determine whether the 83 respondents represented 83 separate agencies (because some agencies sent more than one person to the workshops), it is still significant that the overwhelming majority of workshop participants either had or were considering the development of a client outcome monitoring system. Of particular note is the fact that more than two-thirds (67.4 percent) of the San Francisco workshop participants indicated that their agencies either have a system in place or are considering the development of one. Because the majority of the San Francisco workshop participants were local agency personnel in California, it is clear that a client outcome monitoring system is well supported by local agencies in this locally-administered, state-supervised state.

MONITORING AND EVALUATION: LOOKING AHEAD

Future directions in the monitoring and evaluation of purchased social services must be viewed in the context of a number of factors: (1) the realized and potential impact of Social Services Block Grant and other Reagan initiatives upon the purchase of social services, (2) the federal spending reductions for social services, and (3) the climate of deregulation that currently prevails at the national level.

With passage of the Social Services Block Grant legislation, responsibility for social services was shifted from the federal to the state and local levels. Federal regulatory functions of social service programs were deemphasized and, simultaneously, states began to assume greater responsibility for assessing and responding to the social service needs of their respective populations. In a very real sense, the power struggle for resource allocation with regard to social service programs was shifted from Congress to the various state capitols. However, simultaneous with this shift of responsibility to the state level has come a concommitant federal spending reduction for the social services. Consequently, although states' decision-making authority and control have increased, the resources available to fund and operate social service programs have declined.

In this climate of dwindling resources, it is not likely that the rate of purchase of social services will increase as rapidly as it has in the past and may, in fact, decline if the dollars available for service programs continue to shrink. Public social service agencies will be forced to reduce or hold the line on service levels in order to stay within the parameters of their limited budgets.

Although the rate of purchase of service may not increase in the near future, the need to monitor and evaluate both purchased services and

341

those provided directly will probably intensify in many states. This will result primarily from the political reality of having to allocate scarce resources to meet many competing demands. Under the block grant legislation, the state capitols rather than Congress will serve as the focal point for the allocation of resources. As such, they will most probably become political battle grounds on which various interest groups compete for a share of the limited resources.

As state legislators are faced with balancing the interests of competing groups and making difficult resource allocation decisions, it is highly probable that the issue of accountability will come increasingly to the fore. In many states the legislature is likely to demand more (not less) evaluation data from public social service agencies to assist the legislature in determining the relative effectiveness of various social service programs. It is equally likely that legislatures will also insist that administrative costs be reduced. Thus, public agencies will find themselves in the bind of needing to intensify monitoring and evaluation efforts, but having fewer resources with which to do so. In this climate it is likely that costly, long-term evaluation efforts such as longitudinal studies, may be abandoned in favor of short-term studies that yield quick turnaround results. For example, client outcome monitoring approaches, as one of the less costly evaluative methods, may become more common. There may also be an increase in the number of state studies that compare the effectiveness of services provided directly versus those purchased, because states will need to find more cost-effective methods of delivering services.

Ultimately, however, the level of monitoring and evaluation of purchased services will be determined by the resources available to sustain such efforts. In a national climate of diminishing resources, most states may be forced to expend available monies on direct services and curtail such activities as training and evaluation. Thus, although states may feel the need to expand and intensify their monitoring and evaluation activities in the future, many of them may simply not be able to afford it.

22

The Political Economy of Monitoring: A Contingency Perspective

Bruce S. Jansson

The literature on administration and program evaluation is relatively void of discussion of contract monitoring as an essential human services function. This inattention reflects the mistaken perception that monitoring is a relatively unimportant process that is primarily intended to avert such major scandals as fraud. Public administrators often seem to assume that contracts will automatically be implemented according to expectations. Evaluators tend to perceive monitoring as an uninteresting process involving the inspection of programs to determine their compliance with contract specifications. This process is viewed as less important than evaluation efforts that have as their purpose the determination of the outcomes of contracted programs.

Contract monitoring has, traditionally, been viewed from a limited perspective. This common view holds monitoring to be a reactive process occurring after contracts have been implemented, which seeks to examine compliance in relation to cost, administration, program, and other contract specifications. This restrictive definition is, however, deficient on several counts. First, it suggests that monitors are not included in important decisions in the contract development process. Second, it emphasizes the investigative functions of monitors while downplaying or ignoring their troubleshooting and assistance roles. Finally, this limited view does not emphasize a strategic role for monitors wherein they consider a range of approaches that can be used in pre- and postaward phases to increase the likelihood of superior performance by contractees.

Monitoring is defined broadly in this chapter as a management function that includes formulating strategies in the pre- and postaward phases of the contracting process to increase the likelihood of superior performance by contractees. Monitors have several critical roles. In their preventive role, monitors try to anticipate factors influencing contract performance so that monitoring can be designed as a device to offset the possibility of poor performance. In a trouble-shooting role, monitors analyze factors that impede contract performance during implementation. In strategic roles monitors identify monitoring and contract options in both the pre- and postaward phase that appear likely to increase the quality of contract performance.

Monitors need a framework in which to facilitate identification of those factors that influence contract performance. A political and economic perspective is discussed in this chapter to facilitate identification of funding, administrative, and power realities that impinge upon contract performance. Monitors also need a contingency perspective to move beyond the application of single models by devising and implementing strategies tailored to specific contracting situations. The need to elevate the status and importance of monitors is discussed as a prerequisite if monitors are to assume the several roles.

THE POLITICAL ECONOMY OF MONITORING

Poor performance by some contracted agencies has been recorded in relation to the War on Poverty, Title XX, block grants, Medicaid, economic development, mental health, and other programs (Lourie, in Wedel 1979, 18–29; Lowi 1969; Porter and Warner 1973; Wildavsky and Pressman 1973). Indeed, failure to comply with important contract provisions is not surprising when contractor-contractee relationships are viewed in political and economic terms. Contracting involves the flow of resources, program expectations, and performance requirements from one to another organization. Both contractor and contractee are influenced prior to and during the contractual relationship by numerous forces and beliefs that affect their interactions and shape patterns of dominance, submission, drift, cooperation, negotiation, and deception (Benson 1975).

Staff often try to develop and maintain organizational mission; retain, and where possible extend, organizational autonomy and domain; establish predictable flows of consumers and fiscal resources; and maintain their own distinctive technologies. In the case of cooperative relationships between contractors and contractees, political and economic interests of "both sides" are in balance. Cooperation characterizes inter-organizational relationships (ibid.).

In relationships marked by dominance, however, one of the parties is able to impose its ideology or operational preference modes upon the other, as when, for example, a contractor develops exacting reporting requirements that are rigorously enforced. Dominance often leads to resentment by the subordinate body, particularly when it believes that important political or economic sacrifices have been requested (Williams 1980, 186-189). In such cases grantees may try to use deception, litigation, or power resources to limit the extent of political and economic sacrifices that are required (see chapter 8 for a discussion of the bargaining process).

In relationships marked by "drift," contracts are awarded without sufficient policy or program guidance. Some contracts do not define important objectives or procedures, which may result in the absence of postaward monitoring guidelines and technical assistance capability (Kirschner Associates 1975; Waller 1975). In relationships marked by drift, it is not surprising contractees fail to comply with contractors' expectations particularly when they believe their ideological, political, and economic interests diverge from that of the funding source.

In cases of dominance, deception, and drift, important contract components may not be implemented, particularly when agencies are subject to divergent political and economic forces. Even when a contractor tries to establish dominance, contracters may find ways to circumvent imposed requirements. Divergence of political and economic interests between the two parties is common in the American social welfare state because contracts often bring together markedly different institutional structures. When federal agencies let contracts to state or local public agencies, for example, they expect that policies and regulations enacted in the political environment of the Congress and federal bureaucracies will be applicable and enforceable. But federal policies and regulations often do not coincide with traditional operating modes at state and local levels (Lowi 1969; Wildavsky and Pressman 1973; Williams 1980).

In similar fashion contracts spanning different service sectors are likely to activate divergent political and economic interests. In various welfare reform discussions, for example, federal offices in the (then) Department of Health, Education, and Welfare ultimately rejected the notion of contracting with the Department of Labor for day-care services because they feared it would make needs of children ancillary to job training and placement objectives (Jansson 1975).

Differences between political and economic interests of the two parties are also evident when agencies with different auspices engage in contracting. Although the desire to maintain profits does not necessarily interfere with contract performance, critics fear for-profit agencies will not meet contractual obligations in order to maximize their gains (*Los Angeles Times,* 14 December 1981; Titmuss 1971). Similarly, nonprofit agencies often develop cooperative relationships with public agencies, but are sometimes subject to pressures from their consumers, boards, and staff to provide services that differ from those of public agencies; poor contract performance may be the result when they are asked to provide programs that resemble public models.

The central function of contract monitoring is to develop preventive and postaward processes to increase the likelihood of successfully implementing specific contract provisions. Monitors have to gauge the extent that there are different political and economic interests between the two parties, understand what implications (if any) such divergencies have for contract implementation, and develop corrective strategies. Use of sanctions during the postaward period to secure compliance is, at best, a final recourse, but is hardly a substitute for preventive strategies at earlier points (Herman, in Wedel 1979).

Divergencies: The Case of Public and Nonpublic Agencies

Contract performance is likely to be problemmatic when contractors and contractees have divergent ideological, political, economic, and programmatic interests.

Program and Ideological Divergencies. Public agencies are more likely than not-for-profit agencies to serve consumers who come directly to the agency, live in geographic areas proximate to the agency, and represent minority or low-income groups (Jansson 1979). Public agencies are expected to serve consumers who approach them and who qualify for their services, whereas nonprofit agencies rely heavily upon referrals and appear better able to select consumers who fall within their service priorities. Public agencies are more likely than voluntary agencies to extend organizational resources by providing relatively nonintensive service to a relatively large number of consumers (Neugeboren 1970).

Programmatic differences between public and nonprofit agencies are partially understandable in light of their distinctive positions in the social service delivery system. Public agencies, for example, are charged with administration of public revenues; they must serve those who come for service, focus upon specific catchment or community areas to assure coverage, provide nonintensive services in order to stretch scarce resources to meet existing demands, and target resources to persons with the most pressing problems or to persons who cannot afford alternative services in the private sector (Kupers 1981). In this sense "public mission" is defined by and the result of requirements imposed by funding sources, program mandates, and community pressure.

Programmatic differences between public and voluntary agencies are relevant to the monitoring process because voluntary agencies may resist implementing contract provisions based on conformity to public models. They may lack familiarity with such models or find that they conflict with the ideological preferences of staff. Ideological opposition to specific decision-making, service, or operational approaches may not be readily apparent during the application process, but can impact upon contract implementation even when surface agreement exists.

Political Divergencies. Public executives report that internal planning often has relatively little impact on final decisions and are more likely than nonprofit agency executives to report the influence of external forces on shaping agency policy (Jansson 1979). Likewise, public and nonprofit agencies appear to utilize different sources of information to facilitate decision making. Public agencies are more likely to rely on data from program evaluation and formal planning projects and to allocate staff and budget resources to planning functions. Nonprofit agencies, by contrast, are more likely to make use of policymaking boards in the decision-making process because of legal incorporation requirements and the role of boards for legitimation and fund-raising purposes (Glaser and Sills 1966).

The divergent political environments of public and nonprofit agencies also have important implications for contracting. Executives of nonprofit agencies may resist being monitored because they may perceive it as an unnecessary limitation on their autonomy. Nonpublic agency staff who are not used to providing statistical reports to external bodies—something that public executives take for granted—may withhold required data from monitors. Finally, many nonpublic providers may not implement portions of contracts that require program evaluation, planning, or broadly-based citizen contributions to decision making.

Economic Divergencies. Some nonprofit agencies seek contracts because they want to remedy shortfalls in agency revenue. Although the economic needs of these agencies do not necessarily lead to poor contract performance, they can pose dangers (Porter and Warner 1973). An agency can divert contract revenues to cover overhead and other costs, or the intensity or nature of services given to consumers can be "skimmed" in order to reap "contract surpluses." A counseling agency with a fixed-price contract that is reimbursed for a designated number of clinical hours, for example, might hire lesser qualified staff to stimulate funding surpluses. Agencies may also use "creaming" strategies to select clients who do not require intensive services as do multiproblem families or individuals (*Los Angeles Times,* 5 December 1982). Finally, a contractee may selectively concentrate upon one or several contract requirements to the detriment of others. A health agency might receive a contract to combine provision of various health services with outreach programs, but a monitor may discover subsequently that outreach has been neglected.

Time Perspectives of Agency Officials. The time perspectives of executives need to be examined when gauging the extent to which they may use the various cited strategies. Executives who want ongoing contracts from a funder will generally seek to establish a reputation for fulfilling contract requirements, perhaps even exceeding them despite short-term cash flow problems. In this instance their long-term perspective leads them to resist economic expediency. Officials with short-term perspectives may underperform on contracts because they seek to maximize revenues. Underperformance is even more likely when short-term perspectives are combined with beliefs that it will not be detected, new sources of funds will be discovered so that they will not need to continue to rely on contract revenues, or possible sanctions from the public agency can be countered with political or legal resources.

Interactive Effects. Ideological, political, and economic factors often interact and impact upon the contractual relationship so that it is difficult to disentangle the effects of each (Wilson 1980; Williams 1980). The need to develop preventive monitoring strategies is particularly acute when many factors impede contract performance. The use of fixed-price contracting with agencies whose staff do not place heavy emphasis upon adherence to all contract requirements illustrates these interactive effects. Fixed-price contracts provide agencies with a specified amount of money to provide services and are distinguished from actual cost, incentive, performance, and other kinds of contracts. They are relatively easy to write and allow public officials to identify low bidders, those who can carry out the service at the least cost. The case of a nonprofit hospital that contracted, under fixed-price, to provide medical services to alcoholic patients demonstrates how a combination of economic and ideological factors can frustrate contract performance. Hospital staff took the position that the problems of chronic alcoholics fell beyond the purview of traditional health-care services. Alcoholics were perceived as expensive cases requiring multifaceted services, so staff and administrators referred difficult cases elsewhere. In this and similar cases, monitors need to analyze interactive effects as they might impede contract performance as a prelude to developing preventive contract and monitoring strategies.

CONTINGENCY STRATEGY IN MONITORING

Contract performance, then, hinges upon a variety of ideological, political, economic, and programmatic factors. The monitor wants to gauge the likelihood that specific contracts will be implemented by (1) any providers; (2) specific kinds of providers, such as for-profit, nonprofit, or other public agencies; and (3) specific providers. In the pre-award period, the objective is to develop preventive strategies that decrease potential implementation problems and provide disincentives for poor performance. In the postaward period, the monitor wants to develop data-gathering, inspection, interactional, and technical-assistance tactics that decrease the likelihood of poor contract performance.

Predicting contract performance can be difficult. Although past performance is one indicator of future behavior, contracts themselves can have an important catalytic effect on organizational change as reflected in Zald's (1970a) study of the YMCA, where major system changes occurred following receipt of juvenile delinquency funds. Monitors may also be overly optimistic and accept widely held but erroneous assumptions about specific organizations. Monitors might assume, for example, that the use of public funds by nonpublic agencies would enhance their responsiveness to serving low income groups, especially when compared to the record of nonprofits without such contractual relationships. However, contract agency staff may retain traditional programmatic preferences even when their agencies extensively use public funds.

Another difficulty in predicting contract performance stems from the sheer number of variables that influence the implementation process. Variables germane to preventive monitoring include those that describe:

The nature of the contract tasks or objectives, including their complexity, ambiguity, and scope

The content and form of contracts, including funding mechanisms and clarity

Characteristics of the contractor, including political and economic resources, technical expertise, prior experience with contracting, size, and mission

Monitoring staff, including staff size, position within the bureaucracy, linkages to top decision makers, and skills, orientations, and experience

Characteristics of contracted agencies, including their mission, size, prior experience with contracts, diversification of funding, decision-making patterns, community environment, organizational structure, and financial status

Motivation of contractees in seeking specific contracts, including economic, political, ideological, and other short- as well as long-term orientations

The nature of the contractor-contractee relationship, including the nature and frequency of communication, patterns of autonomy and dominance, use of (or threats of) sanction, and extent and nature of prior relationships

Contractee perceptions of the funding body, including level of trust, fear, and ignorance; and contractor perceptions of the contractee

The divergence between the two parties in mission and contract expectations

The preceding discussion suggests the need to estimate the potential liabilities associated with contracting with particular organizations by analyzing the extent to which specific factors could impede contract performance. Goal deflection costs occur when organizations use public funds in a manner that contradicts public intent regarding service approaches and priorities. Accountability costs can occur when contracted organizations do not use the required information sources. Coordination costs may occur when organizations are asked to participate in efforts to develop referral systems and joint programming, but fail to develop effective agency linkages. Monitoring costs rise when there is resistance to, or nonparticipation in, data gathering and evaluation processes. Consumer utilization costs are encountered to the extent that specific types of clients are excluded from services to which they are entitled by public mandate.

STRATEGY OPTIONS OF MONITORS

Analysis of variables that could imperil contract performance is a precursor to the development of a comprehensive monitoring strategy. As noted earlier, monitors assume a preventive role as they develop strategies in the pre-award phase and a troubleshooting role as they try to improve contract performance in the postaward period.

The Contract. Contract funding mechanisms should be tailored to the nature of the task. Innovative projects that are difficult to "cost out," for example, must often be funded on a cost-plus, rather than fixed-price basis, so that the contractee has the flexibility to develop the program without having to meet the cost standards of more traditional projects (Sammet 1981). In such cases monitors should expend more resources in program inspections to ensure that costs do not become excessive. Monitors also need to participate in decisions regarding the specificity of performance objectives (Waller et al. 1975). When awarding contracts to agencies with no prior experience in providing a service, for example, a public agency might want to be highly specific in stating performance criteria.

Solicitation and Award Strategies. Monitors should have significant roles in shaping decisions about the use of competitive, negotiated, and sole source methods of soliciting candidates for contracts (Cooper

351

1980). A competitive bidding process is useful when contracting relatively routine services that can be delivered by a range of potential providers. Inviting many bidders can, however, have serious shortcomings when the pool of possible providers with the requisite capabilities is small. When political pressures favor the selection of the lowest bidder and few agencies have the competencies to provide the particular service, a negotiated or sole source solicitation process might be preferable to competitive bidding.

Roles in Selection of Contractees. Even after preliminary screening of competitive applicants has been accomplished, monitors should participate in selecting the final contractee(s) (Cooper 1980). When monitors question the performance capability of an applicant, they should urge on-site visits for further assessment. In some cases on-site visits are also important to assess motives of top officials; with for-profit applicants, for example, public officials might look for indications of real or potential creaming, skimming, deletion, and other practices that might be used to enhance short-term revenue at the expense of delivering contracted services. The orientations of top officials are an important influence on how the contract is implemented and cannot always be deciphered in the formal application (Jansson 1980).

Participation by monitors in contractee selection is particularly important when there is concern that inadequate resources will be available for public agency monitoring. In such cases monitors might want to suggest that the public agency choose low-risk contractees, even if they are less efficient or potentially less innovative than others, because postaward monitoring is likely to be superficial.

Monitoring Resources. Monitors need to help top officials in public agencies decide what level of resources to accomplish monitoring functions are needed for specific contracts. Funds devoted to monitoring should be determined in the context of the number and kind of obstacles of contract implementation. When monitors believe that a range of factors inhibits contract performance, they should seek larger resources for monitoring.

Mix of Monitoring Functions. Monitoring budgets should cover some combination of (1) on-site or field functions, (2) information acquisition and processing functions, (3) investigatory functions for problematic contracts, (4) technical assistance functions, (5) community organization functions that include meeting with contractees, and (6) planning and research functions to enable monitors to assume central preventive roles in the preaward phase (Fiene 1981). Monitors need to decide the emphasis to be given to these various functions in specific contracts. In contracts for innovative projects, monitors may wish to stress technical assistance and on-site visits. When public agencies negotiate contracts for relatively standardized services, more attention may be given to data collection and investigatory functions. Public agencies sometimes let contracts to increase "system responsiveness" to some neglected population; in these cases they may wish to devote considerable resources to community organization functions, including meetings between technical assistance staff, providers, and community residents to build commitment and skills (Steinberg 1976b).

Targets of Monitoring. When few resources are allocated to monitoring, scarce resources need to be targeted to grantees who are (1) most in need of technical and other supports and (2) perceived to represent the greatest risks in implementing important contract objectives (Fiene and Nixon 1981). One strategy is to first identify providers who are probably in compliance, based upon their track records and information obtained from on-site visits. Officials in Pennsylvania and four other states developed a brief set of questions that were predictors of contract performance and used this information to divert monitoring resources to problematic providers (Fiene 1981). In many cases, however, public agencies may have no recourse but to spread their scarce monitoring resources to all or most contractees, particularly in the contract start-up phase when tendencies to ignore or downplay some contract provisions may emerge or when there is insufficient data to successfully predict performance.

Relative Emphasis Upon Process and Product. One school of thought suggests that contracts should define specific products or services that are to be provided, but monitors should give contractees relative autonomy in deciding how to achieve these outcomes (Young 1983). In this perspective monitors should not meddle in operations or programs but should focus upon monitoring products or services. A contract to provide health care services to minority groups, for example, might specify the

353

number of black and other persons to be given diagnostic or treatment services, but not specify details of how this will be accomplished.

Although product objectives are often needed, some believe that monitors in the social services often must examine the processes used to achieve objectives (Fiene 1981). In the case of a contracted program to provide health services to minority group members, for example, strategies used to target or draw clients into service could have important impacts on the final product outcomes. Providers could variously rely upon public service announcements, interagency referrals, and community outreach stations to reach neglected populations. The interagency model, however, may not identify those consumers in need of but not currently receiving health-care services.

Program processes should also be examined when program outcomes cannot easily be evaluated, i.e., where program evaluation techniques have limited use or are not feasible. In such cases (some would argue in most social programs), program and service processes must be used as a proxy for program effectiveness, albeit a crude and unsatisfactory one (Wholey et. al. 1970). Monitors often have to examine, for example, the extent to which health providers use established protocols when diagnosing and treating ailments, whether providers appear to adapt service technologies to the needs of specific populations such as the poor, and whether staff are given inservice training relevant to the services to be delivered.

In some cases monitors also need to assess the decision-making and planning processes of contractees. The contractor may want to make providers more responsive to specific populations by requiring that community advisory boards be developed. Or it may want providers to develop needs assessment or other planning projects. Here, monitors may want evidence that contractees are adhering to these decision-making approaches.

The extent to which process or products are emphasized in monitoring depends, as in other contingency decisions, upon the nature of the contracted tasks. In the case of tangible resources like "delivery of 10,000 meals to elderly recipients in their homes," monitors may wish to emphasize products. In other situations, as in the "provision of child development services that draw into service parents of children from disadvantaged families," considerable attention may be given to program

354

processes. Although program processes may be more difficult to monitor than products, they are crucial elements of many social services and should not be ignored because of the difficult task they pose.

When process does become a monitoring concern, the level of standards must be resolved. Some public agencies insist only upon minimum licensing standards (Fiene 1981). Fiscal realities pose difficult issues. If monitoring resources are minimal and contracts are of the fixed-price variety, it may be futile to devise relatively high standards, because they are unenforceable and may not be feasible (for contractees) to implement. It is also difficult to establish standards if no statutory basis exists, because providers may question their legality.

Tradeoffs During Implementation. When contracts specify a number of programmatic, efficiency, and other objectives, monitors need to decide when to relax, maintain, or increase expectations with respect to each. In many cases contractees cannot achieve all objectives simultaneously. A contract may specify the number of consumers to be served, but monitors may decide to relax this requirement during the initial period of implementation to facilitate program planing. Insistence that all contract provisions be accomplished can be dysfunctional. Standards affecting the health and safety of consumers must be in place from the outset, but others can initially receive less emphasis. In other cases monitors may decide that certain contract requirements need greater attention than originally contemplated, whether because they are being ignored or because they now appear to have more relevance to program outcomes. Monitors should always be closely linked to top officials in the public agency so that their decisions carry high-level sanction, particularly when modifications in contracts are contemplated.

Participatory Strategies. Meetings of contractees, monitors, and technical assistance staff can be a valuable resource for sharing information and pinpointing issues (Steinberg 1976b). Contractees may resent monitors who never consult them.

Monitors may decide to hold meetings with several contractees. In some circumstances, however, public officials may not want extensive communication between contractees as when, for example, the development of different approaches to fulfilling contract obligations rather than

355

standardization is desired. They also need to consider how to structure meetings to increase motivation and to address difficulties in contract implementation.

Data Collection Strategies. Monitors can emphasize on-site visits that result in narrative reports covering numerous aspects of project implementation (Waller et al. 1975). Such reports may be useful when contracts specify tasks that cannot be standardized and where specific performance objectives are absent. In other cases, as with the contracted day-care programs in Pennsylvania, instrument-based monitoring is used. This approach relies on the use of standardized and structured instruments during on-site visits and is predicated on the existence of numerous licensing, contract, and regulatory provisions that allow officials to develop checklists. Monitors also need to decide the extent to which they can rely on information supplied by contractees or whether they must obtain data firsthand. When contractees are not implementing important contract provisions, extensive on-site visits are indicated; in these cases monitors may want to insist that contractees supply considerable data—and at frequent intervals—to ensure accountability.

Structural Considerations. Some monitors believe that technical assistance and investigatory functions should be separated to decrease the perception that program suggestions are coercive (Williams 1980). In this perspective compliance-checking and technical assistance functions are incompatible.

Suppose, however, that a monitor is monitoring agencies in rural settings whether it may be economical and efficient to combine the two functions. The case for combining these functions also applies when contractees are close to full compliance and need only relatively brief technical assistance to attain full compliance, so that emphasis can then be placed on the program-enhancing aspects of monitoring. Monitors who possess technical knowledge of programs can also gauge with sensitivity if a contractee is making substantial progress in improving programs or if sanctions are needed to secure compliance.

Some commentators argue that licensing, sanitation, fire, contract, auditing, and other inspections should be consolidated in one department. This may be a sensible policy if and when it eases reporting burdens on contractees and prevents imposition of conflicting standards. In some cases, however, multiple inspections may have positive results. With for-profit nursing homes that have fixed-cost contracts, for example, it may be advantageous for several officials who have different perspectives to visit facilities in order to ensure that cost-saving practices detrimental to their residents are not occurring.

Alternative Models of Monitoring. A distinction is useful between technical, developmental, and advocacy models. In the technical model, monitors emphasize the development of relatively complex and sophisticated sources of information, including financial, administrative, and service statistics (Dunn 1981). In developmental models the monitor is perceived to be a facilitator who establishes collaborative relationships with contractees. The gradual development of the skills of grantees is stressed (Steinberg 1976b). In the advocacy model, monitors may start from the negative premise that contractees are impervious to specific needs of consumers and that ongoing surveillance is required. Accordingly, the use of sanctions and political strategies to secure compliance is emphasized (Townsend 1971). In some cases advocacy monitoring is conducted by persons who are outside the bureaucracy, as illustrated by a Florida social worker who sought to make the state bureaucracy responsive to the needs of the elderly (Bell and Bell 1981).

Research is needed to define alternative monitoring models with greater precision. Rather than using a single approach, monitors should select that combination of models that appears most useful with specific contracts. When contractees are committed to fulfilling contract objectives but require technical assistance in order to do so, a developmental model is useful. Technical models can be used when the contract calls for the provision of tangible and standardized services, or when public agencies have already developed specific programs that they want contractees to implement according to a predetermined plan. Advocacy models are appropriate when contractees may be impervious to important needs of consumers or motivated by short-term financial objectives to the detriment of adequate service delivery.

EMPOWERING MONITORS

In order to assume the preventive, troubleshooting, and strategy roles discussed in this chapter, monitors need to 1) possess ongoing linkages with top management; 2) have a major consultation role in devising pre-award strategy; 3) assume a variety of technical assistance, investigation, and liaison functions during the postaward period; and 4) assist top management with strategy concerning ongoing negotiations with contracted agencies. Their perspectives should also be called upon in the initial decision as to whether to engage in purchase of service arrangements, because contracting agencies usually have the option to provide services directly if political, economic and capability factors suggest that this is the most positive option in a specific instance.

To assume such pivotal roles in the contracting process, monitors need prominent status within the public agency and sophistication in organizational theory, consultation, negotiation, and law. A number of case studies suggest, unfortunately, that monitors often do not hold prominant positions within their agencies or possess the knowledge and skills necessary to aid in strategy development (*Los Angeles Times,* 5 December 1982; Waller et al. 1975; Williams 1980). Apart from case studies, empirical data are lacking about the required attributes of monitors, their ideal location within agencies, or their roles; this dearth of information itself reflects the lack of visibility of monitors.

The failure to define or operationalize a major role for monitors in many contracting agencies stems from a number of realities. First, monitoring has not received sufficient attention from theoreticians. Many program evaluators view monitoring as an uninteresting compliance-checking function that does not use sophisticated research techniques (Wholey et al. 1970). A case can be made that monitoring should receive as much attention as evaluation because it is an ongoing and necessary function in all service-delivering programs.

Monitoring also suffers from definitions that are too restrictive or too expansive. Restrictive definitions limit the monitoring role to postaward investigation of compliance (McLaughlin 1978). When defined in expansive terms, which includes program evaluation functions within its domain, monitoring loses a distinctive focus (Dunn 1981). A middle-range definition is needed that identifies the distinctive management and consultative functions of monitors but does not merge the role of monitors and evaluators. Unlike evaluators who seek to assess program impacts, monitors assume primarily administrative functions in planning and overseeing program implementation. Rather than serving as neutral experts and consultants, positions frequently assumed by evaluators, monitors are integral to the administrative process. Further, they need to be seen by contractees as facilitators, a perception difficult to achieve when it is believed that monitors also evaluate their programs. A good case can be made, then, that monitoring deserves and needs independence from program evaluation functions and roles.

It is not uncommon to simplistically ascribe to monitoring in social services many concepts that are drawn from defense contracting. To some auditors, accountants, and attorneys, for example, the development of well-constructed contracts obviates the need for extensive monitoring because, afterall, contracted parties receive "clear instructions" (Young 1982). Others believe that monitors are primarily auditors who use fiscal information to determine whether contract obligations are being met. In contracts for the manufacture of hardware such as machinery, a simplistic view of monitoring may be appropriate. However, the monitoring process is necessarily more complex in health, social, and rehabilitative services where it is often difficult to specify with precision either process or outcome. In many cases monitors and contracted parties engage in simultaneous learning about implementation issues and problems. Further, fiscal criteria rarely provide a reliable basis for analyzing contract performance and can, indeed, lead to goal displacement. Thus, a contractee may hold unit costs below a certain level, but fail to provide services to multiproblem families.

Finally, political pressures often mitigate against the development of monitoring processes. Officials with an antiregulatory ethos are likely to perceive monitors as unnecessarily restricting the autonomy of contractees (Stigler 1975). Trade and professional associations lobby legislators and governmental officials to restrict efforts to subject them to external pressures. During periods of budget cutbacks, a tendency exists to cut indirect services like monitoring that do not themselves involve distribution of resources or services to consumers.

Simple remedies to the residual status of the monitoring function do not exist. Articulation of an independent discipline of monitoring, however, would be a good beginning. If public agencies reduce the size of their own programs as they increasingly turn to the purchase of services, they will need a highly trained corps of monitors who can help them translate public objectives into operational, contracted programs. Indeed, use of contracting in absence of monitoring represents abdication of the public trust.

359

23

Monitoring Strategies in Purchase of Service Contracting

Kenneth R. Wedel and Nancy Chess

This chapter addresses a number of practical issues involved, in the monitoring of purchase of service contracts and examines the strategic elements involved. A series of questions form the subject headings for this discussion, beginning with consideration of the definition of monitoring.

WHAT IS MONITORING?

Monitoring consists of the review and documentation of service delivery activities that are intended to meet defined ends. A definition of monitoring for contracted services is provided by Kettner and Martin (1985, 71): "Monitoring is defined as the periodic review and documentation of the contractor's progress in fulfilling the stated terms and conditions of the contract, the identification of areas where corrective action is required, and follow-up to insure that corrective action is successfully taken." Included in the process of monitoring should also be the detection and reporting of successful activities that reflect positively upon the contracted services program.

Monitoring involves several components, including quality control. The task is to review the services being delivered at regular intervals to determine whether they meet the standards originally established. Both empirical and normative strategies are available; empirical quality standards are based on averages and ranges of practice considered to be acceptable, and normative quality standards are based on exemplary practices in the field (Wedel 1979). The relative success of these strategies will depend on the extent to which objectives and standards are clearly stated in the written contract from the beginning.

Monitoring also includes the systematic, periodic review of management systems and services to ensure compliance with contract requirements, laws, regulations, and agency policies. Monitoring can assist in the detection and, often, the prevention of problems. To be effective, the monitoring function must have the commitment and support of management and can be seen as a management tool.

It is in the best interest of both the funding agency and the contracted organization to fully recognize respective roles and responsibilities and ensure that systems and safeguards are in place for effective follow-through. It is in the review and oversight role, a component of the monitoring function, that the desire of contracted agencies to self-police and the demands of lawmakers and the general public for accountability, cost effectiveness, prudent management, and assurances of wise and honest expenditures of tax dollars can be balanced.

WHY MONITOR?

Funding agencies must, as need dictates, require corrective action by contracted agencies to improve performance and plan for more effective programs in subsequent operations. They have the responsibility to develop and use procedures so that the information collected and assessments made are fed into ongoing program planning and the selection of contract service providers. Program assessment data may be provided to administrators and governing or citizen boards to aid in their decision making and accountability reports. The monitoring effort therefore ensures accountable management through a continued compliance check in accord with appropriate guidelines.

The purpose of monitoring must be communicated to, and understood by, all involved parties. An effort should be made to dispell any fears associated with the monitoring process and instead interpreted as a facilitative device. If the monitoring process is seen only as a control mechanism, the contracted service provider is likely to react defensively and with resistance. The positive results that may accrue from this process are as important to communicate as the possible imposition of negative noncompliance sanctions.

Monitoring contracts is often specified by law, including the following:

Federal law and regulations. As an example, the Comprehensive Employment and Training Act (CETA) regulations specified that a monitoring unit be established as part of the prime sponsor's internal program management procedures. This unit was to be independent of and not accountable to any unit being monitored. CETA regulations specified that this monitoring unit would periodically monitor and review through on-site visits, program data, all program activities and services, and program management practices supported with funds under the act. Under Title XX regulations, states were required to monitor services, but given considerable latitude in how and by whom these services would be monitored.

State regulations and standards. State licensure laws often provide standards that must be maintained. Contracts that clearly identify objectives provide measurable guidelines for the monitoring process. State funding agencies usually provide policy and procedural manuals for the administration and provision of services. The manual provides a resource identifying standards and policies to be reviewed in the monitoring process. Finally, contracted service providers can be expected to document supporting evidence of compliance with their own policies and regulations.

WHAT SHOULD A MONITORING SYSTEM ACCOMPLISH?

A monitoring system is designed to track activities and indicate areas in which assistance is necessary to ensure that contracted services are properly managed and implemented. The on-going monitoring of activities accomplishes the following purposes:

1. Ensures that reports (both operational and fiscal) are accurate
2. Forecasts program and fiscal trends
3. Ensures contract compliance
4. Identifies management and programmatic areas where corrective action is needed
5. Identifies corrective action steps, in a realistic time frame, to effectively address and overcome identified problems

The monitoring function is best implemented in accord with a set of objectives outlining its purposes and scope of activity. A suggested list of such objectives might include the following:

1. To ensure that federal, state, and local regulations are being met

362

2. To ensure that licensing standards (where applicable) are being met
3. To ensure that providers meet eligibility requirements to provide services in accord with policies and regulations
4. To ensure that clients are eligible to receive services
5. To ensure that clients' needs and service goals are congruent with service plans
6. To ensure that services for which reimbursement is claimed have been authorized and have been delivered
7. To ensure that the quantity and quality of services meet established standards to enhance clients' functioning
8. To ensure that accountability for expenditures is maintained
9. To ensure that the provider is in compliance with all contract terms, including the type and amount of services provided at an approved cost to eligible clients

WHAT IS TO BE MONITORED?

Program/professional performance. A central concern in contract implementation is the extent to which specified services are provided to identifiable clients. Direct observation is one method to monitor services. Attention is given to service goals and objectives, as well as applicable regulations and standards. The monitor reviews (a) supervision, (b) client/participant involvement, (c) physical plant (equipment, building locations), and (d) terms of the contract (compliance).

Administrative/management capability. This monitoring aspect includes a review of overall agency operations with specific attention to personnel policies and procedures in place and degree of compliance with stated standards, including the agency's affirmative action plan and grievance procedures. Determination of the contract service provider's compliance with acceptable personnel practices includes exploration of such questions as, does the agency ensure equal opportunity based on objective personnel policies and practices for recruitment, selection, promotion, classification, compensation, performance evaluation, and employee-management relations? Are these evaluations current? Are merit raises based upon these performance evaluations?

Recording systems. Data concerning services requested, services provided, and follow-up must be readily available to the monitor. Accurate program reports should be current, and all reporting requirements should be met by the agency.

Training and professional development. Both training and professional development should be addressed in the monitoring process. Consideration should be given to the decisions made about the allocation of training resources in relation to demonstrated training needs of staff.

Fiscal responsibility. Proper fiscal management is a necessity. Funding agencies are authorized to legally commit funds for expenditures within contract limitations. These obligations involve the legal reservation of funds, supported by documentation, to cover payment for goods or services rendered. Direct cost items (e.g., staff, payroll, telephone, rent, printing) are also legitimate expenditures in most contracts.

Funding agencies, contract service providers, and subcontractors are responsible for internal controls to safeguard cash and properties purchased with contract funds. Is there a check for accuracy and reliability of accounting data? Are budgets provided? The system needs to provide fiscal controls that include accounting procedures to track receipts and expenditures in accord with contract budget categories. Financial reports must be current and accurate and an audit provided annually. The agency should give evidence that it is operating efficiently. Fiscal procedures need to be on file, and the system should provide controls for the prevention of illegal or unauthorized transactions. Goods and services paid for require receipts. The fiscal operation must supply sufficient, competent, and relevant evidence for an auditor to reach a judgment.

WHO WILL DO THE MONITORING?

The monitoring function may be spelled out in the agency's operating procedures, but not all service funding agencies provide explicit guidelines. Public agency personnel may conduct the monitoring. In some cases funding agencies and contract service providers may adopt a team approach. In other instances monitoring is contracted out to a third disinterested party.

HOW IS THE PROGRAM TO BE MONITORED?

The monitoring flow chart in figure 23.1 illustrates the "how" of monitoring a program. Funding agency regulations may or may not pre-

Figure 23.1. **Monitoring Flow Chart**

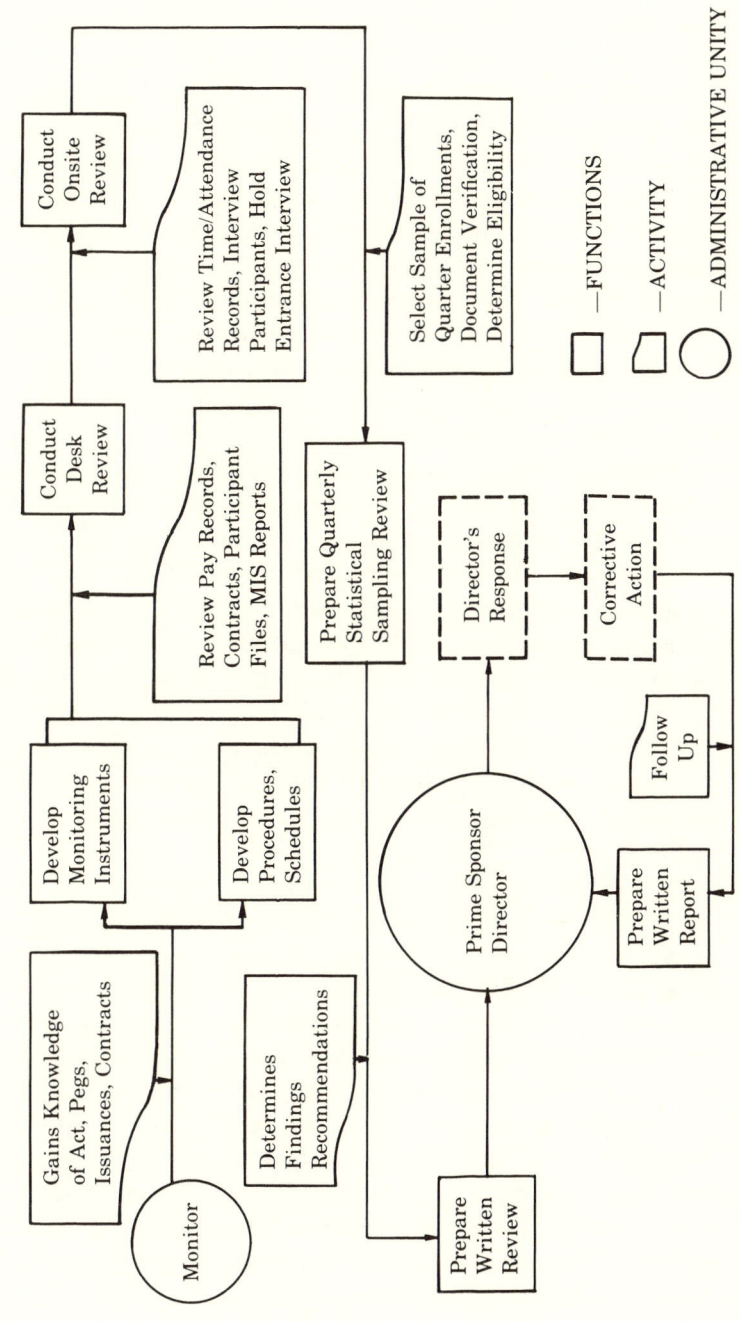

□ —FUNCTIONS

⬠ —ACTIVITY

○ —ADMINISTRATIVE UNITY

scribe a preferred way to monitor. In actuality, it is difficult to prescribe one best way for all consequences. In developing a rational approach, there should be room for variation.

Documented data provided by the monitor form the bases for professional judgments. The data gathering might include review of quarterly and annual reports, on-site observation of the physical plant and actual service delivery, and review of client records. Regardless of how the monitoring is conducted, it is important that all parties understand the procedures to be followed. In order to facilitate cooperation, an initial meeting should take place with the key actors to explan the monitoring process. Confidentiality is a very important aspect of this process.

Techniques and Approaches

Numerous techniques and approaches are available for the monitoring process. Instruments, in the form of checklists, are most useful in site visits. In-depth interviews with management, workers, and clients as well as review of eligibility documentation may also be used. Other source documents to be reviewed are attendance records, expenditure reports, and tracking procedures. When the program being monitored has a management information system (MIS) in place, the availability of data is probably increased. For many contracted service providers, however, data collection will depend on resourceful monitoring practices.

Constructed measures (survey instruments) can be developed for use in organizing, conducting, and reporting all monitoring activities. A necessary prerequisite for the monitor is a working knowledge of the laws and regulations, contracts, plans, policies, and procedures of the funding agency and contracted service provider. References, such as specific regulations, should accompany each survey question as a means to conserve time and provide clarification during the actual monitoring process. A checklist can be especially helpful for compliance survey instruments. On the survey instrument, a yes answer represents compliance, a no answer represents noncompliance, and an N.A. represents nonapplicable. To utilize this checklist, working papers are organized to identify specifically and succinctly the findings to support the noncompliance results. The working paper also contains recommendations for corrective action. Other materials can be referenced on the working paper and attached as on appendix. Often, these other documents are retained in the monitor's files as support documentation for each report.

When testing instruments are used with clients, pre- and posttest results can be incorporated within the written report. Performance, retention, and recidivism rates may also be included in the report. The survey instruments constructed for client feedback usually involve personal interviews. However, client satisfaction in itself should not be regarded as a sufficient measure of progress unless client satisfaction is the goal of the service. If not, then client satisfaction data alone may be a questionable indicator of results. Client satisfaction measures, however, can be helpful as a means to locate trouble spots, obtain practical suggestions about how services can be improved, and as a check against the data collected from other sources (Reid and Smith 1978).

Data Collection

An effective MIS can be utilized to provide information to help determine whether the program is in compliance with regulatory provisions. When monitoring agencies have a sophisticated MIS availability, data collection includes some special considerations.

The data collection activity includes such questions as:

Are the documents that make up the participant record arranged for convenient use by administrative and operations staff?

Are all required eligibility items included on the participant forms?

Are all items required for reporting included on the forms?

Is there an established schedule and system for forms transmittal?

Is there a system in place for eligibility review, verification, and application update?

Are reports prepared properly, accurately, and in a timely manner?

Is there a system in place for tracking the progress of participants (clients) through the program?

Does the MIS provide summaries and reports that can be used to determine whether the program is in compliance with regulatory provisions related to levels of service?

Financial Information

Standards for a sound fiscal information system have been specified by the U.S. Office of Management and Budget (OMB) in Circular A-102. Financial records enable evaluation of the effectiveness of the program; provide information for auditing according to generally accepted accounting principles; and help the agencies to fulfill all financial reporting requirements on a timely, accurate, and accrued expenditure basis.

Financial management monitoring includes the examination of fiscal record-keeping systems to determine whether the required elements of those systems are in place. Reviewing fiscal documents to determine the accuracy of records may be very time-consuming, however, and a sampling approach should provide the information needed. The following questions are related to the financial management systems:

1. Are the financial reports directly traceable through the fiscal records to the source document?
2. Are costs being properly accrued?
3. Are the records accounting properly for all program income spent?
4. Are the records properly accounting for property?
5. Have adequate levels of internal control been established to safeguard assets?

Quantitative Data Review

Quantitative data review is the analysis of individual or aggregate numerical data to determine the degree to which the program is achieving previously established goals and objectives and is in compliance with regulations. Much of these data can be obtained from program or fiscal records. The purpose of the quantitative data review is to identify on a regular basis the status of the program. Specifically, this review is designed to

1. Identify potential or existing problems as well as accomplishments,
2. Indicate necessary corrective action, and
3. Identify and prioritize areas for further questioning during on-site review.

The monitoring approach will likely utilize both desk and on-site review techniques. The monitor reviews the organizational structure, relationships between units within the organization, outputs and flow of information, and provisions for training and technical assistance. Source documents include the plan of operation, procedure manuals and documents, interoffice and other correspondence, organizational charts, job descriptions, and other documents related to each administrative system.

WHEN SHOULD MONITORING TAKE PLACE?

A contract may specifically outline when monitoring is to be scheduled. Again, regulations may specify special emphasis areas for monitoring and plans for frequency. Federal personnel often provide spot-check monitoring of agencies. Regularly scheduled monitoring provides required data, but occasional spot checks often uncover serious problems. Continuous on-site monitoring reports, spot-check visits, information and data generated from records and reports all document the delivery of services. Special requests may be made by federal or state bodies as well as political personnel for monitoring data, leading to more involved and in-depth information discovery processes.

An important issue to consider is the amount of time available for monitoring. Ongoing comprehensive monitoring processes may be very effective. However, for agencies with large numbers of clients, periodic checking may prove to be economical with little sacrifice in accuracy. An important consideration is the fact that monitoring can be very expensive. How long will the process take? How often will it be done? The monitors' handbook should spell out the procedures. There will be exceptions to several practices when administration requests more in-depth findings, such as when contracts are being renegotiated or when the plan of operation is being modified.

HOW IS THE REPORT WRITTEN?

In preparing monitoring reports, the associated activities include analysis of data collected; identification and documentation of findings, including descriptive information about problem areas and accomplishments; and development of recommendations, for corrective action.

The reexamination of programs and activities with previously noticed deficiencies is a necessary and important follow-up activity. Identifying specific names and pointing fingers at individuals should be avoided. The contract service provider is ultimately responsible for corrective action. The use of inflammatory words and/or coined phrases, such as "totally unacceptable, paper shuffling," should also be avoided. List the most significant problems where the greatest improvement is possible. Present findings in order of importance—ignore minor or infrequent problems that require no significant correction. Don't nitpick; if problems have

369

already been corrected, say so. Describe the nature of the monitoring review in general, the purpose, and the results. Don't rely on verbal communications and commitments. Document findings and recommendations.

What is defective or deficient? Are the problems isolated or widespread? State the cause (the underlying reason why the condition occurred) and the reasons for the condition. What criteria (measuring standards) or standards of performance are being used, e.g., laws, regulations, experience, contracts? Finally, describe the corrective action to be taken, giving the contract service provider latitude to adopt or pursue alternatives. In addition to matters of non- or partial compliance, such reports might identify commendable or exemplary activities or services that the monitor considers worthy of special note.

Contracted service providers should review all monitoring reports submitted by the monitor, acknowledge receipt of reports, and make required responses within the designated time frame. When the contracted providers utilize monitoring reports as input for program planning, the basic goals of monitoring have been fulfilled. In summary, the development of written monitoring reports will enable providers not only to improve the overall quality of services, but also to document program operations and answer inquiries from outside parties.

FROM MONITORING TO IMPACT EVALUATION

Although monitoring is a process to facilitate constructive outcomes, impact evaluation can be used to determine whether the benefits achieved outweigh the costs involved. States, in cooperation with local jurisdictions, are increasingly faced with pressures to justify services rendered. Accountability for the overall performance of social services funded through public allocations will continue to be a topic of considerable interest to taxpayers, public officials, and politicians. Policies and programs will be examined to ascertain their impact upon individuals and families. Which programs maintain and increase the capacity of individuals and family to perform the basic social functions—socialization, social protection, social control and provision of basic necessities? We hope priorities will be given to initiating and expanding programs that are most effective in preventing impairments and strengthening individual and family life. Monitoring purchased services should assist in determining these priorities.

370

24

Evaluating Contracted Health and Human Services: Public Policy Perspectives

Mark Schlesinger and Robert A. Dorwart

The past 20 years have seen a massive expansion of publicly funded but privately provided services. Health-care spending under medicare and medicaid is approaching $100 billion annually. State contracting for mental health and social services has been estimated to be of roughly equal magnitude (Schlesinger, Dorwart, and Pulice, forthcoming). These programs were enacted in the 1960s and early 1970s, a period in which the principal concern of policymakers was to encourage access to care (Davis and Schoen 1978; Demone and Schulberg 1984). As a result of significant and unexpected increases in program costs, however, both legislators and the general public have increasingly sought assurance that this money is being well spent.[1]

In theory, formal evaluation of the efficacy and efficiency of government-purchased services can provide such assurances. In practice, requiring broad-scale assessments can have serious liabilities. Careful program evaluation is expensive (Tatara and Pettiford, this volume) the more complex the program, the more complicated—and therefore costly—the evaluation. In an era of limited government budgets, it is fiscally infeasible to evaluate all ongoing programs. To require that public agencies purchase only those services that have been proven effective, then, may overly limit the discretion of the purchasing agencies and tend to exclude from funding the most complicated interventions. In addition, for many services, such as mental health or hospice care, it is difficult or impossible to accurately place a value on benefits. To require that the government purchase only those services with "proven" benefits would favor those services with readily measured benefits, to the detriment of those with equally valuable, but harder to measure, outcomes (Sharfstein, Muszynski, and Myers 1984).

Given these limitations, policymakers are faced with a set of difficult questions: To what extent must government formally evaluate the services it purchases in order to be a reasonable prudent buyer?[2] To what extent can government rely on alternatives to evaluation that might promote equally well the same societal goals? This chapter is intended to provide some insights into these questions. We begin by considering more carefully the goals of program evaluation in the context of purchase of service (POS) contracting. In the subsequent section, the strengths and limitations of evaluation in the context of contracting programs for health and human services are reviewed in more detail. Direct evaluation of program effectiveness is then compared with other strategies for ensuring that purchased services are efficiently and efficaciously delivered. These include systems that encourage competition or limit contracts to particular types of providers. It is our contention that each of these strategies has advantages and disadvantages and that POS systems will function best if methods of assuring quality and efficiency are matched to the characteristics of the services that are purchased. The chapter concludes with a brief discussion of directions for future research and public policy.

THE GOALS OF PROGRAM EVALUATION UNDER POS

The political pressures that have prompted more efforts to evaluate contracted services typically take the form of fairly simple questions: Are the services being provided effective? Are such services being provided in the least costly manner possible? Responding to these pressures, formal program assessments in health and human services have focused on two areas: measures of client outcomes and benefit-cost analyses.

Client outcomes and benefit-cost analyses are important criteria for measuring program performance. They do not, however, capture all the important aspects of program effectiveness. Most contemporary program assessments, whether of publicly provided or contracted services, focus solely on outcomes at a particular time. They rarely include more dynamic aspects of performance: the propensity to innovate, the ability of the program to adapt to changing conditions or its responseness to the concerns of various outside groups, including public officials or private interest groups. For example, a review of self-evaluation and quality assurance programs in community mental health centers found that only 4 percent of the evaluations incorporated citizen input, even though such input was required by law (Landsberg et al. 1978). These dynamic considerations, which have been variously labeled "accountability," "responsiveness," "public control," and "fiduciary responsibility," are important to meeting a number of socially desired goals (Dinkel, Zinober, and Flaherty 1981; Chelimsky 1981).

> Translated into question form, the public choice question is as follows: Does the delivery system provide the public with flexibility to modify its choices or are future choices set by "fixed or sunk" costs? . . . Public control is the ability of the public to control the utilization of program resources for the purposes intended by the public in making the resources available . . . the concept of public control does provide a focus on the conceptual features of a rational system. (Wedel and Harcastle 1978, pp. 181–182)

A second shortcoming in the goals of contemporary evaluations has been the failure to assess programs within the context of the larger political systems in which they operate. This is a particularly serious limitation in the assessment of contracted services. POS systems typically operate within a particularly politicized environment. The development of contracting leads to the growth of private provider groups that have become a major political force in many states. The use of contracting is favored by many for ideological as well as practical reasons (Savas 1981). Political and ideological considerations constrain what is practical within a POS system. Consequently, it is important to consider both how particular contracted services and the process of evaluation in itself fit into these constraints (Meyers 1981).

The next section reviews the strengths and weaknesses of client outcome studies and benefit-cost analyses, virtually the only methods now used for the assessment of either contract or noncontract services. This review focuses on their ability to accurately assess the efficacy and efficiency of contracted services. Subsequent consideration is given to the effectiveness of program assessment from a larger system-based perspective, examining, as well, alternative ways of structuring POS arrangements that might serve as substitutes for expanding formal program evaluation.

It has become common practice to deplore the limited ability of administrators of publicly financed programs to assess the effectiveness of the services they purchase (Meyers 1981; Savas 1981). Across-the-board requirements for program evaluation are typically advocated as a remedy (Chelimsky 1981; Frankfather 1981). Although these concerns are understandable and the recommendations well-intended, requiring formal evaluations as a prerequisite for purchasing serves may have in-advertent and perhaps undesirable consequences. To see why, it is useful to review the strengths and weaknesses of contemporary methods of evaluation and to consider how these methods might be incorporated into a contracting system for health and human services.

Assessing Methods of Program Evaluation

Assessments of Client Outcomes. In the past decade, there has been an impressive growth in the range and sophistication of methods to assess client outcomes in health and human services (Donabedian 1980). These have focused on four types of outcomes (Binner 1980; Schainblatt and Hatry 1979):

Client distress, including symptoms and use of services
Social functioning, including interactions with others, ability to work, and capacity to perform various activities of daily living
Client satisfaction, including perceived outcomes of services and assess-ments of the accessibility and convenience of treatment
Family and social burden, including perceived stress on the part of family members or other care givers, demands on the time of family members, and monetary costs of formal and informal care

The refinement of these concepts and the development of scales on which to measure these outcomes have vastly increased our ability to measure program performance. However, this experience has also made clear a number of limitations with the methods of assessment now in use.

First, because the assessment of human services inevitably requires some subjective measures, biased responses from those judging may seri-ously distort evaluations. On one hand, providers of services are an im-

374

portant source of information about program effectiveness. For example, the best-informed respondent to assess certain aspects of mental health care is the client's therapist. Therapists' assessments of client well-being, however, are shaped by the ongoing relationship with their client, their professional training, and their desire to have their clients grow healthier and the program overall succeed (Endicott and Spitzer 1976; Schainblatt and Hatry 1979; Frankfather 1981; Windle and Sharfstein 1981).

On the other hand, outcome assessments must incorporate, at least to some extent, the judgments of the clients themselves. "Quality" for many human services is idiosyncratic: methods of care preferred by some clients may be disliked by others with apparently identical health and social needs. For example, nursing homes favored by some residents as homelike and family-oriented may be seen by others as intruding on their privacy.

The reliability of clients' judgments, however, depends both on the clients' competence to assess services and their knowledge of available alternatives. All too often, clients of health and human service programs lack the information or ability to make adequate comparative assessments. As a result, their assessments of the services they receive are often positively biased. The clients of publicly financed services—typically the poor and minorities—are generally the least informed and therefore the most likely to give biased responses.[3]

In addition, client outcome studies tend to place greater emphasis on the outcomes experienced directly by the client as opposed to those borne by the family, the extended care network, or society as a whole. This is due in part to the greater availability of measures of client well-being, as well as the greater difficulty in identifying those who bear the social costs and measuring the intensity of their concerns (Schainblatt and Hatry 1979).

Positive biases in provider and client responses create an overly favorable image of many evaluated programs, reducing the effectiveness of formal evaluation as a method of screening out ineffective services. In addition, because outcome studies systematically understate certain costs and benefits (e.g., those widely diffused throughout the community), they favor types of services that have benefits concentrated on clients and costs that are diffused (American Psychiatric Association, Commission on Psychotherapies 1982; Glass, McGaw, and Smith 1981). Similarly, client assessments will be favorably biased toward those services about which clients are least well-informed and thus least able to make reliable comparisons with alternative types of care.

Benefit-Cost Analysis. Benefit-cost analysis was initially developed in the 1930s as a method of evaluating water resource projects conducted by the U.S. Army Corps of Engineers. It is based on two principles: that the appropriate standard for program assessment is a comparison of the aggregate societal costs and benefits produced by the program and that these costs and benefits can be measured and evaluated in terms of a single scale, typically monetary. As the cost of public programs has become a greater concern of policymakers, benefit-cost analysis has increasingly been used in program evaluation. During the 1970s, for example, the number of benefit-cost studies of health care programs grew exponentially (Office of Technology Assessment 1980a).

The increased use and refinement of benefit-cost analyses has improved assessments of program performance in several ways. First, it has highlighted the importance of the indirect costs and benefits created by programs, apart from the direct costs and benefits to the clients (Weisbrod 1983). Second, it has increased awareness of the advantage that may accrue from directing programs to particular target populations for which they are most effective. Studies of hypertension control programs, for instance, have been shown to be as much as ten times more cost effective for some age groups than others (Weinstein and Stason 1976). Finally, it has highlighted the difficulties of comparing the benefits felt by different groups of clients, particularly if some are very old or very young (Avorn 1984).

There are, however, a number of important limitations to benefit-cost methods. These limitations confound the assessment of any program, but are particularly pronounced for health and social services. The shortcomings fall into three broad categories.

First, the complexity of programs may hamper accurate assessments. Virtually any health or human service program involves a complex set of interventions designed to achieve a variety of goals. Day-care programs, for instance, have been designed to socialize and educate children as well as promote their parents' ability to seek employment. Benefit-cost analyses, however, are designed to assess programs within a single, aggregrate measure of performance. This can lead to a number of problems. By combining multiple outcomes within a single measure, a particularly strong

376

or weak performance in one dimension may obscure positive or negative results in a number of other dimensions.

Similarly, aggregate assessments hide the links between particular aspects of the program and favorable or unfavorable outcomes. For example, programs for deinstitutionalizing the chronically mentally ill may prove successful only if they include the provision of housing services. Unfortunately, to determine which aspects of a complicated program are important to its success, it is necessary to evaluate literally dozens of different permutations of the program, each combining a particular subset of the interventions that are a part of the overall program. Rarely, if ever, do the resources exist for such a complex evaluatory scheme. As a result, few past evaluations of health and human service programs have provided much insight into why particular programs have been successful (Office of Technology Assessment 1980a; Weisbrod and Schlesinger 1981).

Second, program benefits may often be difficult to identify. For many health and social services, there is a lack of consensus among providers about the appropriate methods of caring for clients or even assessing their well-being (Hirschman 1974). Is, for instance, education a necessary component of a high-quality day-care program? What types of outcomes—physiological, psychological or social—are indexes of improvement in the mentally ill? Where little professional consensus exists, evaluators may unintentionally omit whole dimensions of performance that may be important parts of a program's success. The less established a particular area of service delivery or the more innovative a specific service, the less professional consensus is likely to exist. Evaluating such programs will thus likely incorporate a negative bias in measuring outcomes.

Third, even if identified, many of the benefits of program may be difficult to measure.[4] The anticipated benefits of health and human services often involve broad social goals. Education is seen as a means to encourage increased and improved citizen participation, programs for the mentally impaired as a way to provide for the needs of those unable to care for themselves (Frank 1981). Although important, these types of benefits are generally difficult to assess. Many cost-benefit studies will simply omit them, distorting the assessment of the program. Even more sophisticated evaluations, however, will almost inevitably contain a bias toward those dimensions of benefits that are readily measurable. As Fein has noted:

377

"The numbers gain currency . . . a 'climate of opinion' is created: that which is measured is important and vice versa" (Fein 1977).

As with client assessments, these biases of cost-benefit evaluations will lead to more favorable findings for particular types of programs. Innovative programs will likely fare less well than the more standardized, because many of the potential benefits of the former may as yet be unrecognized. Programs that benefit a narrow population and have limited goals will generally appear preferrable to those with diffuse, and therefore hard to measure, benefits. Programs providing services that are sold in private markets will typically be ranked above those with unmarketed benefits, since the former outcomes are more readily assessed in monetary terms.

Program Responsiveness and Accountability. Although the responsiveness of service providers to changing social needs is increasingly seen as an important criterion for selecting a contractor, it is rarely, if ever, incorporated into formal program assessments. This is due in part to the absence of generally accepted norms of "responsiveness." Although there is general agreement that programs that are more responsive to the public interest are preferred to those that are less responsive, both the definition of responsiveness and the determination of the parties that represent the "public" are matters of considerable debate (Wedel and Hardcastle 1978). Although researchers have developed some structural measures thought to be related to the extent of program accountability, there has been little research to date actually linking these measures to subsequent performance.[5] Even if measures could be constructed and validated, assessing these dynamic aspects of program performance requires studying programs over extended periods of time. Limited resources for evaluation and short time-horizons of policymakers limit the use of long-term studies. As a result of these limitations, existing methods of program evaluation understate the social benefits derived from programs that are more responsive to public concerns and overstate the value of programs that have limited public accountability.

Incorporating Evaluation into a Contracting System

In addition to these technical limitations, integrating the evaluation process into a ongoing system of contracting may also limit its use and effectiveness. Applying evaluation methods within a POS system can potentially generate opposition from three sources: the individual providers of service, the set of all provider agencies acting as an interest group, and the administrators of the contracting system.

Any evaluation of a service delivery program will meet with some resistance from providers (Heller, Price, and Sher 1980; Cowen 1978). Evaluation is necessarily intrusive, and the protocols required for an effective evaluation may conflict with the priorities of those delivering services (Binner 1980; Schulberg 1976; Weiss 1976). The evaluation of contracted services may also be seen as threatening to service providers collectively (Meyers 1981; Heller 1980; Weiss 1976). Contracting was specifically intended to limit the public sector's role in favor of greater use of private agencies (Dorwart, Schlesinger, and Pulice, forthcoming). As a result, it created a powerful new interest group that has become adept at lobbying for political support (Schlesinger, Dorwart, and Pulice, forthcoming). Political pressure will thus likely be generated to limit the use of evaluation, particularly when provider agencies have organized collective political representation.

Evaluations may also be opposed by those who administer the contracting system. First, these officials have been charged with operating a system that is based on a number of conflicting goals: reducing costs while increasing quality, increasing competition while fostering continuity of care, promoting private innovation while enhancing public accountability (Schlesinger, Dorwart, and Pulice, forthcoming). As long as these conflicts remain implicit, they do not seriously threaten system maintenance. Evaluations, however, may highlight the conflicts and thus threaten the rationale for continued contracting.

For example, if the services offered by some providers are found to be ineffective, the contract officer is under strong pressure to switch to another provider. In many areas, however, there may be no readily available alternative, so that the administrator is faced with the choice between promoting an evidently ineffective service or discouraging access to any care at all (Horn and Griesel 1977). To avoid this overt conflict, officials responsible for contracting may prefer to conduct no evaluations at all.[6]

Second, requiring that services be formally evaluated may place the burden of assessment on the public sector, putting government explicitly in the role of assuring standards of quality and making government officials politically liable for failures in the POS system. Part of the rationale behind POS rests on the perception that professionals, operating outside the constraints of bureaucracy, are better able than government officials to ensure that services are of acceptable quality (Fisk, Kiesling, and Mueller 1978; Wedel 1974). Under such contracting arrangements, if services are found to be of inadequate quality, officials can point to a failure of professional standards. If, however, the responsibility for quality assurance is placed in the hands of the public agency overseeing the contracting process, inadequate quality becomes a political liability for them (Meyers 1981). Under many circumstances, officials may consider themselves better off without this responsibility and thus not encourage the use of evaluations.

Opposition to the use of evaluations is likely to come from providers who are collectively organized and for whom problems would be created if ineffective services were to be revealed. Consequently, in practice evaluations will be discouraged to a greater extent for some services, particularly those with less tangible outcomes. Subjecting some services to evaluations and not others may be unfair to clients. It may also distort the budget allocation process, causing administrators and legislators to shift funds away from those services that might be revealed as ineffective.

Finally, incorporating evaluations within a contracting system may also alter the ways in which they are conducted. Contracts represent legal commitments between government purchasers and private agencies. The cancellation of contracts on the basis of evaluation data could lead to challenges in the courts. As noted above, many of the most important aspects of assessing health and human services entail subjective judgments. These judgments are vulnerable to legal challenge, because they may be viewed by the courts as sufficiently arbitrary to violate due process protections.

Similar legal contraints have shaped the regulation of health and social service agencies by government. As a result, most past attempts to incorporate outcome measures into the regulation of services have been biased toward the most readily quantifiable, least subjective aspects of service delivery. Regulation of day-care facilities, for instance, has been largely limited to the "physical care and safety" of children, typically involving inspections of the physical plant of the facility (Steinfels 1973, 127). A review of nursing home regulations in the state of New York concluded that of the five hundred items assessed by inspectors, a disproportionate number were based on the physical plant and only thirty had any direct relationship to the care of patients (Moreland Act Commission 1976, 5). In a similar way, ongoing evaluations are likely to gravitate toward the most "objectively" measured dimensions and will thus undervalue programs whose benefits are concentrated in other areas.

ALTERNATIVE MODELS OF GOAL-PROMOTING SYSTEMS

The increased use of more sophisticated methods of program evaluation over the past decade has improved our ability to measure the costs and benefits of health and social programs and to better identify the outcomes that are important but difficult to measure. Nevertheless, the evident limitations of existing evaluation techniques have led many policymakers to conclude that it is unwise to require formal evaluations as a prerequisite for purchasing services. Fewer than half of all human service agencies have regular programs of evaluation (Tatara and Pettiford, this volume); only a small number of states use outcomes as a determinant in allocating mental health care dollars (Schainblatt and Hatry 1979). Even where evaluations are required by law, as under the Community Mental Health Act of 1963, they have had at most a marginal impact on the service delivery system. "A view of the past history of community mental health services makes clear that program evaluation has played only a minor role in the major modifications in services" (Windle and Sharfstein 1981, 514).

Given these limitations, it is natural for policymakers to seek alternatives to formal evaluation that might encourage the providers of contract services to achieve socially desired goals.[7] Three major strategies have been proposed to this end:

Client-based competitive strategies rely on competition among contract providers to encourage more efficient and higher-quality services, with the selection of providers made by the clients being served.

Competitive bidding strategies also use competition to promote social goals, but employ a public agency to choose among potential providers.

Provider screening strategies involve restrictions on the types of agencies that are eligible for contracts, with the intent of limiting

381

> providers to those whose objectives are compatible with broader social goals.

Each of these approaches relies on different actors to encourage behavior that is in the public interest. In competitive models improvements in services are initiated by providers seeking to gain an edge on their competitors and are validated by purchasers choosing among competing agencies. Screening models are designed not so much to change provider behavior as to limit contracting to these providers who are predisposed to act in the public interest, that is, consistent with socially defined goals. Each of these approaches has a number of strengths and weaknesses relative to the methods of program evaluation that were analyzed in the last section.

Client-Based Competitive Strategies. Two approaches have been used to provide clients with choices among publicly financed services. The first is based on an insurance model: government agrees to reimburse providers for the delivery of covered services to eligible populations. To provide eligible persons with an incentive to seek low-cost providers, they are typically required to bear a share of costs through copayments. This approach has been used most extensively to purchase health care; until recently, Medicare and Medicaid paid for all services in this way.

Alternatively, each eligible individual can be provided with a prepaid pool of funds, or voucher. Vouchers are paid to providers in return for the promise to deliver services over a period of time. Because the dollar value of the voucher is set in advance of the delivery of services, unlike the insurance model, vouchers limit government liability for the total cost of the program. As a result, voucher systems are, in this era of limited government budgets, becoming the perferred model for client-based competitive systems.[8] To date, vouchers have been used primarily for food stamps and a handful of demonstration projects (Bendick 1984) but are increasingly advocated for a variety of health and social service programs (Brilliant 1973; Savas 1982; Luft 1984).

Voucher-based competition is believed to promote socially desired outcomes in a number of ways. Theoretically, clients are encouraged to seek the providers who deliver the highest quality services at the least cost in order to secure the best return on their fixed resources (Havighurst 1970). Because the choice of services is at the discretion of the client, providers may be selected to meet time-limited needs and new providers identified as individual needs and preferences change (ibid.). Finally, the need to attract clients creates an incentive for providers to innovate and maintain a minimum quality of services, without the costs of direct government supervision.

> A competitive social service market would require innovative, enterprise-minded social workers who always consider the needs and interests of clients. . . . Such a market system would provide a ready measure of the most obvious dimension of agency success: client satisfaction. Without sophisticated monitoring, the organization would have feedback on the effectiveness of a program—feedback that could not be ignored, as present evaluation data commonly are." (Reid 1972, 52–53)

Although we have relatively little experience with voucher systems, it appears that client-based competition does capture a number of these promised benefits. Vouchers for housing and food had program costs from 10 to 50 percent less than comparable programs in which services were directly provided by the government (Isler 1981; Bendick, Campbell, Bawden & Jones 1976). Vouchers clearly permit greater choice by clients. For example, as the medicare program has begun to experiment with this approach, elders are receiving coverage for an array of services, including dental care, vision, and hearing aids, for which they previously were forced to pay from their own pockets (Iglehart 1985). Finally, there is some evidence that the use of vouchers encourages clients to become more careful and better-informed purchasers of service (Bendick 1984).

Juxtaposed against these benefits, however, are a number of disadvantages. As discussed above, clients often are poorly informed about their needs and about the health and social services available for their use. As a result, their selection of a provider may lead to a mismatch of needs and services. In addition, clients may be unable to accurately assess the claims made by competing providers, putting them at risk of misrepresentation by providers who claim to offer one level of service but actually provide services that are less costly and less efficacious (Morris and Youket 1981; Nelson and Kranhinsky 1973; Pruger and Miller 1973).[9]

Because clients are less informed than providers, there is a fundamental inequality in their relationship. Patients, for instance, cede to their physicians much of the control over how much and what types of health care they receive. This agency relationship inhibits clients from questioning and fully assessing the quality of the services they receive (Krause

1977). This vitiates, at least to some extent, the market forces that encourage providers to deliver less costly and more effective care.

Even when clients have the discretion and information to choose among providers, they often lack the opportunity. Clients can reap the benefits of competition only when they can choose among a number of alternative providers. Many publicly funded programs, however, pay providers at such a low rate or impose so many restrictions and preconditions that many potential providers refuse to participate (Sloan 1984). As the Medicaid experience illustrates, this may so restrict clients' options that they have only the facade of choice (Krause 1977).

The last, and perhaps most serious, limitation of client-based competition mirrors one of the major failings of formal evaluations. Clients' selection among providers will inevitably be based on the costs and benefits they face, not the broaders costs and benefits to society. Thus, services that have broadly diffused community benefits will be avoided in favor of those serving the direct concerns of those choosing the providers. This bias against broad social goals has been strongly reflected in the past performance of voucher systems.

> If the goals of a public program are stated modestly—to deliver a well-defined product to an easy-to-reach clientele in a cost-minimizing way—then redistribution of purchasing power to the clients themselves and allowing consumer choice in private markets seem, in many cases, to offer greater efficiency than direct public provision of a good or service. But such modest goals are not at all characteristic of many of the social programs in which governments become involved. To change the life chances of the disadvantaged; to break down racial, class or cultural ghettos; to alter traditional patterns of living—these are often the long-run objectives of public activities. . . . Whatever gains there might be in efficiency from a privatization strategy such as vouchers must be weighed against possible losses in effectiveness in terms of these larger goals. (Bendick 1984, 163)

Competitive Bidding Strategies. A second method of creating market-based incentives for a POS system involves government's purchase of services from private agencies through competitive bidding. This approach has been favored for some time in contracting for many local government services; as of the mid-1970s, roughly half of all service contracts established by state and local governments were competitively bid (Fisk, Kiesling, and Mueller 1978). It has been used extensively for mental health care and social services (Dorwart, Schlesinger, and Pulice, forthcoming) and more recently extended to general health care, with both Arizona and California incorporating competitive bidding into their Medicaid programs.

In principle, competitive bidding can capture a number of the advantages of client-based competitive models without some of their drawbacks. As with vouchers, competition is thought to encourage providers to become more efficient and innovative to improve the quality of services. "The contract is of limited duration . . . and is awarded competitively. Unlike a city agency, the contractor who wins the award has no assurance that he will continue to do the work forever; he cannot become complacent and must aim for continued or improved efficiency and effective service" (Savas 1982, 147).

Unlike client-based competition, the choice among potential providers is made by public officials. Because they have long experience with purchase of services, public officials may be better able than clients to compare competing programs. As the sole purchaser of services, the contracting agency is given a powerful bargaining position, allowing it to negotiate lower prices. Finally, government officials may have a broader perspective that allows them to better assess the societal costs and benefits of different services as opposed to the purely private costs and benefits perceived by clients.

In practice, competitively bid POS systems seem to have achieved a number of these objectives. They have successfully promoted greater flexibility and regional variation in the purchase of services (Schlesinger, Dorwart, and Pulice, forthcoming). Compared with client-based systems, their greater bargaining power has allowed them to reduce costs. For example, both California and Arizona report lower costs under competitively bid Medicaid arrangements than under the insurance models that had been previously used (Christianson, Hillman, and Smith 1983; Mermelstein 1983).

At the same time, the performance of competitive bidding systems has fallen short of the hopes of many proponents. It has proven difficult to make the bidding process truly competitive. There are often only a few agencies bidding on a given contract (Schlesinger, Dorwart, and Pulice, forthcoming; Giovannoni 1982; Young 1983). Concerns for continuity of care (Freedman and Moran 1984; Demone and Schulberg 1984) also inhibit competition because program administrators may place a higher priority on maintaining existing relationships between clients and providers than on switching to providers with lower bids. Finally, because it has proven difficult for small agencies to expediently bid on requests for proposals because of high overhead costs, the use of competitive bidding may lead to increased concentration of services under the control of a small number of large providers. As a result, there is often little competitive pressure to maintain quality or efficiency.

In addition, purchasing agencies have had a poor track record promoting higher quality services under bidding systems (Schlesinger, Dorwart, and Pulice, forthcoming; Fisk, Kiesling, and Mueller 1978). In fact, to make a bidding system functional, officials have been forced to use a number of procedures that inhibit the innovative delivery of services. To select among competing providers, the administrators of the POS system must compare the performance of the existing agencies with the promises of future performance made by other agencies. In practice, such comparisons have proven difficult and seem to have resulted in as many poor as sound choices (Mollica 1983; Massachusetts Taxpayers Foundation 1980).

As a result, contracting administrators have become "gun-shy," preferring to maintain contracts with existing providers—even if the quality they offer is barely acceptable—rather than risk choosing a new agency without a track record. In addition, contract administrators may place too great an emphasis on costs in selecting among providers because of difficulties in comparing quality. Finally, administrators' inabilities to identify high quality providers have led to legislative demands that the nature and quality of services be specified in ever-increasing detail in the request for proposal and the contract itself (Schlesinger, Dorwart, and Pulice, forthcoming). These detailed written requirements inhibit innovation and limit the flexibility and responsiveness of the contracting program to the individual needs of clients.

Recognizing these limitations, public officials have, in practice, questioned the benefits of market forces in competitive bidding systems. As a result, most, if not all such systems evolve over time to become procedures for negotiating between the public agency purchasing services and private suppliers.[10] The bidding process structures this negotiation but does not necessarily alter significantly the way in which providers are selected. To effectively negotiate, administrators operating the POS system must be able to assess the claims and performance of providers. Thus, the requirements for government evaluation of services may in practice remain as large in an ostensibly competitive bidding system as under systems that rely overtly on formal evaluations.

Provider Screening Strategies. A third alternative to formal evaluation under POS involves selectively contracting with only certain types of private agencies, most commonly restricting contracts to private nonprofit organizations. Restrictions of this type are based on the following rationale: Providers are believed to be motivated by both self-interest and a concern for the public good. Some providers are more concerned with the first goal, others with the second. Nonprofit ownership is perceived to restrict providers' opportunities to further their self-interest by limiting their claim to profits gained from delivering services. As a result, those who are primarily self-interested are predicted to affiliate with proprietary organizations.

> There appears to be a near-consensus among persons who write about day care that private for-profit enterprises and the 'market' are an unsatisfactory way of organizing this activity. Relatedly, there is a deep suspicion of for-profit nursing homes and hospitals. Clearly, profit is being mentally associated with exploitation rather than responsible services. (Nelson and Kranhinsky 1973, 55–56)

To the extent that this model of the role of profit as a motivation for providers is accurate, by contracting only with nonprofit agencies, government is able to preselect providers who are motivated to a greater-than-average extent by social concerns. To this end, much past public policy has been designed to subsidize or otherwise expand the role of private nonprofit agencies. At the federal level, nonprofit organizations have been given preferential subsidies to establish or expand hospitals and nursing homes (Lave and Lave 1974), health maintenance organizations (Luft 1984), day-care centers (Greenblatt 1977), educational training programs (Nielsen 1979), and a variety of other health-care facilities (Clark 1980). A number of states have refused to either certify or issue licenses for proprietary home health agencies (Vladeck 1980), health maintenance organizations (McNeil and Schenkler 1975), and foster-care agencies (Young 1983), though some of these restrictions have been loosened in recent years. In New York State, by law, a hospital cannot be a wholly-owned subsidiary of a for-profit corporation.[11]

If the motivations of providers are related to organizational characteristics, such as ownership form, selective contracting has a number of advantages over other goal-promoting strategies. It avoids the costs of extensive formal evaluations. It places the assessment of quality and other attributes of service in the hands of the providers, rather than poorly-informed consumers. It fosters providers' concerns for broadly diffused community benefits, the types of outcomes that both formal evaluations and individual consumers are least likely to effectively assess.

There is, in fact, evidence that providers' orientation to certain social goals is associated with the ownership of the facility. Surveys indicate that respondents associated with nonprofit organizations are more likely to have a "mission orientation" (Fottler 1981), to be concern with a "social presence" (Rawls, Ullrich, and Nelson 1975), and to willingly sacrifice monetary reward (Weisbrod 1983) than are their counterparts in for-profit firms. It has been argued that nonprofit organizations are more compatible with the goals of most professionals (Majone 1984), and studies have shown that nonprofit organizations are less likely to deliver very low-quality care and are more likely to adopt unprofitable services and serve unprofitable clients (Schlesinger and Dorwart 1984; Schlesinger 1985; Marmor, Schlesinger, and Smithey, forthcoming). By contracting preferentially with nonprofit agencies, states may thus be able to indirectly further these practices.

At the same time, it must be recognized that organizational auspices are an imperfect measure of provider motivation. In a number of past instances, nonprofit organizations have been formed to disguise the pursuit of profits (Oleck 1971). The more nonprofit organizations are subsidized or otherwise favorably treated, the more lucrative it becomes for profit-seeking entrepreneurs to clothe themselves in nonprofit garb. Thus, the potential for sacrificing client welfare to pursue monetary gain is present both in for-profit and nonprofit settings.

Even when providers do not surreptitiously seek monetary rewards, they need not automatically be motivated by broader social concerns. Providers may use the funds that would otherwise have gone to profits to erect elaborate facilities or hire superfluous staff. Evidence from past studies suggests that, for at least some services, costs are higher in nonprofit settings, and this cost difference may reflect this sort of unproductive spending (De Alessi 1980). These cost differences are most likely to emerge for services that are for the most part routine, such as laboratory testing or custodial nursing home care (Schlesinger, Dorwart, and Pulice, forthcoming). For other services, the actions of providers may reflect more the values of professional training rather than those of society as a whole. Clark (1980), for example, has argued that the practice of having some patients in hospitals cross-subsidize the care of others represents a form of taxation without representation, motivated more by the pursuit of professional prestige among physicians than by a concern for the patients receiving treatment.

Providers screening strategies, whether based on the auspices of the contracting agency or other characteristics, thus reduce the costs of directly assessing agency performance but also lessen control over the nature of the services that are purchased. Whether this is an appropriate exchange depends on the costs of assessment, the extent to which the screening characteristic can be circumvented by providers, and the similarity in the nonpecuniary goals of providers and the broader objectives of society.

PROMOTING SOCIAL WELFARE UNDER POS ARRANGEMENTS

Although techniques for evaluating health and human services are continually improving, there remain a sufficient number of technical and institutional constraints to limit the extent and benefits of assessing contracted services. In particular, formal evaluations are weakest at assessing diffuse community benefits, idiosyncratic aspects of quality, and dynamic aspects of program performance, including the propensity to innovate and the extent of public accountability. As a result, ongoing evaluations are biased against programs that perform best along these dimensions. In the face of political pressures to limit public spending, it is likely that providers of contracted services will systematically skimp on these aspects of programs performance in an effort to curb costs, leading over time to a reduction in quality of services (Dorwart, Schlesinger, and Pulice, forthcoming).

A number of system-based reforms have been proposed as alternatives to more comprehensive evaluation of contracted services. These include vouchers, competitive bidding, and preselection of providers. As discussed above, not all of these approaches truly represent viable alternatives to formal evaluation. In practice, most competitive bidding systems, for example, appear to evolve into systems of negotiation in which the assessment of services may play an important role.

Other strategies do seem to offer some advantages over direct evaluation. They do so by shifting the assessment role to other parties, either clients or the providers of services themselves.[12] As a result, both voucher and screening models seem better equipped to adapt services to the varying needs of individual clients. The provider screening approach, through its encouragement of professional incentives, seems to provide greater incentive for innovation.

These advantages, however, are at least in part offset by several shortcomings. Voucher approaches appear to be less effective than formal evaluation in appropriately valuing diffuse community benefits. Screening strategies, by enhancing the discretion of providers, may correspondingly weaken public accountability. They may also be inadequate to address goals, such as cost containment, which are less valued by providers than by society as a whole.

Because each of these broad strategies—comprehensive evaluation, voucher systems, and provider screening—have complementary strengths, the public interest may be best served by POS systems that combine these models. For example, a public agency might evaluate the benefits of various health care services and establish a set of prototype service packages, each of which ensures an adequate minimum standard of health care. Clients might then be given the choice among a number of HMOs, each offering one of these packages. This hybrid approach captures some of the benefits of the voucher system while providing greater protection against underprovision of care than is offered by the free market.

Inevitably, though, public agencies responsible for service contracting must decide which of these general approaches to emphasize. Based on the analysis presented above, it seems clear that the appropriate choice will depend largely on the characteristics of the service being delivered. The more quality depends on the individual preferences of the client, the more one would favor voucher models. Conversely, the greater the asymmetries of information between provider and client, the more either screening or evaluation strategies are preferable. Some general criteria for selecting among approaches are presented in table 24.1. These are meant to be illustrative, rather than exhaustive, but do capture some of the more important selection criteria.

Table 24.1 also identifies some prototype services that may fit into each of these three categories. It is important to recognize, however, that

Table 24.1. **Selecting Among Strategies for Assessing Contract Services**

System model	Service attributes that increase effectiveness of model	Possible examples
Formal evaluations	Standards of quality are uniformly applicable among clients	Services to mentally retarded
		Nursing home care
	There are large economies of scale in assessing quality	
	Public accountability is a primary goal	
Client-based vouchers	Idiosyncratic aspects of quality are important	Child day care
		Routine medical care
	Relatively free entry into market for providers	
		Meals on wheels
	Limited asymmetries of information between the providers and the clients	
	Continuity of care not an important aspect of quality	
Provider screening	Professional incentives compatible with broader social goals	Medical care for severe illness
	Screening characteristics can be readily monitored and enforced	Foster care
		Education and training programs
	Service requires provider discretion rather than routine delivery of care	

many of the services generally grouped together, e.g., as "mental-health care," and which are the responsibility of a single public agency, in fact have quite different characteristics. These differences may call for different contracting strategies. For example, although long-term care, routine physicals, and open-heart surgery are all considered health care, formal evaluations seem most appropriate for the first set of services, voucher-like arrangements for the second, and provider screening for the third. In practice, it may prove difficult for public agencies to adopt a mixture of approaches. If these constraints are sufficiently severe, it may be necessary to sacrifice performance for those services deemed less important, or perhaps to avoid contracting for those services at all.

Improving the Practice of Evaluating Contracted Services. Further research is required to eliminate a number of technical limitations of evaluating health and human services. Among other shortcomings, contemporary methods of program assessment inadequately measure dynamic aspects of program performance, including the role of public accountability and the adoption of innovations and outcomes with diffuse community benefits. These particular weaknesses are important because they can be addressed only to a limited extent using voucher or provider screening strategies. It thus seems appropriate to place the highest priority for future research and demonstration projects in these areas.

Although these technical limitations are of concern, it may be equally important to address a number of the political and legal constraints on program evaluation under POS. This should include efforts to develop standards that incorporate subjective assessments of quality and measures of accountability in ways that are legally enforceable. Efforts should also be made to reduce some of the political barriers to the use of evaluations, so that when evaluations are used, they are used in a relatively even way throughout the system. This requires building a constituency, both within the contracting agency and among providers of services.

Taken together, such technical and institutional changes should increase the use and improve the effectiveness of evaluations of contracted services. At the same time, it should be recognized that the limited capabilities of evaluation programs make it unwise to require evaluations as an across-the-board prerequisite for contracting. Other strategies exist for protecting the public interest and should be employed for those types of services for which formal evaluations are likely to be most biased or otherwise inadequate. Used in conjunction, these various strategies— evaluation, voucher, and selective contracting—should enhance the overall performance of POS systems as a mechanism for delivering health and human services.

Notes

1. Much of the so-called "tax-payer revolt" of the late 1970s and early 1980s stemmed from a popular perception that government programs had become wasteful and inefficient (Courant, Gramlich, and Rubinfeld 1981).

2. Certainly, the private sector does not require comprehensive evaluation. The Office of Technology Assessment (1978) has estimated that less than a fifth of all medical procedures that are routinely reimbursed by private insurers have been proven efficacious in controlled clinical trials.

3. For instance, surveys have revealed that up to one-half the elderly living in the community were unaware of the availability of health and social services they felt they needed (Branch 1978; Holmes, Teresi, and Holmes 1983). Minorities were the least likely to have adequate information.

4. It may also be difficult to accurately assess program costs. Because most health and human services are provided by private nonprofit and public agencies, many of the resources used tend to be undervalued. Public hospitals, for example, are rarely charged the true cost of the building and land they use. The costs of volunteer labor are rarely included in these calculations, though volunteers may actually outnumber the paid staff of providers in many agencies and the social value of their time may in the aggregrate be quite high (Weisbrod and Schlesinger 1981; Office of Technology Assessment 1980a). Although accurately valuing these resources is often problematic in practice, these problems are at least in theory more manageable than those of valuing benefits.

5. For the most part, these studies have focused on the composition of the board of directors of the agency (Provan, Beyer, and Kruytbosch 1980; Pennings 1980) or the extent of citizen participation (Dorwart and Meyers 1981). There have also been some attempts to define "fiduciary responsibility" in terms of the propensity of an agency to offer services that are unprofitable, but have broad community benefits (Schlesinger and Dorwart 1984).

6. Based on a survey of contracting for child welfare services, for example, Giovannoni observed "one reason for not using program people in monitoring was that they are perceived as the users of the services and, very often, are dependent on the service backup. One program monitor observed, 'What can we do when the providers have a monopoly and our clients need the service?" (1982, p. 17).

7. As a short-hand, services that further socially desired outcomes, such as increased accessibility, quality, efficiency, and accountability, will be referred to as "goal-promoting" services.

8. Medicare was recently authorized to enroll beneficaries in health maintenance organizations on a prepaid basis. Roughly half the states have begun to experiment with voucher-based systems under their Medicaid programs (Hekman 1984).

9. One approach to overcoming the problems of misinformation in voucher systems uses clients who are thought to be better informed than are publicly supported clients to act as "proxy shoppers" to protect the interest of their less-informed counterparts. Under this approach, agencies that wish to serve publicly funded clients must attract a minimum number of clients who pay for services from private sources. For instance, health maintenance organizations participating in the Medicare program are allowed to enroll Medicare beneficiaries as only half their patients, in the belief that the half who are younger and privately insured will be better able to assess and avoid low-quality health care. These proxy

shopping requirements can be effective only if private purchasers are in fact better informed about services and, once they have selected a provider, they receive the same quality of service as do their financed counterparts (Rose-Ackerman 1983)

10. For discussions on this evolution in the competitive bidding models used in the Medicaid program, see Christianson, Hillman, and Smith, 1983; and Mermelstein 1983.

11. Not all these restrictions are formalized in law. As Young observed, "in the child-care field . . . federal, state and local funding for residential care may be essentially restricted to nonprofit providers" although there are no legal requirements to do this (1983, p. 150).

12. Variants on these approaches involve the use of case managers or utilization review to assess program performance. Because these are more closely linked to what has been termed here "monitoring" rather than "evaluation," we leave the discussion of these methods to other chapters in this section.

PART SEVEN

Conclusion

In this volume the purchase of health and human services has been explored from a variety of perspectives, ranging from the theoretical and philosophical bases for POS to the actual experiences and their results in implementing this alternative mechanism for delivering services. It has been seen that the ever-increasing use of POS is based on a complex set of factors that involve social values and preferences, political ideology (particularly, perceptions about the role of government), cost, vested interests, and simple pragmatism, among others. These factors have combined, historically and most notably since the 1960s, to significantly favor the use of alternatives to a purely public system of service delivery, of which POS has been seen as the most feasible and, perhaps, the easiest to implement in relative haste.

Experience with the purchasing of services had shown mixed results, a not unusual occurrence in the implementation of many American social policies and practices. Expectations may often exceed potential realities. Disillusionment may quickly set in when the inevitable "quirks" in the system become manifest. The modern media plays an increasing role in identifying and evaluating the implications of these system faults, as evidenced in frequent print and visual media reports of corruption, conflict of interest, cost overruns, and other abuses of contracting. Perhaps inevitably, more attention is given to the faults and failures of contracting than to the more positive outcomes of this system.

There are, indeed, real problems with contracting. Some of these problems may be inherent within the larger American health and social welfare system, where "mixed messages" about goals, range of services, breadth of designated client/patient populations, and even desired outcomes can be easily discerned. As a society, the United States has historically been hesitant, if not reluctant, to establish anything approaching a welfare state. The earliest ideologies promoting the virtues of self-reliance and "pulling oneself up by the boot straps" very much remain strong beliefs, though perhaps not as overt. There is increasing awareness of a growing underclass. Our systems for implementing health and social welfare programs manifest and replicate the ambivalence and uncertainty about their desirability, although need may be less disputed.

The political context in which American social policy systems and programs are devised and implemented, where process and content often accomodate the variety of interests, also suggests that outcomes are likely to deviate from expectations. Expectations, too, are often couched in unrealistically short time intervals and, often, without the necessary financial backing for proper implementation or system evaluation. These characteristics of American social policy apply no differently to the purchase of services than to any other program or system. They are essential features of our political processes.

Criticisms of POS range from the very general (purchase is simply a modification and thus perpetuation of current, inadequate service delivery mechanisms and/or purchase does not go far enough toward privatization because it is based on public funding) to the more specific—lack of standards, lack of long-term planning, lack of coordination between the public and private sector, inadequate staffing of contracted programs, and inaccurate rate-setting procedures, among others. Despite the general and specific charges against POS, what is perhaps most noteworthy is the substantial unanimity about maintaining the system through incremental improvements, rather than discarding it.

Thus, despite the volume and scope of problems with POS, the factors giving rise to its pervasive use combine again to justify and verify its relevance, desirability, and feasibility as a major means to deliver health and human services. Although the weighting of the separate factors promoting the use of POS may have changed (reordering the rationales), the total combination of factors suggests that POS is still a most viable system and one not likely to soon be abandoned. The reason, of course, may simply be the lack of other real alternatives. It may also be that POS continues to satisfy the disparate requirements of a wide segment of the American political and general publics. Both may be true.

It is not likely that we will soon see a major turn away from the popular concept and practice of privatization. To the extent that privatizing remains a high political and social priority, the purchase of services will likely continue to serve as a major means by which to link the public and private systems. Role assignments, of course, will vary and be clarified and changed over time. The concurrent priority placed on decreasing the size and cost of the bureaucracy—at the federal, state, and local levels—will also continue to favor POS. These factors affecting the future use of POS are explored in this chapter as they hinder or promote the role and scope of purchasing services in our health and social welfare system of tomorrow.

25

The Future of Purchase of Service

Harold W. Demone, Jr., and Margaret Gibelman

Forecasting in our volatile environment is replete with complexities. The future of purchase of service (POS) is no less subject to the exigences of the times. If decisions were limited to empirical criteria and matters of cost and effectiveness, most publicly operated services and, virtually all goods would be purchased. It is usually less expensive to purchase services than for government to directly provide them. Purchase encourages more effective quality control and administrative flexibility. In an era in which achieving a balanced budget is among the highest government priorities, cost factors alone would favor the purchase of services.

The preference for purchasing services can be seen in a number of recent policy shifts. Selective changes stimulated by such initiatives as the 1981 and 1986 tax reforms and the recommendations of bodies such as the President's Private Sector Survey on Cost Control (known as the Grace Commission), are likely to stimulate even more transfer of responsibility to the private sector, including management or even ownership of bridges, transportation fleets, airports, and public office buildings. And finally, there is ideology. The increasing disenchantment with government, including criticisms of the vertical monopolistic structure and the immobile bureaucracy, shifts in sovereign immunity rights, and renewed emphasis on federalism all reinforce each other and encourage even more purchase of services.

VARIABLES AFFECTING THE FUTURE

Arguments in favor of and against contracting continue. In some cases the actors are the same; in other instances new groups enter the debate when their interests are involved. Political considerations factor into the equation, as do vested interests. The Reagan administration has perhaps done more to publicize and legitimize privatization than any other public or private force. Although future administrations may not maintain or instill the same fervor about privatizing, the concept, terminology, and practice now pervade our society and several others in the Western world.

Variables affecting the future use of purchase of service include attitudes of public officials; choices made about current, new or emerging service delivery models and arenas of responsibility; role delegation and assignment; ideology; and actual experience. Nor is there great consistency. The several levels of government—federal, state and local (including counties)— are behaving quite differently.

Political Factors. Present predilections are often based upon trends extrapolated from practice over the last twenty to thirty years. These include recent legislation, court decisions, and the preferences and actions of key decision makers, usually with the support of the general public. The same impetus toward increased use of POS at the federal level is also evident in local government. The reactions of state and county governments with regard to POS are much less certain.

The Office of Management and Budget's (OMB) continuing emphasis on contracting, which has spanned nearly thirty years, is illustrated in its April 1982 proposal: "Policies & Procedures for Acquiring Commercial Products and Services Needed By The Government" (*Washington Post*, 16 April 1982). The OMB strongly recommended that federal agencies contract out much of the work currently performed by government. For activities with fewer than ten full-time employees, contract conversion should occur as soon as practical; for larger in-house activities, the government should continue to provide the product or service only if it can do so at a lower total cost than if obtained from the private sector. These pronouncements clearly favor contracting, whereas in the past, the emphasis had been on continuing or sustaining government operations unless there was evidence that the private sector could be more efficient.

In response to this edict by the OMB, the chief of the National Foundation of Federal Employees (a union representing government workers) described the proposed revision of federal contracting policies as a policy shift. His opinion of this alleged shift was strongly negative, noting that such change "is perhaps the most blatant attempt yet to funnel federal

400

revenues to private industry at the expense of the American taxpayers" (*Washington Post*, 18 April 1982).

This opposition and that of like others was of sufficient magnitude and influence that within three months the OMB was claiming that the emphasis on contracting heretofore public functions was "never official", (*Washington Post*, 6 July 1982). Instead, the newly stated priority was now given to searching for a means to reduce contracting paper work, a much more nebulous and politically neutral stance. Nevertheless, the decision to expand contracting, and certainly to continue current patterns in this direction, was not repudiated.

As noted elsewhere in this volume the public employee unions have led the opposition to privatizing public functions. In individual states they have successfully blocked the transfer of resources from public institutions to community-based alternatives. They have stated their opposition publicly. They do possess considerable political influence.

Yet not denying the importance of the negative stands of the public employee unions, we suspect that apathy is the major culprit. It is often too much to engage in the steps necessary to successfully implement the contractual model.

Change often requires more energy and capacity than is available. The *New York Times* reported in a front-page article, "U.S. Pressing Plan to Contract Work," the actions of the Reagan administration to "put new vigor in a thirty-year-old government directive that services be performed by private contractors whenever it is possible to save money that way" (11 March 1985). It was noted that in fiscal year 1980, the federal government spent $100.2 billion in contracting for commercial services (prior to President Reagan's assumption of office). It was estimated that for 1985, the figure would be $173 billion, a 70 percent increase.

Nor is promoting contracting as an alternative to public provision of goods or services exclusive to the executive branch of government. The General Accounting Office (GAO) of Congress is similarly directed. For example, in an August 1982 study, "Civilianizing Certain Air Force Positions . . . ," the GAO found itself in conflict with the Air Force bureaucracy, which favors continuing selected strategic air command support positions under military auspices. The GAO believes that by filling the positions with qualified civilian employees, several advantages would accrue. The Air Force could save money, reduce some military skill shortages, and defer military construction projects.

401

In a 1984 joint study by the Congressional Budget Office and the General Accounting Office, the findings of the president's Private Sector Survey on Cost Control were used as a reference point. Although the study findings challenged the estimated cost savings identified in the president's survey (concluding that the latter's statistics had failed to reflect statutory restrictions on contracting in the Veteran's Administration and the Defense Department), maximum savings were still in the area of $1.1 billion (*New York Times,* 11 March 1985).

State governments appear to be much less certain about the continued or expanded use of POS. Proclamations about the value and necessity of purchasing services seem much less likely to originate from state officials. Given a recent resurgence in interest in "states' rights" (seldom states' responsibilities), the opportunity to exercise the anticipated power and influence associated with block grants appeared to divert attention from maximizing expenditures to building political and bureaucratic bases. On the other hand, state governments are also feeling the pressure to decrease the size of the bureaucracy. The pervasive and ongoing cuts in federal funds available to state governments, as in the elimination of revenue sharing, may also substantially reduce decision-making flexibility and favor the more traditional service delivery patterns. States may now use their own discretion as to whether and how much private providers are to contribute to the cost of contractual arrangements. In theory, the matching formula may vary from contract to contract or among types of contracts. The result is that states have substantially greater leeway to promote a mix of federal and private dollars.

It is not only the philosophy and actions of the Reagan administration that have encouraged states to examine their relationship with the private sector; public opinion also favors a decrease in the size and role of government at all levels. These factors may, in varying degrees, cause many states to at least continue, if not expand, their use of POS.

As noted in chapter 2, the extent of local government interest in POS appears to be growing. Activity is not limited to those middle-sized cities with professional city manager chief executives who are often the leaders in progressive public administration practices. Several examples from New York City and Washington, D.C., suggest POS may not only be good management, but also good politics. In Washington, D.C., a city that relies heavily on POS, even several prolonged scandals regarding contracting have failed to sway the practices of this local government (*Wash-*

ington Post, 23 March 1985; 21 May 1985). A *New York Times* article acknowledged that in New York City, although there is increasing public uneasiness about purchasing public services from the private sector in light of allegations of bribery and fraud, it was proclaimed that "a sharp veering away from privatization would be a disservice to the taxpayers." The authors conclude that "honorably awarded contracts have demonstrably enabled officials across the nation to exploit innovation in the private sector for the public good" (*New York Times,* 15 February 1986).

According to the Federal Procurement Data Center, a division of the General Services Administration, the total value of contracts let by the federal government during fiscal year 1984 totaled $166 billion (*Washington Post,* 20 August 1985). Given the pronounced shift to POS and the large amount of money associated with it, one consistent theme running through many, if not most, of the commentaries about purchase of service is the lack of considered thinking about the matter. Most knowledgeable observers are generally pragmatic. Both those in favor and those uncertain about the use of POS seem to agree that we need to consider more carefully the rationale, process, and implications of alternative choices. One effort to foster and slow the debate simultaneously came from the Reagan administration. The 15 July 1983 *Federal Register* announced the availability of grant funds to explore ideas about alternative financing and delivery mechanisms within the social services that "increase consumer choice, promote competition among providers, and reduce governmental control over decisions for the provision of social services" (p.32391). On the other hand, those opposed to POS in any form do not equivocate and are not interested in such debates.

Ideology. Ideology is another variable concerning the future of POS. Purchase of service is currently in a strong ideological position. It seems to be compatible with both fundamental conservative beliefs and some developing forms of liberalism. Two major phases of liberalism in this country, Jeffersonian and Hamiltonian, each had its inevitable consequences. The Jeffersonian model, although reasonably successful in controlling governmental abuses, failed in its control of private abuses. The Hamiltonian, or big government model, redressed the excesses of the private sector but failed to achieve commonweal.

The identification of bureaucratic "big government" as the problem rather than the solution is a phenomenon that transcends national boundaries. The rejection of "bigness" is occurring not only in the United

States, but in such diverse countries as France, Italy, Spain, West Germany, Brazil, Canada, Great Britain, Mexico, Turkey, Portugal, Ireland, Japan, the Phillipines, Singapore, Malaysia, and even the Soviet Union. Obviously, the desire to "privatize" as an alternative to big government is not necessarily tied to conservative goals in all nations. The common denominator is a significant disenchantment with both the process and achievements of government and a desire to test the feasibility of alternatives by means of a private market strategy. In France pressures are building to sell back to private investors government-owned companies (*New York Times,* 11 September 1986). In Portugal Prime Minister Anibal Cadaco Silda has embarked on a program to reestablish private enterprise as the driving force behind the economy (Boston Sunday Globe, 22 December 1985). In Great Britain Margaret Thatcher has been criticized for failing to successfully implement a privatization program (*Washington Post,* 5 July 1986). In the Soviet Union Mikhail Gorbachev's reform program includes changes that will allow limited private enterprise that will "democratize" and make more flexible the Soviet economy (ibid., 28 November 1986). In Ireland the liberal Fine Gael party advocated greater reliance on the private sector in the 1987 election campaign (*New York Times,* 15 February 1987). In Africa the twenty-nine poorest nations have sold or closed down about 5 percent of the enterprises owned by the several states since 1980. Governments in the poor countries have not found it easy to locate buyers, even for companies that are healthy (Alm 1986).

Purchase of service, although currently supported by conservatives, would have a tenuous future if this were the principle base of support. This nation is basically liberal. In varying degrees we have felt, and acted upon, a sense of responsibility for our brethren. There is also a measurable history of periods of considerable liberal reform separated by shorter periods of conservatism (*New York Times,* 20 September 1980). Jeremy Dentham's statement of "the greatest happiness to the greatest number" is the continuing common objective of our nation.

Liberalism has, historically, reemerged after conservative periods, and it will likely to so in the future. However, in our evolving postindustrialized society, it is unlikely that either liberalism or conservatism will be an exact replication of their recent forms, some of which have been rejected even by their former advocates. Thus, to maximally survive in a viable and legitimate form, POS should satisfy the ideological needs of

404

reformers, moderates, and conservatives. At a minimum, POS should not be opposed by more than one segment of the populace. Given its long but intermittent character, gradual but steady growth in the 1950s and early 1960s, and substantial growth thereafter until the major cutbacks of the Reagan administration, POS seems to have temporarily satisfied the ideological needs of a broad spectrum of the body politic. Such broad-based ideological support is most unusual in our society.

Jansson (1977, this volume) took a novel approach to the public-private ideological issue. Setting aside matters of effectiveness and efficiency, he examined ideology at the administrative level and found that, indeed, there are attitudinal differences between public and private agency executives. He also determined that, in general, these attitudes reflected the missions of their organizations. He concluded that because of the value differences, public officials, prior to entering contractual arrangements, should examine the priorities, service, and decision-making approaches of the POS candidates. Subsequent to contracting, Jansson urges aggressive monitoring, particularly to determine whether minorities or persons with low income are discouraged from using services. Other data suggest that creaming the better clients is controllable, but needs monitoring (Gibelman 1980).

Ideological matters range from a macro view of alternatives to the way organizational employees practice their professions. Successful implementation of any position requires a sensitive understanding of ideology and values.

Role delegation. Another future POS concern is found in the continued debate about the delegation of roles between the public and private sectors. The body of thought publicly and unequivocally opposed to all public purchase of human services is currently dormant. Those favoring the use of a voucher system are intermittently vigorous, but proponents currently lack sufficient consensus to mount a major countervailing force. Concerns, when they surface, seem primarily to center around delineating functions exclusively public from those primarily public: identifying new and better methods to cost and monitor contracts, allocating public sector functions, and protecting the rights of public employees affected by contracting.

Kahn (1972), Jansson (1980) and the American Public Welfare Association Board of Directors (*Washington Report,* 1981), and several authors of articles within this volume (Wolock, Ten Broeck, and McGovern), among others argue for a position that divides responsibility among the sectors. In general, the public sector would serve as planner, resource developer, funder, coordinator, and monitor. At a minimum, it would provide initial gatekeeping functions such as information and referral. The APWA would also require that the public sector provide selective, protective functions.

Virtually all commentators advocating for shared responsibility between the public and private sectors acknowledge implementation problems. Nevertheless, it is argued that, rather than abandon public-private role delegation efforts, the problems can and should be corrected. Taking the implementation experiences and issues as a given, these authors agree that resource allocation, planning, and monitoring are clearly within the purview of the public sector. Information and referral is less obviously a public function. Selective, protective services fall into the ambiguous category. The delegation of roles is fraught with turf and political implications and may not be subject to solely objective classification.

The rationale for any direct service public sector role is unclear. The typical review is more assertive of function than justified. For example, the information and referral program currently operated by public social service agencies was, for many years, a catchall used to cover employees who could not otherwise be included under various federal categories. Until block grants, it was more a payroll than programmatic device and a way to increase the state share of federal dollars. Information and referral (I & R) is also, by definition, a function performed by almost all agencies, individual professionals, newspapers, and other media as a normal, but secondary, part of their responsibilities. It is performed as a principal and primary role by some public social service agencies, especially under Title XX, and by some agencies usually supported by United Way. The proposition that the I & R program performed by the public social service agencies can be comprehensive, inclusive, or well delivered has not been substantiated anywhere in the literature. A new central effort to superimpose another I & R system on a geographic community (it has been tried and failed) seems highly ill-advised. A more responsible objective is for the public human service industry, including rehabilitation, public health, social services, and mental health, among others, to join together in a system that coordinates the existing efforts and fills gaps as needed by subject, content, time, and geography.

According to Bill B. Benton (1981), former deputy director of the Maryland Department of Human Services, the principal future agenda, given budget constraints, is to exercise state leadership. This would be accomplished by implementing an automated social service system and management by objectives. To his counterpart in Connecticut, Hector A. Rivera (1981), the major future objective is to improve program monitoring, fiscal auditing, and state-level planning.

In New Jersey Larry Lockhart, then special assistant to the commissioner, Department of Human Services, described the role of state government as providing resources and acting as a catalyst to strengthen nonprofit organizations (Newsletter, Association for Children, 1983). A surprisingly compatible view of future needs is proposed by John R. Healy, executive director of the Massachusetts Council of Human Services Providers, representing the private sector, responding to criticisms made by the Massachusetts Taxpayers Foundation (1980). The Council of Human Services Providers (Healy, 1981) identified five major problem areas and introduced legislation to resolve these matters: (1) payment procedures; (2) rate-setting; (3) local government relations; (4) monitoring, evaluation, and accountability; and (5) the capacity to finance capital improvements. A 1986 report produced by the Massachusetts Senate Committee on Ways and Means on the need to improve the administration of state-contracted services found massive implementation problems from the perspective of both the state agencies and the providers in such areas as standards, long-term planning, coordination, adequate staffing, and administrative resources and structures. The recommendations are even more detailed and extensive than those set forth in 1981 and, as discussed earlier in this volume, pose the essential question about the adequacy of contracting itself (see McGovern, chapter 17). The answer is clear: even with all of the documented faults of POS, the system should be repaired, not discarded.

Role delegation is a recurrent theme throughout federal and state-initiated studies on the implementation experiences with contracting for services. Although consensus is lacking on exactly what roles are to be delegated to whom, it seems clear that the distribution of roles and responsibilities between the public and private sectors is a fundamental issue in current and future purchase of service arrangements. Of all potential human service roles, there appears finally to be agreement that three are primary government responsibilities: allocation of funds, planning, and monitoring. There are successful examples of contracted

407

planning and monitoring, although the responsibility is exclusively found in the public sector.

Public functions. Further exploration of the three primary public roles (funding, planning, and monitoring) help to clarify their unique characteristics. Despite the occasional mutterings of some ideologues and politicians, no one seriously believes that the private sector can or will fund the bulk of humans services. The securing and allocating of resources is a major governmental activity made possible through its unique taxing authority.

The planning function is sometimes linked to and seen as overlapping that of coordination. In the schema outlined by Pruger and Miller (1973), the public agency plays a much expanded coordinative role. To these authors, "coordination is an efficiency creating mission within a particular system." Basically, it is a method by which to maximize resources and is present-oriented. As coordinator, the public agency would (1) develop and implement a method by which consumers and providers will have the information appropriate to their roles as consumers and providers will have the information appropriate to their roles in a competitive system and (2) stimulate and foster the development of alternative suppliers for each kind of service offered. This view is a rather dramatic extension of the planning role typically assigned to government.

From a futuristic perspective, the expansion of public planning can be easily sanctioned. The development of a competent, sophisticated, planning operation in the public sector seems generally favored by most analysts of public-private relationships. Agreement in principal with this view comes easily. However, the history of public human services planning has shown it to be a rather unique form, quite unlike that generally proposed. Typically, most public human service planning agencies, whether comprehensive or categorical, have had a similar history.

Products of the 1960s and 1970s, these agencies have been found to be highly effective and utilitarian. A caveat is that only a small proportion of agency resources are actually devoted to planning. Instead, the planner tends to be a generalist who troubleshoots. For example, health planners in the 1970s and 1980s were substantially constrained by budgetary factors. They were underfunded, and considerable amounts of their time and effort went into cost containment efforts for others. From their residual resources, crisis response was likely to be the major activity. Planning as a rational, future-oriented activity was given short shrift. We need only look to the rapid demise of educational programs designed to produce planning experts. Urban planning, for example, as a discipline is now largely dormant. Health planning in schools of public health and social planning in schools of social work are similarly constrained.

From the early 1960s through the late 1970s, there was a considerable growth in resources commitment to human services planning in the public sector. This incremental growth was largely stimulated by the federal government in categorical fields, such as health, mental health, recreation, rehabilitation, alcohol and drug abuse, and criminal justice. More systematic and encompassing efforts previously were found in health planning and social services planning. The outcomes have been far different from those envisioned. The ad hoc, time-responsive planning efforts were generally given good grades. When institutionalized, however, governmental human services planning took on its crisis-oriented nature. Thus, although there is general agreement that government agencies should improve their planning capacity, converting a reasonable proportion of existing resources to this purpose will require considerable skill and commitment. Politics runs on short time frames. Crisis management is the rule.

Another public role about which considerable consensus exists is that of monitoring. Those who control the purse strings and who are ultimately accountable must be able to ensure the appropriate use of the funds. The periodic complaints about U.S. Department of Defense procurement and military contractors reinforces the legitimacy and importance of this role. The exact manner in which this function is performed is considerably more flexible. For example, some of the components can be contracted to the private sector. Ultimately, however, monitoring is the means by which to ensure accountability in the use of public funds. Even when some monitoring functions are contracted out, public agencies are likely to specify in detail the procedures to be followed. In fact, newly heard complaints by contracted service providers center around the volume of forms to be completed in the name of monitoring and accountability. Some are concerned with the questionable utility of many monitoring methods. Certainly, there are serious questions about how data derived from the monitoring process are used to improve performance. Paper collection can become an end in itself.

In some states, human services monitors are becoming increasingly skillful. They leave many of the nonprofit organizations substantially dependent on them. Salaries are barely adequate, at best, and maintenance is deferred. Support costs are only partially covered. The margins are tenuous. If they are reduced any more, they will be driven out of business, but this is where the contracting skill manifests itself. The limits are sensed.

The "capture theory," whereby regulatory commissions are captured by the monitored interests, appears not to have occurred among the nonprofits. Perhaps it is limited to the for-profit sector.

Despite the problems associated with the proper implementation of roles delegated to the public sector, the fact remains that their unique characteristics render them within the responsibility of government. The public sector may need help to improve its capacity to carry out these roles, but it cannot abrogate or fully reassign them.

Finally, there is one other uniquely public function of this American society: equity, the exclusive franchise of government. Protecting the rights and welfare of citizens is a responsibility that cannot be delegated. There is no private-sector organization whose primary mission is to protect and to enhance equity for all citizens. In the design, implementation, funding, and evaluation of human services, government must ensure that the principal of equity is upheld.

Regulations. All aspects of human service delivery systems will be affected by recent efforts to reduce the number of regulations supporting our laws. A major component of the 1980 and 1984 presidential campaigns, repeated in many Congressional and state and local political campaigns, was a general criticism of the bureaucracy, with special attention directed to the "bungling" of the regulatory role. In consequence, concerted attempts have been made to reduce the scope and number of regulations governing governmental programs. This deregulation process also extends to purchased goods and services and could result in substantial changes at the state and local levels, with variations abounding. Significant success, especially in the human services, is not visible. For example, in the health and social services controls have expanded. The AFDC and SSI client under the deregulators is likely to experience an even more complicated bureaucratic maze than was heretofore the case. New Jersey's medically needy program for its first seven months cost

410

thirteen dollars in administration for every one dollar in benefits delivered (*New York Times,* 15 February 1987).

Rules and regulations regarding the purchase of human services have heretofore tended to become more codified, more numerous, and more cumbersome from the vantage point of public agencies who must administer POS programs and providers who are bound by the regulations. Lourie (1979) suggests that if public agencies could acquire enough capable staff to visit agencies and provide good technical assistance, overregulation could be controlled. Lacking adequate client information systems, data become confused with information. Data are collected but not used in helpful ways.

Monitoring and accountability in the performance of the regulatory role can occur in a variety of forms. As Lourie (1979) reminds us, our human services industry lacks consistency. The health component is replete with controls, including professional licensure, standards, accreditation, peer review, second opinions, and diagnostic-related groups. In contrast, the criminal justice system and the public social service system have extremely limited external controls, although accreditation for voluntary child welfare and family service agencies has prevailed for some time. Psychologists are licensed in all states, as are nurses. Social workers are now licensed in about 85 percent of the states, and the National Association of Social Workers has a voluntary certification program for its members. When third party fees follow licensure, it is usually accompanied by peer review.

The field of rehabilitation is even more uncontrolled, except for the recent development of an accreditation program for sheltered workshops. Of course, the rehabilitation field does use a case management model, which, when well practiced, compensates for many deficiencies.

All of the major human service professions have national accreditation for their professional schools. Unfortunately, many civil service agencies fail to take advantage of these national standards. In many instances uncredentialed employees are hired for perceived cost savings. Declassification of heretofore professional positions is a trend in several states.

The application of regulatory and standard-setting principles can take several forms. The wealthy, sophisticated service user purchasing professional assistance in the open market ordinarily will look for a person with appropriate professional credentials and board certification or its equivalent. This type of person prefers a graduate from one of the better universities with solid references, experiences, and a university affiliation. The process of selecting an organization to provide services would be similar. If these are the criteria used by the more sophisticated consumers in selecting a professional or organization to service them or their families, it is abundantly sensible to apply the same criteria for or by those who are not as rich and not as sophisticated about such matters.

Dual systems and standards, are, however, characteristic, in part due to the regulatory process. Regulatory excesses are so compounded that even natural allies of government have become increasingly disenchanted with their government colleagues. There are often contradictions in goals. The regulatory system can be stressed to the limit by having to address issues of stricter accountability, human rights, equity, privacy, and creativity as equally legitimate objectives. The General Accounting Office (1982a), among others, urges more flexibility in grant administration.

Examples of regulatory excesses are not difficult to find. Is there a taxpayer without a complaint about the forms supplied by the Internal Revenue Service? On the other hand, there also exist examples of the skilled application of the regulatory apparatus. It may well be that each purchased product or service stimulates its own unique abuses. University-public agency contracts for training have tended to force the production of many unnecessary and unread reports (Gibelman and Humphreys 1982). In the defense industry, abuses may take the form of conflict of interest or cost inflation. In contracting for municipal services, unfair bidding practices and favoritism may be characteristic.

Lourie (1979) suggests that monitoring and accountability in the performance of the regulatory role can occur in a variety of forms. It does not necessarily make for greater efficiency or effectiveness in contract administration to emphasize meaningless and frequent counts of units of service performed under the guise of accountability. More outcome, results-oriented requirements, such as those suggested by Jansson (this volume) offer a worthwhile alternative.

One development of note, evident for several years, is the tension between governmental program and fiscal personnel; these tensions are now complicated by the new quasi-police group of regulators. This significant, continuing struggle within the public sector is now beginning to spill over into the private sector. It is extremely important that private providers of service understand the nature of the fiscal-programmatic conflict, for if the fiscal side wins out, it is likely that many public decisions will be made on grounds inimical to quality client services. On the other hand, the programmatic professionals must develop financial, administrative, and other competencies if they are to effectively maintain their roles and responsibilities. This is analogous to the strains in industry. The target is the "accounting mentality" focusing on short-term profits to the detriment of long-term viability.

With respect to the growing regulatory role within human service agencies, Herman (1979, p. 35) describes the development of a "profession" of state agency regulators. "Their vocabulary is replete with such words as 'surveillance,' 'stakeout,' 'suspect,' and 'suppression of illegal operations.' They may apply these words not to international criminals, but to a day care mother who is licensed to provide services for four children instead of six." Should the public auditor/policeman win a predominant role, the results can be predicted. More layers will be added to the bureaucracy. Whether the stimulus be a public scandal or an intraorganizational struggle for power, the result is typically the same. The cost of the new control mechanism is likely to substantially exceed any anticipated savings, quality will decline, and the public sector will be further impaired and subject to additional criticism.

Some new government directives may be more benign in nature, but hold major ramifications for the future of purchase of service. Rule changes approved by the Office of Management and Budget went into effect on 12 August 1985. The new guidelines revise the measurement tools the federal agency must use when they consider whether to purchase products or services or to maintain the function in-house, utilizing civil servants. Now, fringe benefits are to be calculated into the formula by which private industry versus civil service costs are to be calculated, giving a decided advantage to the private sector. Indeed, the prospects are not encouraging for federal workers. In the case of defense, for example, contractors underbid the government 52 percent of the time, with most of the savings from reduced personnel costs (*Washington Post,* 20 August 1985). Further, according to the guidelines, federal agencies must periodically examine the cost of their support and service functions to assess whether the work can be performed at less cost by private firms.

Because payroll costs are relatively fixed in government, the private sector is at an advantage because it may adjust the number of workers or pay employees less.

The private sector. The future of purchase of service, of course, is not only affected by the rules, regulations and prerogatives of government, but also by the actions, preferences, and political influence wielded by the private sector. A continuing examination of private sector goals and objectives is strongly advised. The private sector needs to consider carefully what roles it wishes to play within human services in relation to the public sector now and in the future.

There is general consensus among commentators on the subject that the reliance on government funds has led to substantial changes in the nature of nonprofit agencies. Such changes are manifest in the voluntary agencies' primary service focus, types of programs offered, mode of operations, and management style. In many cases it can be hypothesized that these are unintended consequences that have occurred on an incremental basis over time. In the quest to initiate, expand, or supplement existing or new programs, voluntary agencies have often entered into a financially dependent relationship with government with little consideration to their long-term impact. Fundamental questions go unanswered: Will a given contract enhance, inhibit, or be neutral with respect to the perceived future directions of the agency? Will the contract augment or inhibit resources? Is a continued relationship with the public sector viable and desirable? Should the private sector contract to conduct a program not in keeping with its objectives but which would provide some financial stability? Even if the contracted program is compatible with objectives, can it be incorporated without major negative consequences to the agency? Is it a good match with the administrative, substantive, and financial capacities of the agencies? These and similar matters have been discussed herein by several authors. The value and importance of these questions to the private sector can not be underemphasized.

An appropriate stance on the part of the private sector may be that of flexibility. As priorities and fads shift and evolve, today's contract may be tomorrow's cancellation. The ability to distinguish between hard and soft money, to start up when funds come slowly, to manage during cash flow difficulties, and to shift resources and staff as the situation demands, requires skillful management and flexible organizations in a stable financial position.

Questions of philosophy and ideology also come into play; it is not merely a matter of the pragmatic contractual relationship. Often, it seems that agencies enter the contracting business without engaging in the appropriate planning processes concerning the desired means and outcomes of such arrangements. Smith (this volume) points to the blurring of the distinctive roles of voluntary agencies that may occur as a result of the intermingling of goals, programs, and funds that are inherent in contracting. Some voluntary agencies have come into existence solely to serve government purposes; if public funds had not been available, the agencies would not exist.

It is not uncommon for public and private agencies to have different constituencies, operating modes, service philosophies, and intervention methods. In fact, it is precisely these distinctions between public and private that make each sector unique. However, these points of difference may lead to problems in the public-private relationship that can affect the implementation of a contracted program and have negative ramifications on agency morale, operating procedures, and the like. Understanding the mission, philosophy, and operating mode of the other organization can enhance the potential for successful partnership arrangements. Conversely, the lack of such clarity and understanding can have unanticipated consequences both for the implementation of a specific contract and the private organization as a whole. It is far better that such matters be addressed and resolved before, rather than after, the fact of contracting.

There is now a relatively long history of contracting between the public and private sectors upon which to base an assessment of these arrangements. Purchase of service has become big news. The *New York Times* and *Washington Post,* two of the major national newspapers, contain numerous and consistent references to issues, probes, and even scandals surrounding federal, state, and local contracting with the private sector. A *Washington Post* (6 July 1982) headline story, "Putting the Government Out Of Business," described a feud between the American Federation of Government Employees (AFGE) and the Reagan administration. Stimulating the article was a General Accounting Office report that cited eighteen examples in which the private sector assumed tasks once performed by the government. Deficiencies were found in six contracted programs. The Office of Management and Budget concluded that the difficulties resulted from the inexperience or unwillingness of government supervisors to make the arrangement more explicit and to monitor more effectively. In 1985 the *Washington Post* (30 June) reported "9 of 10 Top Defense Firms Under Criminal Investigation." The list of allegations included bribery, kickback, false claims, gratuities, bid rigging, cost mischarging, and product substitution. By mid 1988 the scandals in the defense department were headlined daily. In 1983 a *Washington Post* (28 November 1983), headline read: "GAO Investigates Social Science Grant Program." Here, it was reported that a social science grant program administered through the Office of Human Development Services let contracts for projects rated as the lowest of their class, but some highly ranked proposals were not funded. The potential for "impropriety" was under investigation to determine whether the selection process was tinged with favoritism or conflict of interest.

A major outcome of the Iran-Contra Operation by the Reagan administration was the privatization of American foreign policy according to many critics. Individual profit-oriented entrepreneurs with nominal checks and balances were negotiating exchanges and committing the American government to policy positions. "The result, the critics say, was a parallel government with its own treasury, air-force, envoys, communications network and chain of command, accountable to neither the State Department nor the Congress" (*New York Times,* 20 January 1987).

Frustrated by his government, the president contracted out several key foreign policy operations by converting the National Security Council into a quasi free-standing government. Even the most severe critics of government have not recommended contracting the military or foreign policy.

The message is very clear: When government fails to function as desired, try the private sector.

The above examples are but a few of a large number, nor are they limited to the federal government. Allegations about the New York and Washington, D.C., governments occur regularly in those same two newspapers. They serve to indicate that implementation problems have occurred within the government agency, the provider agencies, and in the relationship between the two. Not surprisingly, the highest number of allegations are found within the defense industry; the sheer volume of defense contracting and the relatively longer history with such arrangements would suggest a proportionately higher number of real or alleged incidents of wrongdoing. Contracting within the human services, however, has not been immune from "bad press." And although problems are also reported far more often than success stories (it is the nature of the American press), it may be fair to conclude that pragmatism, ideology, interests, and politics may have as much to do with the continuation and expansion of purchase of service as actual positive experiences.

The criticisms of, and problems with, contracting have led to some proposals to improve or modify the system. At the more conservative end, Congress has taken an active stance to revise federal procurement policies and procedures. Essentially, such changes would leave the purchase of service system intact, but tighten those aspects of the system that have been identified as problematic. More extreme is the 1986 declaration by the director of the Office of Personnel Management (OPM) that the "Reagan administration's efforts to contract out government services to private industry have failed" (Havemann, 1986). The OPM proposed that federal employees be given as much as 49 percent of the stock in new companies that provide the privatized services as a means by which to reduce opposition to contracting, open new opportunities for business, improve productivity, and save taxpayers' money. According to the OPM, the chief cause of the failure of privatization lies with the opposition of federal employees who are concerned that they will lose their jobs to contractors.

One option that has been suggested to the current POS system is to bypass agencies altogether and encourage contracting with individual private practitioners. An 23 August 1984 *Federal Register* announcement called for proposals for demonstration projects "to increase productivity and efficiency in the use of POS resources by use of performance contracting with individual private practitioners rather than with other public or non-profit agencies . . . the results should be able to provide local agencies with alternative approaches they could use for types of cases for which private clinicians are the preferred approach, the quality control and management approaches most effective, and the type of fiscal incentive methods that seem most able to insure desired outcomes at the preferred level of quality." The rationale offered for such demonstrations and potential applications is offered by the Office of Human Development Services in a delineation of the problems related to POS contracting. They cite as examples the lack of public agency control, inadequate monitoring of the contract agency, overly broad discretion for contract agency to select the type of client they will serve, and conflict of goals between the public and the contracted agency. Despite the search for alternatives, however, the resources, vested interests, and political popularity associated with purchase of service will likely perpetuate the current system.

PURCHASE OF SERVICE: LOOKING AHEAD

Despite positive statements of objectives and an underlying aura of support for purchase of service on the part of public and private officials, the latter part of the Carter administration and the Reagan administration tested prevailing assumptions and practices. The degree to which POS can withstand the exigencies of fiscal retrenchment and policy alterations has been put to the test.

Contracting arrangements have been significantly impacted by policy decisions made in Washington. For example, in one state purchase of service was a widely used practice to secure training for employees of public social service agencies. The federal government supplied 75 percent of total expenditures, with the contracted agencies providing a 25 percent match. When the available funds were reduced by approximately 50 percent in 1979, the state agency unilaterally terminated, within a one-month period, all its contracts, with one small exception. The state agency's own internal training operation, which consumed about 50 percent of the original allocation, was reduced slightly. In effect, the state agency's response to federal fiscal retrenchment was to preserve its internal resources while eliminating all of its contracts. Matters of competence, quality, efficiency, effectiveness, and other measures of outcome quickly became irrelevant. The bureaucracy protected its own. Contracting was designed to operate quickly, and it did so, even if in a negative way.

When contracting is initiated in a new service field, the public-private partnership may be on tenuous ground. Lacking entrenched interests to help secure future contracts, cost containment efforts may result in the termination of newer contract arrangements. For example, group-care homes, which received a great impetus as a result of deinstitutionalization in the late 1960s and 1970s, stimulated the development of private-sector operated, public-sector financed arrangements. Yet in 1982, barely a decade and a half after its beginning, the funding base was in jeopardy (Hart 1982).

Massachusetts may well be the major state user of contracts. In 1980 about 1,800 voluntary agencies were contractually involved with the

418

commonwealth. Of a sample of 400 studied provider agencies, over 270 (70 percent) had serious cash flow problems. Of those who were able to establish lines of credit, the average interest cost in 1980 exceeded seven thousand dollars per agency. Time devoted to cash flow management concerns created by the commonwealth's incapacity to manage itself effectively exceeded eighteen hours of executive time per week/per agency (Healy 1981).

In Massachusetts the State Rate Setting Commission had a curious practice that served to discourage contracted agencies from other fund raising activities. The commission deducted income generated from philanthropy from the service rate, a procedure designed to guarantee continuing dependence on the public agency, continuing cash flow problems, and reduced innovativeness, flexibility, financial contributions, and client services. (Following more than a decade of complaints, the provision was finally amended.)

The relative dependence of voluntary agencies on government contracts will, in large part, be affected by external stimuli, including the status of the general economy. The 1981 Economic Recovery Tax Act has had a mixed effect on giving by corporations. Since it reduced corporate tax rates and overall tax liability, the real cost of corporate contributions increased. In compensation it raised the maximum deduction for corporate contributions from 5 to 10 percent of pretax net income (Fosler 1981). The Tax Reform Act of 1986 promises to further substantially impair philanthropy. It has been predicted, for example, that the new tax law will result in a reduction of gifts of charity of $11.8 billion a year, representing a cut in giving of 20 percent. At the same time, the Reagan administration is urging nonprofit organizations to carry a larger share of the burden of financing human services (*Washington Post,* 4 February 1985).

The 1986 Tax Reform Law affects charitable giving in a number of ways. Beginning in 1987, no tax deductions for charitable donations were allowed on the short form of the IRS 1040 tax return. Although people do not give to causes of their choice solely due to tax considerations, such deductions are at least one important motivator. In a phase-in plan, maximum tax rates for individuals and corporations are also decreased. As a result, the tax "write-off" incentive for corporations and individuals who itemize is decreased. Changes also affect gifts of tangible personal property to public charities and gifts of appreciated property to private

419

foundations and alters the treatment of all revisionary trusts (Weithorn 1986).

In the face of such anticipated loss of fiscal resources, voluntary organizations are now faced with the very real and intractable dilemma of maintaining, if not increasing, the services offered with substantially fewer dollars. It would not be surprising if the voluntary sector was forced to rely even more heavily upon purchase of service arrangements.

Prospects. Given the widespread view that the public monopoly over selected services has been the major source of their undoing, a private monopoly should not be proposed as a replacement. Fortunately, separation of planning, financing, and monitoring from service delivery has several systemic virtues, role separation being the principal asset. Monopolies and vertical organizations are generally viewed with suspicion, if not disfavor. In combination, they are strongly ill-advised. Although separation of functions and role delegation appear to be one viable alternative to monopoly, Wedel (1976) appropriately notes that overdependence in the contractual relationship on the part of either partner appears to be undesirable. Striking a balance between autonomy and monopoly on the one hand and role delegation and dependence on the other is not a simple task. Clouding the picture are the array of external variables affecting purchase of service, as well as, separately, public and voluntary social welfare systems.

Bell (1967) described four major forces of change in the United States: (1) technological developments; (2) the diffusion of goods and privileges throughout our society; (3) structural changes, particularly the centralization of the political system and the husbanding of human capital; and (4) the relationship of the United States to all other countries.

The future of purchase of service would seem to be remarkably dependent on each of the propositions set forth by Bell. POS is a technology and concurrently is sensitive to other technological developments that impact on its effectiveness. To the degree that such arrangements are successful, they will enhance the diffusion of goods and services throughout our society. Certainly, the expansion of POS signifies structural changes in both the public and private sector. It offers the public administrator organizational flexibility and, when successful, utilizes human capital more successfully than available alternatives. POS is neutral with regard to the matter of political system centralization and is void of major foreign relations significance, although most of the major western countries are simi-

420

larly engaged. The International Monetary Fund Guidelines has now encouraged private investment and governmental budget reductions through privatization (*New York Times,* 4 October 1986). It thus appears that POS is internally consistent with most great forces of change in our society. Integration is feasible.

If left unhindered by major external variables, it is likely that the use of purchase of service arrangements will continue to grow throughout this century. There are, of course, potential barriers. Fear of job loss, loss of authority and control, lethargy, and a genuine fear of and antagonism to change are formidable foes. Even proponents of POS may not always be helpful to its growth. Having it claimed as an essential tool of privatization and then having privatization claimed by the political conservatives as ideologically pure will not sit well with those who define themselves otherwise. The bureaucrats who manage the contracts and who are generally linked and committed to their success have their own way of undermining these same positives. They tolerate the abuse by defense contractors and, at the same time, underbudget and overregulate the day-care providers, driving them into lower-quality programming and the use of less well-trained personnel. In both cases goals of efficiency and effectiveness are abused. Excesses of abuses may well lead to more serious consideration of alternatives.

Purchase of service remains a major financing and service delivery mechanism that represents an option to a purely public or private service delivery system. It suggests a blend of service providers, each doing what it is best able to do. Pluralism is an important underlining conceptual base by which to mold purchase of service arrangements. When clear, unequivocal answers are not available, alternative modes of delivery may be advisable. At such times, interorganizational relationships may take many forms, none of which is necessarily better than the other. Experience must be the judge as well as the particular consequences and preferences of the environment and actors involved. It may well be better that several alternative routes be attempted simultaneously.

In this search for more effective, efficient, and viable solutions to financing and delivering human services, it is important to recognize that all presently known options may be considered temporary in nature. It was disappointment with the results of public actions that caused a decided preferential shift to the private sector. Eventually, disenchantment with the performance of the private sector may emerge, and the cycle continues. Similarly, political ideology and fundamental beliefs about who should be doing what in this society are subject to change. The half century or so of politization in the Western world, as described by Drucker (1968), has led to the increased interest in privatization; the pendulum, however, may swing back, and we should expect new patterns to emerge in the future.

Arthur Schlesinger (1986) plots thirty-years cycles of alternating periods of conservatism and liberalism in our society. Practices based on private interests and retrenchment alternate with freedom, equality, and social responsibility. Lekachman (1987), examining the nation after Reagan, is much more pessimistic. He sees post-Reagan American as a playground for the rich, not an accomodating place for the vulnerable and poor. Among the phenomenon likely to continue to grow, according to Lekachman, will be privatization, a development he equates with unemployment, militarization, and the triumph of plutocracy.

In the meantime the realities of our political system, the policies set forth by our government, the preferences articulated by our human service administrators and managers and even the actions of the direct service workers will affect the future of purchase of service. Such arrangements have a strong past, a stronger present, and indications are that these trends will not soon abate.

422

Bibliography

Abell, D. F. 1980. *Defining the business: The starting point of strategic planning.* Englewood Cliffs, N.J.: Prentice-Hall.

Ahlbrandt, R. S., Jr. 1974. Implications of contracting for public services. *Urban Affairs Quarterly* 9:337–359.

Alm, R. 1986. When the government sells out. *U.S. News and World Report,* 10 November, 63–64.

Altman, S. H. 1986. *Will the medicare prospective payment system succeed? Technical adjustments can make the difference.* Berkeley: University of California, School of Public Health.

American Bar Association. 1980. *The model procurement code for state and local government.* Washington, D.C.

———. 1981. *Model procurement code for state and local government; Summary of legislative activity.* Washington, D.C.

American Psychiatric Association, Commission on Psychotherapies. 1982. *Psychotherapy research: Methodological and efficacy issues.* Washington, D.C.: American Psychiatric Association.

American Public Welfare Association. 1981. Administration seen shifting more services to private hands. *Washington Report,* June, 1.

———. 1981a. *A study of purchase of social services in selected states* (final report). Washington, D.C.

———. 1981b. Policy statement on social services. *Public Welfare* 39:44–46.

Anderson, W. F. et al., eds. 1972. *Managing human services.* Washington, D.C.: International City Management Association.

Anthony, R. N. and G. A. Welsch. 1981. *Fundamentals of management accounting.* Homewood, Ill: Richard D. Irwin.

Association for Children of New Jersey. 1983. Human services representative makes comments. *Newsletter* 6 (1):3.

Austin, D. 1982. Monitoring the impact of changes in social programs. In M. Gibelman (ed.), *Proceedings of an invitational symposium on evaluation and assessment in the human services: A progress report.* Washington, D.C.: National Conference on Social Welfare.

Avorn, J. 1984. Benefit and cost analysis in geriatric care. *New England Journal of Medicine* 310:1294–1301.

Baligh, H. H. and L. E. Richartz. 1967. *Vertical market structures.* Boston, Mass.: Allyn & Bacon.

Bartlett, H. M. 1970. *The common base of social work practice.* Washington, D.C.: National Association of Social Workers.

Bassoff, B. Z. and S. Ludwig. 1980. Interdisciplinary education for health care professionals. *Health and Social Work* 4:58–72.

Beck, B. 1971. Government contracts with the non-profit social welfare corporations. In B. L. R. Smith and D. C. Hague, eds., *The dilemma of accountability in modern government: Independence versus control.* N.Y.: St. Martins Press.

Bell, D. 1967. The year 2000. Trajectory of an idea. *Daedulus* 96:639–651.

Bell, W. G. and B. L. Bell. 1981. Monitoring the bureaucracy. In M. Mahaffey and J. W. Hanks, eds., *Practical politics: Social work and political responsibility.* Silver Spring, Md.: National Association of Social Workers.

Bendick, M., Jr. 1984. Privatization of public services: Recent experience. In H. Brooks, L. Liebman, and C. S. Schelling, eds., *Toward efficiency and effectiveness in the WIC delivery system.* Washington, D.C.: Urban Institute.

Bendick, M., Jr., T. H. Campbell, D. L. Bawden, and M. Jones. 1976. *Toward efficiency and effectiveness in the WIC delivery system.* Washington, D.C.: Urban Institute.

Benson, J. K. 1975. The interorganizational network as a political economy. *Administrative Science Quarterly* 20:229–249.

Benson, J. K. et al. 1973. *Coordinating human services: A sociological study of an interorganizational network.* Mo.: Regional Rehabilitation Research Institute.

Benton, B. B. 1981. Purchase of service: A management challenge for state government. *New England Journal of Human Services* 1:48,50.

Benton, B. B., R. Millar, and T. Feild. 1978. *Social Services: Federal legislation vs. state implementation.* Washington, D.C.: Urban Institute.

Berkowitz, S. 1963. Public subsidies of private programs. *Social Work* 8:106–108.

Bernstein, B. E. 1980. Lawyer and social worker as an interdisciplinary team. *Social Casework* 61:416–422.

Bienen, L. 1980. Rape III—National developments in rape reform legislation. *Women's Rights Law Reporter* 6:171–213.

Binner, P. R. 1980. Program evaluation. In S. Feldman, ed., *The administration of mental health services,* 2d ed. Springfield, Ill.: Charles Thomas Publisher.

Blacker, E. July 1983. Personal communication.

Bloom, B. L. and H. J. Parad. 1976. Interdisciplinary functioning: A survey of attitudes and practices in community mental health. *American Journal of Orthopsychiatry* 46:669–677.

Booz-Allen and Hamilton. 1971. *Purchase of service: Study of the experiences of three states in purchase of service under the provision of the 1967 amendments to the Social Security Act.* Washington, D.C.: U.S. Department of Health, Education, and Welfare, Social and Rehabilitation Services.

Boston Sunday Globe, 12 June 1985; 22 December 1985.

Boulding, K. E. 1973. Intersects: The peculiar organizations. In Conference Board, ed., *Challenge to leadership.* N.Y.: Free Press.

Bowers, G. E. and M. R. Bowers. 1976. *The elusive unit of service.* Human Services Monograph Series, no. 1 (Sept.). Rockville, Md.: Project Share.

Bracht, N. F. and S. Briar. 1979. Collaboration between schools of social work and university medical centers. *Health and Social Work* 4:72–91.

Branch, L. G. 1978. *Boston elders: A survey of needs.* Boston, Mass.: Commission on Affairs of the Elderly, Area Agency on Aging, Region VI.

Brilliant, E. 1973. Private or public: A model of ambiguities. *Social Service Review* 47:384–396.

Brintnall, M. 1981. Caseloads, performance, and street-level bureaucracy. *Urban Affairs Quarterly* 16:281–298.

Brodyaga, L. et al. 1975. *Rape and its victims: A report for citizens, health facilities and criminal justice agencies*. Washington, D.C.: National Institute of Law Enforcement and Criminal Justice.

Bromley, D. G. and F. J. Weed. 1978. The vanishing sociology-social work alliance: A study in the politics of professionalism. *Journal of Sociology and Social Welfare* 5:168–187.

Brown, J. 1940. *Public relief, 1929–1939*. N.Y.: Henry Holt & Co.

Burian, W. 1970. *Purchase of service in child welfare: A problem of interorganizational exchange*. Ph.D. diss., University of Chicago.

Burns, E. M. 1956. *Social security and public policy*. N.Y.: Columbia University Press.

Buttrick, S. M. 1970. On choices and services. *Social Service Review* 44:427–433.

Caine, L. V. 1983. Letter to the editor. *Chronicle of Higher Education* (6 April):34.

California Tax Foundation. 1981. *Contracting out local government services in California*. Sacramento, Calif.

Capoccia, V. A. 1978. *Public planning for social services: An analysis of the design of social service delivery systems under the Title XX amendments to the Social Security Act of 1974*. Ph.D. diss., Brandeis University, Waltham, Mass.

Carr, J. J. 1979. An administrative retrospective on police crisis teams. *Social Casework* 60:416–422.

Center for Women Policy Studies, The Resource Center on Domestic Violence 1980. *Federally funded projects on domestic violence*. Rockville, Md.: National Clearinghouse for Domestic Violence.

Center, L. J. 1979. *Summary report: Evaluation of the national elderly victimization prevention and assistance program*. Washington, D.C.: National Council of Senior Citizens.

Chelimsky, E. 1981. Making block grants accountable. In E. R. House, S. Amthison, J. A. Pearsol, and H. Preskill, eds., *Evaluation Studies Review Annual* 7:633–664.

Children's Defense Fund. 1978. *Children without homes*. Washington, D.C.

Christianson, J., D. Hillman, and K. Smith. 1983. The Arizona experiment: Competitive bidding for indigent medical care. *Health Affairs* 2:88–103.

Chronicle of Higher Education, 10 July 1985.

Chu, F. D. and S. Trotter. 1974. *The madness establishment*. N.Y.: Grossman.

Cicchetti, D. and J. L. Aber. 1980. Abused children-abusive parents: An overstated case. *Harvard Educational Review* 50:244–254.

Citizen participation in urban renewal. 1966. *Columbia Law Review* 66:485–607.

Clark, R. C. 1980. Does the nonprofit form fit the hospital industry? *Harvard Law Review* 93:1416–1489.

Clearinghouse on Child Abuse and Neglect. 1986. *Discretionary and state discretionary grants: profiles for fiscal year 1985.* Washington, D.C.: National Center for Child Abuse and Neglect.

Clotfelter, C. T. and C. E. Steuerle. 1981. Charitable contributions. In H. Aaron and J. Pechman, eds., *How taxes affect economic behavior.* Washington, D.C.: Brookings Institution.

Cloward, R. A. and I. Epstein. 1965. Private social welfare's disengagement from the poor: The case of family adjustment agencies. In M. N. Zald, ed., *Social welfare institutions: A sociological reader.* N.Y.: John Wiley & Sons.

Cohen, H. 1980. *You can negotiate anything.* Secaucus, N.J.: Lyle Stuart.

Cole, E. P. 1970. Voluntary agencies in the purchase of care and services. In I. R. Winogrand, ed., *Purchase of care and services in the health and welfare fields.* Milwaukee: University of Wisconsin School of Social Welfare.

Comprehensive Employment and Training Act, 87 *stat* 839. 28 December 1983.

———. (a), 87 *stat* 839, sec. 105(a)1(D), 28 December, 1983.

———. (b), 87 *stat* 839, sec. 105(a)3(A). 28 December, 1983.

Comptroller General. 1979. *Grant auditing: A maze of inconsistency, gaps, and duplication that needs overhauling.* Report to the Congress by the comptroller general of the U.S. Washington, D.C.: Government Printing Office, 15 June.

———. 1982. *Less sole source: More competition needed in federal civil agencies contracting*, PLRD 82.40. Washington, D.C.: Government Printing Office.

Cook, F. L. et al. 1981. *Setting and reformulating policy agendas: The case of criminal victimization of the elderly.* N.Y.: Oxford University Press.

Cook, K. S. 1977. Exchange and power in networks of interorganizational relations. *Sociological Quarterly* 18:62–82.

Cooper, P. 1980. Government contracts in public administration. *Public Administration Review* 40:459–468.

Copeland, W. C. 1976. *Audit-proof contracting for federal money for children's services.* Washington, D.C.: CWLA Hecht Institute for State Child Welfare Planning.

Coughlin, B. J. 1961. Private social welfare in a public welfare bureaucracy. *Social Service Review* 35:184–193.

———. 1965. *Church and state in social welfare.* N.Y.: Columbia University Press.

Courant, P. N., E. M. Gramlich, and D. L. Rubinfeld. 1981. Why voters support tax limitation amendments: The Michigan case. In H. F. Ladd and T. N. Tideman, eds., *Tax and expenditure limitations.* Washington, D.C.: Urban Institute.

Cowen, E. L. 1978. Some problems in community program evaluation research. *Journal of Consulting and Clinical Psychology* 46:792–805.

Cruthirds, C. T., Jr. 1972. *The community action program agency and voluntary delegate organizations: Issues in interorganizational contracting.* Ph.D. diss., Tulane University, New Orleans.

Davidson, R. H. 1972. *The politics of comprehensive manpower legislation.* Baltimore, Md.: Johns Hopkins Press.

Davis, K. and C. Schoen. 1978. *Health and the war on poverty: A ten year appraisal*. Washington, D.C.: Brookings Institution.

De Alessi, L. 1980. The economics of property rights: A review of the evidence. In R. O. Zerbe, ed., *Research in Law and Economics*, vol. 2. Greenwich, Conn.: JAI Press.

deHoog, R. H. 1984. *Contracting out for human services*. Albany: State University of New York Press.

Demone, H. W., Jr. and M. Gibelman. 1983. Alternative service delivery strategies: Factors in states' decision making. *Journal of Sociology and Social Welfare* 10:326–338.

Demone, H. W., Jr., and H. C. Schulberg. 1984. Human services and health administration education: Management development issues. *Journal of Health Administration Education* 3:186–211.

Department of Social Services. 1985. *Fiscal year 1986 budget request*. Commonwealth of Massachusetts.

Derthick, M. 1975. *Uncontrollable spending for social service grants*. Washington, D.C.: Brookings Institution.

Dinkel, N. R., J. W. Zinober, and E. W. Flaherty. 1981. Citizen participation in community mental health center program evaluation: A neglected potential. *Community Mental Health Journal* 17:45–65.

Donabedian, A. 1980. *The definition of quality and approaches to its assessment*, vol. 1. Ann Arbor, Mich.: Health Administration Press.

Dorwart, R. A. and W. R. Meyers. 1981. *Citizen participation in mental health*. Springfield, Ill.: Charles C. Thomas.

Dorwart, R. A., M. Schlesinger, and R. T. Pulice. Forthcoming. Privatizing public mental health care: The case of purchase of service contracting in Massachusetts. *Hospital and Community Psychiatry*.

Dowling, W. L. 1974. Prospective reimbursement of hospitals. *Inquiry* 11.

Drucker, P. F. 1968. *The age of discontinuity*. N.Y.: Harper & Row.

Dunn, R. 1981. *Public policy analysis*. Englewood Cliffs, N.J.: Prentice-Hall.

Edwards, S., B. Benton, R. Millar and T. Feild. 1978. *The purchase of service and Title XX*, Working Paper 0990–18. Washington, D.C.: Urban Institute.

Edwards, G. C., III, and I. Sharkansky. 1978. *The policy predicament*. San Francisco: W. W. Freeman.

Elazar, D. 1962. *The American partnership*. Chicago, Ill.: University of Chicago Press.

Elkin, R. 1980. *A human service manager's guide to developing unit costs*. Falls Church, Va.: Institute for Informational Studies.

Emerson, R. 1962. Power-dependence relations. *American Sociological Review* 27:31–41.

Endicott, J. and R. L. Spitzer. 1976. Clinical evaluation of patient outcome. In E. W. Markson and D. F. Allen, eds., *Trends in mental health evaluation*. Lexington, Mass.: Lexington Books.

Etzioni, A. 1972. The untapped potential of the "third sector." *Business and Society Review*: 39–44.

427

———. 1975. Alternative conceptions of accountability: The example of health administration. *Public Administration Review* 35:279–286.

Evan, W. 1966. The organization-set: Toward a theory of interorganizational relations. In J. Thompson, ed., *Approaches to organization design*. Pittsburgh: University of Pittsburgh Press.

———. 1972. An organization-set model of interorganizational relations. In M. Tuite, R. Chisholm, and M. Radnor, eds., *Interorganization decision making*. Ill.: Aldine Publishing.

Family Violence Prevention and Services Act of 1984. *P.L.* 98–457.

Fanshel, D. and E. Shinn. 1978. *Children in foster care: A longitudinal investigation*. N.Y.: Columbia University Press.

Federal Register, 15 July 1983; 23 August 1984.

Fein, R. 1977. But on the other hand: High blood pressure, economics, and equity. *New England Journal of Medicine* 296:751–753.

Feine, R. 1981. *A conceptual framework for monitoring children's services*. Washington, D.C.: Children's Services Monitoring Consortium.

Fiene, R. and M. G. Nixon. 1981. *An instrument-based program monitoring system: A new tool for day care monitoring*. Washington, D.C.: Children's Services Monitoring Consortium.

Fine, S. H. 1981a. *A concept sector in the economy*. Paper presented at the joint conference of the American Marketing Association/European Society of Opinion and Marketing Research: Paris, France.

———. 1981b. *The marketing of ideas and social issues*. N.Y.: Praeger.

Fisher, R. and W. Ury. 1983. *Getting to yes*. N.Y.: Penguin Books.

Fisk, D., H. Kiesling, and T. Mueller. 1978. *Private provision of public services: An overview*. Washington, D.C.: Urban Institute.

Fitch, L. C. 1974. Increasing the role of the private sector in providing public services. In W. D. Hawley and D. Rogers, eds., *Improving the quality of urban management*. Beverly Hills, Calif.: Sage.

Florestano, P. S. and S. B. Gordon. 1980. Public vs. private: Small government contracting with the private sector. *Public Administration Review* 40:29–34.

Folks, H. 1902. *The care of destitute, neglected and delinquent children*. N.Y.: Macmillan.

Forman, L. H. 1976. Physician and the social worker. *American Family Physician* 13:40–93.

Fosler, S. 1981. Public and private roles in providing community services. *Congressional Record*, S15778–S15781, 16 December.

Fottler, M. 1981. Is management really generic? *Academy of Management Review* 6:1–12.

Frank, R. G. 1981. Cost-benefit analysis in mental health services: A review of the literature. *Administration in Mental Health* 8:161–176.

Frankfather, D. L. 1981. Welfare entrepreneurialism and the politics of innovation. *Social Service Review* 55:129–146.

Freedman, R. I. and A. Moran. 1984. Wanderers in a promised land: The chronically mentally ill and deinstitutionalization. *Medical Care* 22:12, Special supplement.

Frieden, B. and M. Kaplan. 1976. *Community development and the model cities legacy* (working paper no. 42). Cambridge, Mass.: Joint Center for Urban Studies of MIT and Harvard University.

Frost, P. J. 1978. On the folly of rewarding "A" while hoping for "B." In P. J. Frost, ed., *Organizational Reality*. Santa Monica, Calif.: Goodyear Publishing.

Garrick, M. A. and W. L. Moore. 1979. Uniform assessments and standards of social and health care services. *Social Service Review* 53:343–357.

Gates, B. L. 1980. *Social program administration: The implementation of public policy*. Englewood Cliffs, N.J.: Prentice-Hall.

Geiser, R. 1973. *The illusion of caring: Children in foster care*. Boston, Mass.: Beacon Press.

Geissler, E. M. 1965. When you eye public money. *YMCA Magazine*. May:9ff.

General Accounting Office. 1982a. *Civilianizing certain Air Force positions could result in economies and better use of military personnel* (Acc. No. 119163). Washington, D.C.: Government Printing Office.

———. 1982b. *NSF experiment with research grant administration promising changes needed to assure accountability* (Acc. no. 119421). Washington, D.C.: Government Printing Office.

———. 1984. *States use several strategies to cope with funding reductions under social services block grant* (Report no. GAO/HRD 84–69–8). Washington, D.C.: Government Printing Office.

Ghezzi, S. G. 1983. A private network of social controls: Insurance investigation units. *Social Problems* 30:521–531.

Gibelman, M. 1980. Title XX purchase of services: Some speculations about service provision to the poor. *Urban and Social Change Review* 13:9–14.

———. 1981. Are clients served better when services are purchased? *Public Welfare* 39:26–33.

Gibelman, M. and N. Humphreys. 1982. Contracting for educational services: The impact on schools of social work. *Journal of Continuing Social Work Education* 2:3–10.

Gil, D. G. 1970. *Violence against children: Physical abuse in the United States*. Cambridge, Mass.: Harvard University Press.

———. 1976. *The challenge of social equality*. Cambridge, Mass.: Schenkman.

Gilbert, N. 1977. The transformation of social services. *Social Service Review* 51:624–641.

———. 1983. *Capitalism and the welfare state: Dilemmas of social benevolence*. New Haven, Conn.: Yale University Press.

Ginsburg, S. G. 1981. Negotiating budgets: Games people play. *Inc.* (September).

Giovannoni, J. 1982. *Perspectives on the purchase of services from the public and private sectors*. Report to the Region IX Child Welfare Training Center. Los Angeles: University of California at Los Angeles.

Glaser, W. and D. Sills, eds. 1966. *The government of associations*. Totowa, N.J.: Bedminster Press.

Glass, G. V., B. McGaw, and M. L. Smith. 1981. *Meta-analysis in social research.* Beverly Hills, Calif.: Sage.

Goodsell, C. T. 1983. *The case for bureaucracy.* Chatham, N.J.: Chatham House.

Government Employees Council, AFL-CIO. 1962. Presentation of the Government Employees Council, AFL-CIO to the Executive Branch in Reference to Bureau of the Budget Bulletin. Washington, D.C.

Gramlich, E. M. and P. P. Koshel. 1975. *Educational performance contracting. An evaluation of an experiment.* Washington, D.C.: Brookings Institution.

Green, J. W. 1978. The role of cultural anthropology in the education of service personnel. *Journal of Sociology and Social Welfare* 5:214–229.

Greenblatt, B. 1977. *Responsibility for child care.* San Francisco: Jossey-Bass.

Greenley, J. R. and S. A. Kirk. 1973. Organizational characteristics of agencies and the distribution of services to applicants. *Journal of Health and Social Behavior* 14:70–79.

Gundersdorg, J. 1977. Management and financial control. In W. F. Anderson, B. J. Frieden, and M. J. Murphy, eds., *Managing human services.* Washington, D.C.: International City Management Association.

Gurin, A. and B. Friedman. 1980. *Contracting for services as a mechanism for the delivery of human services: A study of contracting practices in three human service agencies in Massachusetts.* Waltham, Mass.: Brandeis University, The Florence Heller School for Advanced Studies in Social Welfare.

Guttman, D. and B. Willner. 1976. *The shadow government: The government's multi-billion dollar giveaway of its decision-making powers to private management consultants, "experts," and think tanks.* N.Y.: Pantheon Books.

Hall, R. and J. Clark. 1974. Problems in the study of interorganizational relationships. *Organizations and Administrative Science* 5:45–60.

Hall, R. et al. 1977. Patterns of interorganizational relationships. *Administrative Science Quarterly* 22:457–474.

Hamlin, R. 1963. *Voluntary health and welfare agencies in the United States.* N.Y.: Schoolmasters' Press.

Hamos, J. E. 1980. *State domestic laws and how to pass them: A manual for lobbyists.* Domestic Violence Monograph Series 2. Rockville, Md.: National Clearinghouse on Domestic Violence.

Hanrahan, J. D. 1977. *Government for sale: Contracting out, the new patronage.* Washington, D.C.: The American Federation of State, County, and Municipal Employees.

Hart, A. F. 1982. Uneasy public-private partnerships for social services: Massachusetts as a case in point. *Conference Bulletin, National Conference on Social Welfare* 85:13ff.

Hartman, A. 1979. *Finding families: An ecological approach to family assessment in adoption.* Beverly Hills, Calif.: Sage.

Hartogs, N. and J. Weber. 1978. *Impact of government funding on the management of voluntary agencies.* N.Y.: Greater New York Fund/United Way.

———. 1979. *Managing government funded programs in voluntary agencies.* N.Y.: Greater New York Fund/United Way.

430

Hasenfeld, Y. 1972. People processing organizations: An exchange approach. *American Sociological Review* 37:256–263.

Hatry, H. P. 1982. *Alternative service delivery approaches involving increased use of the private sector.* Unpublished manuscript. Washington, D.C.: Urban Institute.

————. 1983. *A review of private approaches for delivery of public services.* Washington, D.C.: Urban Institute.

Hatry, H. P. and E. Durman. 1985. *Issues in competitive contracting for social services.* Falls Church, Va.: National Institute of Governmental Purchasing.

Havighurst, C. C. 1970. Health maintenance organizations and the market for health services. *Journal of Law and Contemporary Problems* 35:716–734.

Healy, J. R. 1981. Purchase of service: A management challenge for state government. *New England Journal of Human Services* 1:51–52.

Hekman, E. L. 1984. *State efforts at health care cost containment.* Denver: National Conference of State Legislatures.

Heller, K., R. H. Price, and K. J. Sher. 1980. Research and evaluation in primary prevention: Issues and guidelines. In R. H. Price, R. F. Ketterer, B. C. Bader, and J. Monahan, eds., *Prevention in mental health: Research, policy, and practice,* vol. 1. Beverly Hills, Calif.: Sage.

Herman, M. 1979. Purchase of service contracting: Promise or threat to social agencies? In K. R. Wedel, A. J. Katz, and A. Weick, eds., *Social services by government contract: A policy analysis.* N.Y.: Praeger.

Hewes, L. I. et al. 1979. Issues and problems of voluntary social service organizations in federal assistance. In *Managing Federal Assistance in the 1980's.* Washington, D.C.: Office of Management and Budget.

Hiestand, O. W. 1979. Blueprint for improving public procurement. *Contract Management* 19:6–9.

Hill, W. G. 1971. Voluntary and governmental financial transactions. *Social Casework* 52:356–361.

Hilman, A. 1960. *Neighborhood centers today: Programs for a rapidly changing world.* N.Y.: National Federation of Settlements.

Hinderlang, M. J. 1976. *Criminal victimization in eight American cities: A descriptive analysis of common theft and assault.* Cambridge, Mass.: Ballinger.

Hirschman, A. 1974. Exit, voice and loyalty: Further reflections and a survey of recent contributions. *Social Science Information* 13:7–26.

Hoffman, E. 1979. Policy and politics: The child abuse prevention and treatment act. In R. Bourne and E. Newberger, eds., *Critical perspectives on child abuse.* Lexington, Mass.: Lexington Books.

Holmes, D., J. Teresi, and M. Holmes. 1983. Differences among black, hispanic and white people in knowledge about long-term care services. *Health Care Financing Review* 5:51–67.

Horn, L. and E. Griesel. 1977. *Nursing homes: A citizen's action guide.* Boston, Mass.: Beacon Press.

Hoshino, G. 1979. Correspondence to Leonard Schneiderman, Chairman, NASW Task Force on Social Services, 8 October.

———. 1982. Local welfare departments: What is their future role? *Human Development News*, April.

Housing and Community Development Act of 1974, 88 *stat* 633, sec. 104(b)(2), 22 August (a).

———. 88 *stat* 633, sec. 101(c)(4), 22 August, (b).

Iglehart, J. K. 1985. Medicare turns to HMOs. *New England Journal of Medicine* 312:132–137.

Isler, M. L. 1981. Policy implications: Moving from research to programs. In R. L. Struyk and M. Bendick, Jr., eds., *Housing vouchers for the poor: Lessons from a national experiment*. Washington, D.C.: Urban Institute.

Jacobs, D. 1974. Dependency and vulnerability: An exchange approach to the control of organizations. *Administrative Science Quarterly* 19:45–59.

James, L., Jr. 1980. *Department of social services 1980 quality assurance report*. Wisconsin: Milwaukee County Department of Social Services.

Jansson, B. S. 1975. *Politics of selected children's programs*. Ph.D. diss., University of Chicago.

———. 1979. Public monitoring of contracts with nonprofit organizations: Organizational mission in two sectors. *Journal of Sociology and Social Welfare* 6:362–374.

———. 1980. Policy dissonance and executive preferences: Implications for reform. *Administration in Mental Health* 7:175–186.

———. 1982. Ecology of preventive services. *Social Work Research and Abstracts* 18:14–22.

Johnson, A. 1959. Public funds for voluntary agencies. *Social Welfare Forum*. N.Y.: Columbia University Press.

Kahn, A. J. 1972. Public social services: The next phase. *Public Welfare* 30: 15–25.

———. 1973. *Social policy and social services*. N.Y.: Random House.

Kamerman, S. B. 1983. The new mixed economy of welfare. *Social Work* 28:5–10.

Kamerman, S. B. and A. J. Kahn. 1976. *Social services in the United States: Policies and programs*. Philadelphia: Temple University Press.

Katz, A. J. 1979. Quality of service professionalism and the purchase of service factor. In K. R. Wedel, A. J. Katz, and A. Weick, eds., *Social service by government contract: A policy analysis*. N.Y.: Praeger.

Kempe, C. H. and R. E. Helfer, eds. 1972. *Helping the battered child and his family*. Philadelphia: J. B. Lippincott.

Kettner, P. M. and L. C. Martin. 1985. Issues in the development of monitoring systems for purchase of service contracting. *Administration in Social Work* 9:69–82.

———. 1987. *Purchase of service contracting*. Beverly Hills, Calif.: Sage.

Kimmich, M. H. 1985. *America's children: Who cares?* Washington, D.C.: Urban Institutes.

Klein, F. 1977. Developing new models: Rape crisis centers. *Feminist Alliance Against Rape*, July–August.

Kramer, R. M. 1964. *An analysis of policy issues in relationships between governmental and voluntary social welfare agencies.* Ph.D. diss., University of California at Berkeley.

———. 1966. Voluntary agencies and the use of public funds: Some policy issues. *Social Service Review* 40:15–26.

———. 1979. Public fiscal policy and voluntary agencies in welfare states. *Social Service Review* 53:1–14.

———. 1981. *Voluntary agencies in the welfare state.* Berkeley: University of California Press.

Kramer, R. M. and P. Terrell. 1982. *Human service contracting in the San Francisco Bay Area.* Berkeley: Institute of Governmental Studies, University of California Press.

Krause, E. A. 1977. *Power and illness: The political sociology of health and medical care.* N.Y.: Elsevier.

Kupers, T. A. 1981. *Public therapy.* N.Y.: Free Press.

Landsberg, G., R. Hammer, and W. Neigher. 1978. *Analyzing the evaluation activities in CMHCs in NIMH Region II.* Paper presented at the 1978 annual meeting of the National Council of Community Mental Health Centers, Kansas City, Mo.

Largen, M. A. 1981. Personal interview with Susan Freinkel, 25 February.

Lave, J. R. and L. B. Lave. 1974. *The hospital construction act.* Washington, D.C.: American Enterprise Institute.

Leaning, J. 1983. The national seashore as motel owner. *Cape Cod Business Journal* (July):8, 10–11.

LeGrand, J. and R. Robinson, eds. 1984. *Privatisation and the welfare state.* London: George Allen & Unwin.

Lekachman, R. 1987. *America after Reagan.* N.Y.: Macmillan.

Levenson, R. 1977. Can private social services substitute for public employees? *Public Personnel Management,* 139–148.

Levy, R. L., R. Lambert, and G. Davis. 1979. Social work and dentistry in clinical, training and research collaboration. *Social Work in Health Care* 5:177–185.

Litwak, E. et al. 1970. *Towards the multi-factor theory and practice of linkages between formal organizations.* Washington, D.C.: U.S. Department of Health, Education, and Welfare.

Litwak, E. and H. J. Meyer. 1966. A balanced theory of coordination between bureaucratic organizations and community primary groups. *Administrative Science Quarterly* 11:35–58.

Los Angeles Times, 14 December 1982; 10 December 1982.

Lourie, N. V. 1979. Purchase of service contracting: Issues confronting the government-sponsored agency. In K. R. Wedel, A. J. Katz, and A. Weick, eds., *Social services by government contract: A policy analysis.* N.Y.: Praeger.

Lowe, J. L. and M. Herranen. 1984. Conflict in teamwork: Understanding roles and relationships. *Social Work in Health Care.*

Lowi, T. 1969. *End of liberalism.* N.Y.: Norton.

Luft, H. 1984. On the use of vouchers for medicare. *Milbank Memorial Fund Quarterly* 62:237–250.

Lurie, A. 1977. Social work in health care in the next ten years. *Social Work in Health Care* 2:419–428.

Majone, G. 1984. Professionalism and nonprofit organizations. *Journal of Health Politics, Policy and Law* 8:639–659.

Manser, G. 1974. Further thoughts on purchase of service. *Social Casework* 55: 421–427.

Mansfield, H. C. 1971. Independence and accountability for federal contractors and grantees. In B. L. R. Smith and D. C. Hague, eds., *The dilemma of accountability in modern government.* N.Y.: St. Martin's Press.

Marmor, T. R. and J. A. Morone. 1980. Representing consumer interests: Imbalanced markets, health planning, and the HSAs. *Milbank Memorial Fund Quarterly* 58.

Marmor, T. R., M. Schlesinger, and R. W. Smithey. Forthcoming. Nonprofit organizations and health care. In W. W. Powell, ed., *Between the public and private: The nonprofit sector.* New Haven Conn.: Yale University Press.

Massachusetts Taxpayer's Foundation. 1980. *Purchase of service: Can state government gain control?* Boston, Mass.

McLaughlin, C. P. 1978. Productivity and effectiveness in government. In J. Sutherland, ed., *Management handbook for public administrators.* N.Y.: Van Nostrand Reinhold.

McNeil, R. and R. Schenkler. 1975. HMOs, competition and government. *Milbank Memorial Fund Quarterly* 53:195–224.

Mencher, S. 1967. *Poor law to poverty program.* Pittsburgh: University of Pittsburgh Press.

Mermelstein, R. 1983. Cutting health care costs in California. *Law, Medicine and Health Care* 11:177–181.

Meyers, W. R. 1981. *The evaluation enterprise.* San Francisco: Jossey-Bass.

Miller, L. and R. Pruger. 1978. Evaluation in care programs: With illustrations in homemaker-chore in California. *Administration in Social Work* (Winter) 2: 469–478.

Miller, S. M., A. A. de Vos van Steenwijk, and P. Roby. 1970. Creaming the poor. *Transaction* (June) 7:39–45.

Mindlin, S. E. and H. Aldrich. 1975. Interorganizational dependence: A review of the concepts and a re-examination of the findings of the Ashton Group. *Administrative Science Quarterly*, 382–392.

Mintor, E. 1965. Voluntary and public relationships in family service. *Social Work Practice*, 41–54. N.Y.: Columbia University Press.

Mirengoff, W. 1976. *The comprehensive employment and training act.* Washington, D.C.: National Academy of Sciences.

Mollica, R. 1983. From asylum to community: The threatened disintegration of public psychiatry. *New England Journal of Medicine* 308:367–373.

Moore, J. 1986. Personal interview, 11 July.

Moreland Act Commission. 1976. *Long term care regulation: Past lapses, future prospects.* Summary report of the New York State Commission on Nursing Homes and Residential Facilities. Albany: State of New York.

Morris, R. and P. Youket. 1981. The long-term care issue: Identifying the problems and potential solutions. In J. J. Callahan and S. S. Wallack, eds., *Reforming the long-term care system.* Lexington, Mass.: Lexington.

Musolf, L. V. and H. Seidman. 1980. The blurred boundaries of public administration. *Public Administration Review* 40:124–130.

Nader, R. 1976. Introduction to *The Shadow Government.* D. Guttman and B. Willner. N.Y.: Pantheon Books.

Nagi, S. Z. 1974. Gate-keeping decisions in service organizations: When validity fails. *Human Organization* 33:47–58.

Nathan, R. et al. 1977. *Bloc grants for community development.* Washington, D.C.: Government Printing Office.

National Commission on Children in Need of Parents. 1979. *Who knows? Who cares? Forgotten children in foster care.* N.Y.: Institute of Public Affairs.

National Institutes of Health. 1982. *Guide for grants and contracts* 11 (5 November): 3. Washington, D.C.

Nelson, B. J. 1978. Purchase from the private sector: Technique and theory. *Productivity improvement handbook for state and local governments.* N.Y.: John Wiley.

Nelson, R. and M. Kranshinsky. 1973. Two major issues of public policy: Public subsidy and organization of supply. In D. Young and R. Nelson, eds., *Public policy for day care of young children.* Lexington, Mass.: Lexington.

Neugeboren, B. 1970. *Psychiatric clinics: A typology of service patterns.* Metuchen, N.J.: Scarecrow Press.

Newman, E. and J. Turem. 1974. The crisis of accountability. *Social Work* 19:5–12.

New York Times, 23 November 1979; 20 September 1980; 5 October 1980; 13 October 1980; 19 June 1981; 31 August 1981; 19 October 1981; 30 November 1981; 3 April 1982; 20 June 1982; 6 March 1983; 6 June 1983; 12 June 1983; 14 November 1983; 11 March 1985; 28 April 1985; 28 May 1985; 2 February 1986; 15 February 1986; 4 October 1986; 7 December 1986; 20 January 1987; 15 February 1987.

Nielson, W. E. 1979. *The endangered sector.* N.Y.: Columbia University Press.

Nierenburg, G. I. 1973. *Fundamentals of negotiating.* N.Y.: Hawthorne Books.

O'Connell, B. 1976. Accepting tax dollars. Voluntary agencies must ask: What price independence? *Foundation News* (July/August):16–20.

Office of Human Development Services, Administration for Public Services. 1976. *Social services, USA* (DHHS). Washington, D.C.: Government Printing Office.

Office of Management and Budget. 1979. Uniform administrative requirements for grants-in-aid to state and local government, Circular A–102. *Federal Register* (October 22) 44:205.

Office of Personnel Administration. 1979. Title 5, *Code of Federal Regulations* (Part 900, Subpart F), 44 (34), February 16. Washington, D.C.: Government Printing Office.

Office of Technology Assessment (U.S. Congress). 1978. *Assessing the efficacy and safety of medical technologies.* Washington, D.C.: Government Printing Office.

———. 1980a. *Methodological issues and literature review.* Background paper no. 1 to the implications of cost-effectiveness analysis of medical technology. Washington, D.C.: Government Printing Office.

———. 1980b. *The efficacy and cost effectiveness of psychotherapy.* Background paper no. 3 to the implications of cost-effectiveness analysis of medical technology. Washington, D.C.: Government Printing Office.

Office of the Secretary, U.S. Department of Health and Human Services, OHDS. 1980. *Annual Report to the Congress on Title XX of the Social Security Act, Fiscal Year 1979.* Washington, D.C.: Government Printing Office.

———. 1981. *Annual Report to the Congress on Title XX of the Social Security Act, Fiscal Year 1980.* Washington, D.C.: Government Printing Office.

Oleck, H. 1971. Proprietary mentality and the new nonprofit corporation laws. *Cleveland State Law Review* 20:145–168.

Orlans, H., ed. 1980. *Non-profit organizations: A government management tool.* N.Y.: Praeger Publishers.

O'Sullivan, E. 1978. What has happened to rape crisis centers? A look at their structure, members and funding. *Victimology: An International Journal* 3: 45–62.

Ostrom, V. 1974. *The intellectual crisis in American public administration.* University, Ala.: University of Alabama Press.

Pacific Consultants. 1979. *Title XX purchase of service: A description of states' service delivery and management practices.* Washington, D.C.: U.S. Department of Health, Education, and Welfare, Administration for Public Services.

Pacific Consultants. 1979. *Title XX purchase of service: The feasibility of comparing costs between direct delivery and purchased services.* Washington, D.C.: U.S. Department of Health, Education, and Welfare, Administration for Public Services.

Palmer, J. L. and I. V. Sawhill. 1982. Perspectives on the Reagan experiment. In J. L. Palmer and I. V. Sawhill, eds., *The Reagan experiment.* Washington, D.C.: Urban Institute.

Pelton, L. 1981a. Child abuse and neglect: The myth of classlessness. In L. Pelton, ed., *The social context of child abuse and neglect.* N.Y.: Human Sciences Press.

———. 1981b. *Situational influences, personalistic attributions, and client perspectives in child welfare cases.* Unpublished manuscript. Trenton, N.J.

Pennings, J. 1980. *Interlocking directorates.* San Francisco: Jossey-Bass.

Perlmutter, F. 1971. Public funds and private agencies. *Child Welfare* 50:264–270.

Perrow, C. 1961. Goals in complex organizations. *American Sociological Review* 26:854–865.

Pfeffer, J. and G. Salancik. 1978. *The external control of organizations: A resource dependence perspective.* N.Y.: Harper & Row.

Phillips, M. H. 1978. The communication school: A partnership between a school and child welfare agency. *Child Welfare* 57:83–91.

Physicians' Task Force on Hunger in America. 1985. *Hunger in America: The growing epidemic.* Boston, Mass.: Harvard University School of Public Health.

Porter, D. O. and D. C. Warner. 1973. How effective are grantor controls? The case of federal aid to education. In K. E. Boulding, M. Plaff, and A. Plaff, eds., *Transfers In an Urbanized Economy.* Belmont, Calif.: Wadsworth.

Pressman, J. L. and A. B. Waldavsky. 1973. *Implementation.* Berkeley: University of California Press.

Proven, K., J. Beyer, and C. Kruytbosch. 1980. Environmental linkages and power in resource-dependence relations between organizations. *Administrative Science Quarterly* 25:200–225.

Pruger, R. and L. Miller. 1973. Competition and the public social services. *Public Welfare* 31:16– 25.

Purcell, F. P. 1964. The helping professions and the problems of the brief contact in low income areas. In F. Riessman, J. Cohen, and A. Pearl, eds., *Mental health of the poor.* N.Y.: Free Press.

Randolph, J. L. 1976. *Interagency coordination and purchase of service agreements: A study of public-private dilemmas.* Ph.D. diss., University of Utah, Salt Lake City.

Rawls, J. R., R. A. Ullrich, and O. T. Nelson. 1975. A comparison of managers entering or re-entering the profit and nonprofit sectors. *Academy of Management Journal* 18:616–622.

Reagan, M. D. 1965. *Politics, economics, and the general welfare.* Chicago: Scott Foresman.

Reichert, K. 1982. Human services and the market system. *Health and Social Work* 7:174.

Reid, P. N. 1972. Reforming the social services monopoly. *Social Work* 17:44–54.

Reid, W. J. 1964. Interagency coordination in delinquency prevention and control. *Social Service Review* 38:418–428.

Reid, W. J. and A. D. Smith. 1978. Obtaining the consumer's point of view. In W. C. Sze and J. G. Hopps, eds., *Evaluation and accountability in human service programs.* Cambridge, Mass.: Schenkman.

Report of the Blue Ribbon Commission on the Future of Inpatient Mental Health Services in Massachusetts. 1981. *Mental health crossroads.* Boston, Mass.: Author.

Rice, R. M. 1975. Impact of government contracts on voluntary social agencies. *Social Casework* 56:387–95.

Riggs, F. W. 1964. *Administration in developing countries: The theory of prismatic society.* Boston, Mass.: Houghton Miflin.

Rivera, H. A. 1981. Purchase of service: A management challenge for state government. *New England Journal of Human Services* 1:50–51.

Rivlin, A. 1971. *Systematic thinking for social action*. Washington, D.C.: Brookings Institution.

Roberts, M. 1981. *An organizational analysis of a purchase of service program between public and private child welfare agencies*. Ph.D. diss., University of Texas, Austin.

Rodgers, B. 1976. *Cross-national studies of social service systems: United Kingdom reports*, vol. 1. N.Y.: Columbia University School of Social Work.

Rogers, D. and J. Molnar. 1975. *Interorganizational relations among developing organizations: Empirical assessment and implications for interorganizational coordination*. Ames: Iowa State University.

Rondell, F. and A. M. Murphy. 1974. *New dimensions in adoption*. N.Y.: Crown Publishers.

Rose-Ackerman, S. 1983. Social services and the market. *Columbia Law Review* 83:1405–1438.

Rosenbaum, N. 1981. Government funding and the voluntary sector: Impacts and options. *Journal of Voluntary Action Research* 10:82–89.

Rosenberg, G. and A. Weissman. 1981. Marketing social services in health care facilities. *Health and Social Work* 6:13–20.

Rosenthal, H. 1977. Testimony of Harold Rosenthal, Director, Division of Youth and Family Services, 11 March. N.J.: House Committee on Select Education: Hearings to extend the Child Abuse Prevention and Treatment Act.

Rosner, D. 1980. Gaining control: Reform, reimbursement and politics in New York's communities, 1890–1915. *American Journal of Public Health* 20: 533–542.

Rothman, J. et al. 1983. *Marketing human service innovations*. Beverly Hills, Calif.: Sage.

Rubenstein, H. 1975. Purchase of services: An unexamined assumption and the dilemmas of practice. *Public Welfare* 33:47–51.

Rudman, S. 1970. Controversial revenue sharing regs have farreaching implications. *Grantsmanship Center News* 20:46–48.

Sager, A. 1983. Drastic treatment needed in urban health care. *Brandeis Review* 3:13–18.

Salamon, L. M. 1984. Nonprofit organizations: The lost opportunity. In J. K. Palmer and I. V. Sawhill, eds., *The Reagan record*. Washington, D.C.: Urban Institute.

Salamon, L. M. and A. J. Abramson. 1982. The nonprofit sector. In J. L. Palmer and I. V. Sawhill, eds., *The Reagan experiment*. Washington, D.C.: Urban Institute.

Sammet, G. 1981. *Subcontract management handbook*. N.Y.: AMACOM.

Savas, E. S., ed., 1977. *Alternatives for delivering public services*. Boulder, Col.: Westview Press.

———. 1977. Policy analysis for local government: Public vs. private refuse collection. *Policy Analysis* 3:44–74.

———. 1979. Public vs. private refuse collection: A critical review of the evidence. *Urban Analysis* 6:1–13.

438

————. 1981. Intra-city competition between public and private service delivery. *Public Administration Review* 41:46–52.

————. 1982. *Privatizing the public sector: How to shrink government.* Chatham, N.J.: Chatham House Publishers.

Schainblatt, A. H. and H. A. Hatry. 1979. *Mental health services: What happens to the clients?* Report No. UI 1185–3–1. Washington, D.C.: Urban Institute.

Schechter, S. 1982. *Women and male violence: The visions and struggles of the battered women's movement.* Boston, Mass.: South End Press.

Schelling, T. C. 1963. *The strategy of conflict.* Cambridge, Mass.: Harvard University Press.

Schlesinger, A. 1986. *The cycles of American history.* N.Y.: Houghton-Mifflin.

Schlesinger, M. 1985. The rise of proprietary health care. *Business and Health* 2:7–12.

Schlesinger, M. and R. A. Dorwart. 1984. Ownership and mental health care: A reappraisal. *New England Journal of Medicine* 311:959–965.

Schlesinger, M., R. A. Dorwart, and R. T. Pulice. Forthcoming. Competitive bidding and states' purchase of services: The case of mental health care in Massachusetts. *Journal of Policy Analysis and Management.*

Schorr, A. L. 1970. The tasks for voluntarism in the next decade. *Child Welfare* 49:425–434.

Schulberg, H. C. 1976. The changing environment and purposes of mental health program evaluation. In E. W. Markson and D. F. Allen, eds., *Trends in mental health evaluation.* Lexington, Mass.: Lexington Press.

Schwartz, E. E. and M. Wolins. 1958. *Cost analysis in child welfare services*, Children's Bureau Publication 366. Washington, D.C.: Government Printing Office.

Scott, R. A. 1967. The selection of clients by social welfare agencies: The case of the blind. *Social Problems* 14:248–257.

Selig, M. K. 1963. The challenge of public funds to voluntary agencies. *Journal of Jewish Communal Services* 39:368–377.

————. 1973. New dimensions in government funding of voluntary agencies: Potentials and risks. *Journal of Jewish Communal Services* 50:125–135.

Sharfstein, S. S., S. Muszynski, and E. Myers. 1984. *Health insurance and psychiatric care: Update and appraisal.* Washington, D.C.: American Psychiatric Association.

Sharkansky, I. 1979. *Wither the state? Politics and public enterprise in three countries.* Chatham, N.J.: Chatham House Publishers.

————. 1980a. Government contracting. *State Government, 55.*

————. 1980. Policymaking and service delivery on the margins of government: The case of contractors. *Public Administration Review* 4:116–123.

Shearing, C. D. and P. C. Stenning. 1983. Private security: Implications for social control. *Social Problems* 30:493–506.

Shepsle, K. W. 1980. The private use of public interest. *Society* 17:35–41.

Skolnik, A. M. and S. R. Dales. 1977. Social welfare expenditures: Fiscal year 1976. *Social Security Bulletin* 40 (1):3–20.

Slack, I. 1979. *Title XX at the crossroads*. Washington, D.C.: American Public Welfare Association.

Sloan, F. A. 1984. State discretion in federal categorical assistance programs: The case of Medicaid. *Public Finance Quarterly* 12:321–346.

Smith, B. L. R. 1971. Accountability and independence in the contract state. In B. L. R. Smith and D. C. Hague, eds., *The dilemma of accountability in modern government: Independence versus control.* N.Y.: St. Martin's Press.

Smith, B. L. R., ed. 1975. *The new political economy: The public use of the private sector.* N.Y.: John Wiley & Sons.

Smith, B. L. R. and D. C. Hague, eds. 1971. *The dilemma of accountability in modern government: Independence versus control.* London: Macmillan.

Solomons, D. 1965. *Divisional performance: Measurement and control.* Homewood, Ill.: Richard D. Irwin.

Southern Wisconsin Colony and Training School, Union Grove. Memorandum of 8 October 1975.

Staff. 1985. *Concentrated course in government contracts.* Denver, Col.: University of Denver, College of Law and Federal Publications.

State of Wisconsin, Joint Committee for Review of Administrative Rules. Correspondence of 18 July 1978.

State of Wisconsin Purchase Contract, Agreement Number Dc-I-c-65. 29 November, 1977, with attachments.

Stein, J. H. 1979. *Anti-crime programs for the elderly: Combining community crime prevention and victim services.* Washington, D.C.: National Council of Senior Citizens.

Steinberg, R. M. 1976a. *Grants regulations and accountability procedures related to performance deflection in planning and implementating services to the aging.* Ph.D. diss., University of California, Los Angeles.

————. 1976b. A longitudinal analysis of 97 area agencies on aging: A study of funding regulations, program agreements, and monitoring procedures. In U.S. Congress, House Subcommittee on Aging, Committee on Human Resources. *Hearings on the Older Americans Act of 1978.* Washington, D.C.: Government Printing Office.

Steinfels, M. 1973. *Who's minding the children?* N.Y.: Simon and Schuster.

Stigler, G. 1975. *The citizen and the state.* Chicago, Ill.: University of Chicago Press.

Stoesz, D. 1981. A wake for the welfare state: Social welfare and the neoconservative challenge. *Social Service Review* 55:398–410.

Terrell, P. 1979. Private alternatives to public human services administration. *Social Service Review* 53:56–74.

————. 1977. *The social impact of revenue sharing.* N.Y.: Praeger.

Titmuss, R. 1971. *The gift relationship.* N.Y.: Pantheon.

Touche, Ross and Co. 1972. *Cost analysis of social services.* U.S. Department of Health, Education, and Welfare. Washington, D.C.: Government Printing Office.

Townsend, C. 1971. *Old age: The last segregation.* N.Y.: Grossman.

440

Turner, J. B., ed. 1977. *Encyclopedia of social work*, 17th ed. Washington, D.C.: National Association of Social Workers, Inc., 1532–1533.

United Community Planning Corporation and Massachusetts Association of Mental health. 1983. *More than shelter: A community response to homelessness.* Boston, Mass.: Author.

U.S. Congress, House of Representatives, Committee on Post Office and Civil Service. 1977. *Contracting out of jobs and services.* Washington, D.C.: Government Printing Office.

U.S. Congress, House of Representatives, Select Committee on Aging, Subcommittee on Housing and Consumer Interests. 1976. *Elderly crime victimization hearings.* Federal Law Enforcement Agencies, LEAA and FBI. 94th Congress, 2d Session.

U.S. Congress, Senate, Subcommittee on Employment, Manpower, and Poverty, Committee on Labor and Public Welfare. 1972. *Hearings on Senate Bill 1243, the Manpower Revenue Sharing Act of 1971.* 92d Congress, 2d sess., 8 March.

U.S. Department of Transportation. 1979. *Elderly and handicapped transportation: Eight case studies.* Washington, D.C.: Public Technology.

U.S. Office of Personnel Management. 1980. *Types of government contracts.* Washington, D.C.: The Management Training Center, Upward Mobility Series.

United Way of Los Angeles. 1981. *United Way: A study of contracting problems between government agencies and non-profit organizations in California.* Mimeo.

University of Denver. 1985. *Flyer.* Denver: College of Law and Federal Publications, Inc.

Victims of Crime Act of 1984, *P.L.* 98–473.

Vladeck, B. C. 1980. *Unloving care: The nursing home tragedy.* N.Y.: Basic Books.

Waller, J. D., D. MacNeil, J. W. Scanlon, F. L. Tolson, and J. S. Wholey. 1975. *Monitoring for criminal justice planning agencies.* Washington, D.C.: U.S. Department of Justice, National Institute of Law Enforcement and Criminal Justice.

Wall Street Journal, 29 July 1981.

Walsh, A. H. 1978. *The public's business: The politics and practices of government corporations.* Cambridge, Mass.: MIT Press.

Wamsley, G. and M. Zald. 1973a. The political economy of public organizations. *Public Administration Review* 33:62–73.

———. 1973b. *The political economy of public organizations: A critique and approach to the study of public administration.* Lexington, Mass.: Lexington Books.

Warner, A. G. 1894. *American charities: A study in philanthropy and economics.* N.Y.: Thomas Y. Crowell.

Warner, A. B., S. E. Queen, and E. B. Harper. 1930. *American charities and social work.* N.Y.: Thomas Y. Crowell Company.

Washington Post, 25 August 1981; 11 October, 1981; 16 April 1982; 6 July 1982;

441

18 April 1982; 28 November 1983; 20 December 1984; 4 February 1985; 23 March 1985; 7 May 1985; 21 May 1985; 30 June 1985; 9 July 1985; 20 August 1985; 21 November 1985; 30 March 1986; 5 July 1986; 21 July 1986; 2 August 1986; 28 November 1986.

Washington Star, 27 January 1981.

Wedel, K. R. 1974. Contracting for public assistance social services. *Public Welfare* 32:57–62.

———. 1976. Government contracting for purchase of service. *Social Work* 21: 101–105.

———. 1979. Purchase of service contracting: A state of the art review. In K. R. Wedel, A. J. Katz, and A. Weick, eds., *Social services by government contract: A policy analysis.* N.Y.: Praeger.

———. 1980. Purchase of service contracting in human services. *Journal of Health and Human Resources Administration* 1:327–341.

Wedel, K. R. and D. Hardcastle. 1978. Alternatives to monolithic public social services. *Midwest Review of Public Administration* 12:177–188.

Wedel, K. R., Katz, A. J., and A. Weick, eds., 1978. *Proceedings of the national institute on purchase of service contracting.* Lawrence: University of Kansas School of Social Welfare.

———. 1979. *Social services by government contract: A policy analysis.* N.Y.: Praeger.

Wedemeyer, J. M. 1970. Government agencies and purchase of social services. In I. R. Winogrand, ed., *Proceedings of the first Milwaukee Institute on a social welfare issue of the day: Purchase of care and services in the health and welfare fields.* Milwaukee: The University of Wisconsin.

Weick, A. 1979. Title XX as a new context for social service planning. In Wedel, K. R., A. J. Katz, and A. Weick, eds., *Social services by government contract: A policy analysis.* N.Y.: Praeger.

Weinstein, M. et al. 1979. *Title XX: Comparing the costs of alternative delivery systems.* Berkeley, Calif.: Pacific Consultants.

Weinstein, M. C. and W. B. Stason. 1976. *Hypertension: A policy perspective.* Cambridge, Mass.: Harvard University Press.

Weisbrod, B. A. 1983. A guide to benefit-cost analysis as seen through a controlled experiment in treating the mentally ill. *Journal of Health Politics, Policy and Law* 7:808–845.

Weisbrod, B. A. and M. Schlesinger. 1981. Benefit-cost analysis in the mental health area: Issues and directions for research. In T. G. McGuire and B. A. Weisbrod, eds., *Economics and mental health.* National Institute of Mental Health series EN no. 1, DHHS publication no. ADM 81–1114. Washington, D.C.: Government Printing Office.

Weiss, C. H. 1972. *Evaluating action programs: Reading in social action and evaluation.* Boston, Mass.: Allyn & Bacon.

———. 1976. The three faces of evaluation: Policy, program and the public. In E. W. Markson and D. F. Allen, eds., *Trends in mental health evaluation.* Lexington, Mass.: Lexington.

Weithorn, S. S. 1986. *Impact of tax reform legislation on charitable planning: Steps to take in 1986.* N.Y.: National Health Council.

Werner, R. M. 1961. *Public financing of voluntary foster care.* N.Y.: Child Welfare League of America.

Whiteneck, G. G. 1975. *The state-of-the-art in defining social services, developing service units, and determining unit costs, with an annotated bibliography.* Denver, Colo.: Denver Research Institute, University of Denver.

Wholey, J. S., J. W. Scanlon, H. G. Duffy, J. S. Fukumoto, and L. M. Vogel. 1970. *Federal evaluation policy.* Washington, D.C.: Urban Institute.

Wickenden, E. and W. Bell. 1961. *Public welfare: Time for a change.* N.Y.: New York School of Social Work.

Wiebe, G. D. 1951. Merchandising commodities and citizenship on television. *Public Opinion Quarterly* 15:679–691.

Wildavsky, A. and J. Pressman. 1973. *Implementation.* Berkeley: University of California.

Wilensky, H. L. and C. N. Lebeaux. 1965. *Industrial Society and Social Welfare,* 2d ed. N.Y.: Free Press.

Williams, C. K., N. F. Bracht, R. A. Williams, and R. L. Evans. 1978. Social work and nursing in hospital settings: A study of interprofessional experiences. *Social Work in Health Care.* 3:311–322.

Williams, W. 1980. *Government by agency.* N.Y.: Academic Press.

Wilson, J. Q., ed., 1980. *The politics of regulation.* N.Y.: Basic Books.

Windle, C. and S. S. Sharfstein. 1981. Mental health service policy and program evaluation: Living in sin? *Health Policy Quarterly* 1:73–90.

Wisconsin Department of Health and Human Services. Memorandum of 11 July 1978.

Wolock, I. and B. Horowitz. 1978. *Child maltreatment records in a public child welfare agency.* Unpublished manuscript. New Brunswick, N.J.: Rutgers University Graduate School of Social Work.

Wood, C. T. 1982. Relate hospital charges to use of services. *Harvard Business Review* 60:123–130.

Woodrow, R. J. 1977. *Federal grants and contracts to colleges and universities.* Mimeo. Cambridge, Mass.: The Sloan Commission on Government and Higher Education.

Young, Arthur and Co. 1982. *Contracting out: An option for local government.* A Symposium. Long Beach, Calif.

Young, D. 1978. Contracting out for services. In M. Murphy and T. Glynn, eds., *Human services management: Priorities for research.* Washington, D.C.: International City Management Association.

———. 1983. *If not for profit, for what?* Lexington, Mass.: Lexington Books.

Young, D. W. and A. Brandt. 1977. Benefit-cost analysis in the social services: The example of adoption reimbursement. *Social Service Review* 51:249–264.

Young, D. W. and S. J. Finch. 1977. *Foster Care and non-profit agencies.* Lexington, Mass.: Lexington Books.

Young, D. W. and R. B. Saltman. 1982. Medical practice, case mix, and cost containment. *Journal of the American Medical Association* 247:801–805.

Yuchtman, E. and S. Seashore. 1967. A system resource approach to organizational effectiveness. *American Sociological Review* 32:891–903.

Zald, M. 1970a. *Organizational change: the political economy of the YMCA*. Chicago, Ill.: University of Chicago Press.

———. 1970b. A framework for comparative analysis. In M. Zald, ed., *Power organizations*. Tenn.: Vanderbilt University Press.

Index

DATE DUE

GAYLORD

PRINTED IN U.S.A.